Recent Advances in

Paediatrics

Recent Advances in Paediatrics 17
Edited by T. J. David

ISBN 0-443-06184-X
ISSN 0-309-0140

Look out for *Recent Advances in Paediatrics* 19 in January 2001

NUMBER
18

Recent Advances in
Paediatrics

Edited by

T. J. David MD PhD FRCP FRCPCH DCH

Professor of Child Health and Paediatrics,
University of Manchester;
Honorary Consultant Paediatrician,
Booth Hall Children's Hospital,
Royal Manchester Children's Hospital and St Mary's Hospital,
Manchester, UK

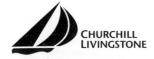
CHURCHILL
LIVINGSTONE

EDINBURGH LONDON NEW YORK PHILADELPHIA SYDNEY TORONTO 2000

CHURCHILL LIVINGSTONE
An imprint of Harcourt Brace Publishers Limited

Robert Stevenson House, 1–3 Baxter's Place, Leith Walk, Edinburgh, EH1 3AF

© Harcourt Brace Publishers Limited 2000

First published 2000

ISBN 0-443-06430-X

ISSN 0-309-0140

British Library Cataloguing in Publication Data
A catalogue record for this book is available from the British Library

Library of Congress Cataloging in Publication Data
A catalog record for this book is available from the Library of Congress

Commissioning Editor – Ellen Green
Project Editor – Michele Staunton
Project Controller – Frances Affleck
Designer – Sarah Russell

The
publisher's
policy is to use
paper manufactured
from sustainable forests

Printed in China

Contents

Preface

The aim of *Recent Advances in Paediatrics* is to provide a review of important topics and help doctors keep abreast of developments in the subject. The book is intended for the practising clinician, those in specialty training, and doctors preparing for specialty examinations. The book is sold very widely in Britain, Europe, North America and Asia, and the contents and authorship are selected with this very broad readership in mind. There are 10 chapters which cover a variety of general paediatric, neonatal and community paediatric areas. As usual, the selection of topics has veered towards those of general rather than special interest.

This year, two chapters are considerably more extensive than usual. Paul Brand's explanation of the practical interpretation of lung function tests is long because the author was specially asked to provide a set of worked examples. The other longer chapter is a comprehensive review of retinal haemorrhages, with special reference to the shaken impact syndrome. There is arguably no paediatric subject of quite such importance that has been addressed so confusingly in the literature to date. The remit of Dr Alex Levin, whose observations have had such a singular impact on our understanding, was to comprehensively cover every aspect of this topic, which resulted in an exceptionally lengthy chapter.

The final chapter, an annotated literature review, is a personal selection of key articles and useful reviews published in 1998. Comment about a paper is sometimes as important as the original article, so when a paper has been followed by interesting or important correspondence this is also referred to. As with the choice of subjects for the main chapters, the selection of articles has inclined towards those of general rather than special interest. There is, however, special emphasis on community paediatrics and medicine in the tropics, as these two important areas tend to be less well covered in general paediatric journals. Trying to reduce to an acceptable size the short-list of particularly interesting articles is an especially difficult task. Each topic in the literature review section is asterisked in the index, so selected publications on (for example) child abuse can be identified easily, as can any parts of the book that touch on the topic.

I am indebted to the authors for their hard work, prompt delivery of manuscripts and patience in dealing with my queries and requests. I would also like to thank my secretaries Angela Smithies and Val Smith, and Gill Haddock of Churchill Livingstone (Harcourt Publishers Limited) for all their help, and my wife and sons for all their support.

2000   **Professor T J David**
E-mail: tjd@netcomuk.co.uk
University Department of Child Health, Booth Hall Children's Hospital, Manchester M9 7AA, UK

Contributors

Geraldine B Boylan MSc
Research Fellow, Neonatal Unit, King's College Hospital, London, UK

Paul L.P. Brand MD PhD
Consultant Paediatric Pulmonologist, Isala Clinics, De Weezenlanden
Hospital, Zwolle, The Netherlands

Sangkae Chamnanavanakij MD
Research Fellow, Department of Pediatrics, Division of Neonatal-Perinatal
Medicine, University of Texas Southwestern Medical Center, Dallas, Texas,
USA

T.J. David MD PhD FRCP FRCPCH DCH
Professor of Child Health and Paediatrics, University of Manchester;
Honorary Consultant Paediatrician, Booth Hall Children's Hospital, Royal
Manchester Children's Hospital and St Mary's Hospital, Manchester, UK

Dominic A. Fitzgerald MBBS PhD FRACP
Paediatric Respiratory Physician, The Royal Alexandra Hospital for Children,
Sydney, Australia

Dirk Huyer MD
Director, Suspected Child Abuse and Neglect Program, The Hospital for Sick
Children and Assistant Professor, Department of Pediatrics, University of
Toronto, Toronto, Ontario, Canada

Alex V. Levin MD FRCSC
Staff Ophthalmologist and Assistant Professor, Department of
Ophthalmology, The Hospital for Sick Children, University of Toronto,
Toronto, Ontario, Canada

Karen A McLeod BSc MD MRCP
Senior Registrar in Paediatric Cardiology, Department of Cardiology, Royal
Hospital for Sick Children, Yorkhill, Glasgow, UK

Thomas H. Ollendick PhD
Heilig-Meyers Professor of Psychology, Child Study Center, Department of Psychology, Virginia Polytechnic Institute and State University, Blacksburg, Virginia, USA

Jeffrey M. Perlman MB
Professor of Pediatrics and Obstetrics/Gynecology and Clinical Director of Special Care Nurseries, Department of Pediatrics, Division of Neonatal-Perinatal Medicine, University of Texas Southwestern Medical Center, Dallas, Texas, USA

Isabelle Rapin MD
Professor of Neurology and Pediatrics (Neurology), Saul R. Korey Department of Neurology, Department of Pediatrics, and Rose F. Kennedy Center for Research in Mental Retardation and Human Development, Albert Einstein College of Medicine, Bronx, New York, USA

Janet M Rennie MA MD FRCP FRCPCH DCH
Consultant and Senior Lecturer in Neonatal Medicine, King's College Hospital, London, UK

Stephen M. Schexnayder MD
Associate Professor of Pediatrics and Internal Medicine, University of Arkansas for Medical Sciences and Arkansas Childen's Hospital, Little Roak, Arkansas, USA

Laura D. Seligman MS
Clinical Psychology Intern, The Kennedy Krieger Institute, Johns Hopkins Medical School, Baltimore, Maryland, USA

Hiran C. Selvadurai MBBS
Fellow in Paediatric Respiratory Medicine, The Royal Alexandra Hospital for Children, Sydney, Australia

Michelle Shouldice BScH MSc MD FRCPC
Clinical Fellow, Division of Pediatric Medicine, University of Toronto, The Hospital for Sick Children, Toronto, Ontario, Canada

John B.P. Stephenson MA DM FRCP FRCPCH
Professor and Consultant in Paediatric Neurology, Fraser of Allander Neurosciences Unit, and EEG Department, Royal Hospital for Sick Children, Yorkhill, Glasgow, UK

John B.P. Stephenson Karen A. McLeod

CHAPTER 1

Reflex anoxic seizures

This chapter is about reflex anoxic seizures as first described in these terms in 1978:[1]

> *In a typical case, an unsteady toddler on his own trips and falls. His mother hears a bump but no succeeding cry and hurries to him. She finds her child lying deathly still with eyes fixed upwards, lips dusky. As she lifts him, he abruptly stiffens into rigid extension with jaw clenched and hands fisted, gives a few jerks, and after what seems an age (but in fact is less than half a minute) relaxes limply with an absent far-away look. Then he opens his eyes, at once recognises his mother, cries a little, and drifts off to sleep, his face distinctly pale.*

In the succeeding 21 years, reflex anoxic seizures (RAS) have been increasingly recognised, but still run the risk of being diagnosed as epilepsy or temper tantrums. Such confusion arises in part because of the 'lack of a universal descriptive name to label the attacks'.[1] Therefore, it is important to look at the terminology before going into the clinical details.

TERMINOLOGY

To find publications on RAS in databases such as Medline, one has to search not only under 'reflex anoxic seizures' but under 'breath-holding spells' and 'syncope'. The most popular synonyms for RAS are pallid breath-holding spells[2] and pallid syncope[3] or pallid infantile syncope.[4] Other terms which

John B.P. Stephenson MA DM FRCP FRCPCH
Professor and Consultant in Paediatric Neurology, Fraser of Allander Neurosciences Unit, and EEG Department, Royal Hospital for Sick Children, Yorkhill, Glasgow G3 8SJ, UK (for correspondence)

Karen A McLeod BSc MD MRCP, Senior Registrar in Paediatric Cardiology, Department of Cardiology, Royal Hospital for Sick Children, Yorkhill, Glasgow G3 8SJ, UK have been used include vagal attack[1] vagocardiac syncope[5] infantile vaso-vagal syncope[6] and infantile neurocardiogenic syncope.[6] In the original RAS paper,[1] 'white breath-holding' was added to the title at the insistence of one of the referees, but RAS are only superficially similar to the cyanotic breath-holding spells[7] of the prolonged expiratory apnoea[8] variety.

To many people, seizure means epileptic seizure such that the use of RAS to label non-epileptic events has quite reasonably been criticised.[9] However, such criticism ignores the existence of anoxic seizures (fainting fits, non-epileptic convulsive syncope) and of anoxic-epileptic seizures.[5,10] If one looks carefully at the clinical features, a lot of this confusion evaporates, so we will include genuine if anonymised case histories in the next section (the histories incorporate parents' descriptions).

CLINICAL FEATURES

There may not be a fundamental difference between RAS in infants and toddlers as previously described,[1,5] and the cardio-inhibitory syncope of older children.[5,10] Nonetheless, it may help to describe them separately.

Reflex anoxic seizures

Episodes begin from infancy onwards, usually in response to an unpleasant stimulus such as bumping the head. The first such case from our institution in which short latency cardiac asystole was confirmed in a natural episode in the child's home was published as case 9.29 in 1990.[5]

Case 1

A 2-year-old boy had increasingly frequent episodes of loss of consciousness with rigidity, beginning at age 9 months. Although the onset was not always witnessed, all those which were began after he bumped his head or face. He would give a brief cry and then go rigid, with back arched, head back, arms twisted, and legs tremoring. His teeth seemed to be clenched very hard, but there was no breath-holding apparent. He had begun to wet himself during each attack. Usually, he was a ghastly pale colour afterwards. The frequency was now at least once a day. Postictal sleep or somnolence disrupted family life. His 5-year-old sister had recently begun similar attacks after pain or bump. After 48 h with an EEG/ECG monitor attached he had two typical RAS with 14 and 22 s asystole recorded together with the typical slow–flat–slow EEG appearance of an anoxic seizure. Daily atropine (as atropine methonitrate) reduced the number of episodes to one per month; he relapsed when the medication was briefly withdrawn, and responded again when the atropine was re-introduced.[11]

Recently the use of videorecording and particularly the availability of continuous loop cardiomemo ECG recorders (see Event monitoring in the Diagnosis section below) which can be worn for long periods in the child's home have expanded our ideas about what RAS are. These monitors which are attached to the chest not only pick up the ECG signal and so reveal the asystole but also detect rapid expiratory grunting when that is present, together with the intense EMG activity which signals the tonic component of the anoxic seizure. Ictal recordings (that is, recordings during an attack) have demonstrated that rapidly repeated expiratory grunts may or may not coincide with cardiac asystole in RAS. This expiratory grunting does not appear to play any important part in the induction of the syncope and anoxic seizure, but it confuses doctors because it looks like 'breath-holding'. A good illustration of this follows.

Case 2

A girl aged 30 months presented with a history of RAS since age 4 months, at first only due to pain, later when upset or angry. 'You can see the silent cry' preceded opisthotonic rigidity. Ictal cardiomemo recordings (Fig. 1.1) showed repeated expiratory grunts while she was already asystolic. Urinary incontinence was not recognised until she was out of nappies. Because of the disruption to her life (episodes occurring 3 or 4 times a day meant that she was most of the time asleep including on Christmas Day) she was entered into a blinded study of cardiac pacing (*see* Cardiac pacing in the 'Management' section), and is now (age 5 years) symptom free.

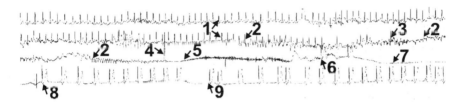

Fig. 1.1 Example of one of the RAS recorded by a cardiomemo event recorder King of Hearts recorder. Solid arrows guide the reader through the changes seen, each number pointing to key features. Continuous recording over 2 min is shown, each line representing 30 s of ECG. (**1**) ECG normal rate, base-line unremarkable; (**2**) signals of rapid expiratory grunting at first before and soon after cardiac asystole, appearing as a jagged 'saw-toothed' artefact on the baseline; (**3**) asystole after transient bradycardia; (**4**) signal of event button pressing. (**5**) onset of EMG signal of tonic anoxic (non-epileptic) seizure; (**6**) return of systole after prolonged asystole; (**7**) quiescent phase of limp post-ictal phase, with disappearance of EMG; (**8**) post-ictal bradycardia. (**9**) loss of P-waves from continued vagal efferent discharge (nodal rhythm).

One of the best published descriptions of syncopes in general[12] (which deserves to be read by all clinical doctors) includes emphasis on two less well known manifestations which may also be recognised in RAS.[5] These are first automatisms and secondly hallucinations or out-of body experiences. Recognition that these phenomena can occur should prevent the easy mis-diagnosis of epilepsy and the psychological after-effects of the hallucinations may need attention. Automatisms are discussed now, and hallucinations and out-of body experiences in the section on Cardioinhibitory syncopes below.

Automatisms

A good example is case 4.9 in Fits and Faints.[5]

Case 3

A 30-month-old girl was known to have RAS as were her sister and cousin. All three had had anoxic seizures reproduced by ocular compression in the EEG department. She was referred again because of what appeared to be a different type of attack over the past several months which was thought to be 'undoubtedly epileptic'. Episodes were induced by rather minor stimuli such as her father raising his voice. The most recent episode, precipitated by being told to hurry up, was typical. She first looked dazed and then slumped. Her eyes went funny and she stiffened up, made a slavering noise, opened her eyes wide and stared, and kept putting her hand to her mouth and making mouth and lip movements for what appeared to be several minutes until she came out of the attack, crying and looking white. This history was written down in the mother's words before the next stage in the investigation which was ocular compression under EEG and ECG control. This induced an asystole of 26 s with 17 s of flat EEG followed by prolonged slow activity. The resultant anoxic seizure was characterised by upward deviation of the eyes, flexion, a moan, extension, full extension, staring, a snort, another noise, a jerk, another extension and a dazed appearance. Then, there were lip movements and further staring and an 'ooh ooh' noise, and then putting her hand to her mouth, looking up and putting her tongue in and out, looking about slightly and looking at her mother but not clearly knowing her, touching the electrodes crying a little and scratching her ear, looking at her mother crying and indistinctly speaking, rubbing her eyes, holding out her arms and making gurgly vocalisation and more tongue movements, protruding and licking her lips, and poking her mouth and teeth with her fingers. After about 6 min, she was back to normal. Her mother said that this was identical in every way to the episodes which she had observed at home.

It was important in this situation to have written down the history in detail before the attempted replication by ocular compression.

Cardio-inhibitory syncopes of older children

We do not know how many varieties of cardio-inhibitory syncopes there are nor whether the cardio-inhibitory syncopes of older children such as venepuncture fits have the same basis as RAS.[13] However, there is no doubt that RAS may persist into later childhood and adolescence. Even though the frequency may become much less, reducing to perhaps once every 6 months, the syncopes tend to be more distressing, particularly if accompanied by urinary incontinence, as is often the case. The following example[10] illustrates the transition from infantile onset RAS to short latency pain-induced cardioinhibitory vasovagal syncope to blood-illness-injury phobia in adolescence.

Case 4

A 13-year-old girl had her first episode at the age of 10 months after a very slight bump to her head. The attacks were similar from then on, except that the severity had tended to increase. Currently there would be a latency of 10–20 s during which she might say 'oh mum I've hurt myself'. By this time the blood would have drained from her face and she would fall as if dead, going totally rigid and making a noise like a cackle or gurgle, with her hands and feet turned in and her back sometimes forming the shape of an arc. Sometimes her arms would jerk, not violently, and her legs would look as if she was pedalling a bicycle, but on other occasions she would thrash as if having a 'full seizure'. She would then again look like death and wake up as if coming out of a very deep sleep. She would be disorientated and not know what had happened or where she was for a couple of minutes before coming to and wanting to lie down and have a proper sleep. From about the age of 7 years, she began to describe an aura. She would hear a noise like high pitched screaming and would sometimes hear a voice which she could not describe precisely. Sometimes she would see red, a colour she does not like, and sometimes there would be hallucinations such as of a train rushing towards her. Her mother said that the triggers of her RAS had changed over the years. After the first episode which followed a head bump, all the episodes in early childhood followed small pains like a finger being bent back. Later she began to develop the same reaction to seeing a minor injury such as a scab which had come off a wound. Then she developed inevitable syncope at the sight of blood. Finally merely the thought of self-injury was a sufficient trigger. On the evening before her consultation she was told (wrongly) that her eyeballs would be pressed down and within 2 min she was stiff and snorting. A family history of syncope of any kind was denied, but later the mother admitted to several faints in adolescence and in pregnancy. She had not mentioned these because she did not have a 'fit'.

In addition to the progression from RAS to more recognisable vasovagal syncope (albeit clearly cardio-inhibitory) the above case shows how there may be an aura suggesting partial epilepsy and also illustrates how a family history may be denied.

Hallucinations and out-of-body experiences

According to Lempert,[12] hallucinations and out-of-body experiences occur at the end of a syncope rather than at the beginning as in an epileptic aura. Some such phenomena associated with RAS may not be that rare.[14] Descriptions include passing into a dark tunnel and being hurtled towards a light, the tunnel being frightening but the white light nice, like a Christmas light.[14] An example in an older child follows:[5]

Case 5
A 12-year-old girl had three identical episodes including one induced by a hamster bite. She passed out, growled in her throat, went very tense and rigid with slight body spasms (a few jerks) and then came round talking gibberish, a horrible white colour. Later, she said that she had had a dream about firemen spraying blood out of a hose. Her mother also appeared in the dream.

Older children with RAS or cardio-inhibitory vasovagal syncope who have syncopes in school not uncommonly say that, for a short while afterwards, they believe that they are at home in bed dreaming that they are at school.

DIAGNOSIS

History, history, history, history, history

False diagnoses of epilepsy are common in adults[15] and in children,[16] the major errors relating to vasovagal syncope and to RAS. In diagnosis, the clinical history is all, or nearly all. How to take a history of a paroxysmal disorder has been elaborated at length previously,[5] but there are some points which deserve special attention.

Prolonged interrogation

'The diagnosis is as good as the history. The objective is to elicit a sequence which, replayed in the mind's eye, is as good as or better than a split-screen video recording with full polygraphy. With experience, a few minutes may be enough for a watertight history, but your author still finds that an hour may be necessary, first to disentangle, and then to weave the threads of a true likeness of the hitherto undiagnosed seizure'.[5]

Individual assessment

Obviously, the general paediatric evaluation is of some importance in determining the significance of a paroxysmal event, but beware particularly the temptation to be swayed towards a diagnosis of epilepsy simply because the child has some sort of brain disorder. If a child with hydrocephalus has a tonic seizure, there is no difficulty in inferring that this means high intracranial pressure rather than epilepsy, but one should remember that having, for example, athetoid cerebral palsy does not make one immune from having RAS.

Family history

Syncopes in first degree relatives are often denied completely at first. Fainting during pregnancy or when having blood taken, often do not seem to count in parents' minds. One may have to press the question, specifically asking about these settings. Be sceptical of the history of 'known epileptic' in a parent, bearing in mind that the diagnosis of epilepsy is wrong in 25–50% of cases.[5,15]

Setting

It may seem obvious, but if a child has a tonic seizure with or without urinary incontinence in church, in school assembly, standing to read in the classroom, or kneeling for a haircut, then the diagnosis is cardio-inhibitory syncope. Beware, however, excited outdoor activities with chasing games or an episode in sleep, a setting for a long QT syndrome anoxic seizure.

Stimulus

One expects RAS to be triggered by something unpleasant or surprising, albeit the stimulus is not always obvious. Epileptic seizures are not triggered by pain or by brief head bumps, but one has to know this to make the diagnosis of RAS. The following example[10] illustrates this well:

Case 6

A consultant (adult) neurologist wrote to the family doctor: 'Thank you for asking me to see this 7-year-old young man. As a toddler, he began to have attacks of loss of awareness, rigidity and eye rolling which would be induced by minor knocks. This has continued and recently an episode occurred in which he had an undoubted tonic/clonic seizure with incontinence of urine. Curiously, as far as I can tell from mother's account, every attack has been triggered by a minor bump on the head and he has never had an attack out of the blue. He had difficulties at birth. The family history is clear except for a convulsion in the mother when she was tiny, about which there is no further information. It seems to me that this boy is having some sort of reflex epileptic seizure and my inclination would have been to start treatment with sodium valproate. In fact, mother told me that he is attending the paediatric department at [an English hospital] and that he was started on Epilim just a couple of weeks ago. Even though two EEGs have been normal, I do not doubt that he has an epileptic tendency and I am sure that he should be on treatment for at least a couple of years free from attacks.'

Anoxic seizures (as these were) triggered only by head bumps are not a feature of cyanotic breath-holding spells nor of long QT syndrome: rather they are the typical manifestation of RAS. Had the stimulus, on the other hand, been exertion or extreme emotion or an unexpected sound[17] such as a doorbell suddenly ringing or an episode in sleep then alarm bells for one of the long QT syndromes[18] should ring in the paediatrician's mind.

For completeness, one should mention another type of seizure reported in one out of 70 sport related concussions, the so-called concussive convulsions. Conceivably, these head bump triggered non-epileptic seizures occur in children as well as in adults. If so, they would be distinguished from RAS by their very short latency, less than 2 s, as compared to the usual RAS latency of 10 s or so.

Aura

The very young child will of course not be able to describe warning sensations. Older children may experience abdominal pain at onset.[5] The typical transient blacking out which accompanies the light-headed type of dizziness may at first be denied. Sensitive and persistent questioning may be needed to elicit this diagnostic information. Sometimes, the parent is certain that the child had a warning but, nonetheless, cannot remember it afterwards. A more complex aura[14] should not shift the diagnosis to epilepsy if other features are concordant with syncope.

Onset

Although it is often the case that the first motor event in RAS or in the similar fast onset cardio-inhibitory syncopes of older children is a limp falling to the floor, this is not necessarily so. It is important to recognise that an individual may fall stiffly with stiff legs in a syncope[12] and that such does not imply an epileptic convulsion.

Ictal course

It may take a great deal of effort to elicit all the features described in RAS[5] and other syncopes.[12] The most obvious characteristics are stiffenings of a somewhat 'decerebrate' appearance, with irregular non-rhythmic jerks and spasms totalling perhaps not more than 10 and lasting usually not more than about half a minute. A snorty vocalisation which occurs at the end of the tonic phase should be remembered by the parent. It is important to remember that urinary incontinence is common in RAS and in similar neurocardiogenic syncopes. In infancy and toddlerhood this may not be noticed because of nappy wearing. In later years, wetting is, of course, an upsetting and socially disabling symptom.

Immediate postictal state

Young children may remain unrousable for over an hour after RAS (Lobban, personal communication), but commonly there is a brief look of anxious recognition before sleep takes over. In older children, confusion rarely lasts more than a few minutes.

History from a second witness

Once a child has started nursery or gone to school, it is essential to interview the witness who has seen the event. Telephone interviews are usually sufficient, but, on occasion, it may be necessary to meet the witness(es) so that the use of miming may be employed, or videotapes of different kinds of syncope and epileptic seizures shown for identification.

Videorecording

The use of a camcorder is really an extension of the history, giving both auditory and visual information. As indicated above, even if it is not possible to capture the beginning of an attack, successful videorecordings of other children with known RAS are available (e.g. from the RAS support group) for parents to compare with their own child's attacks.

Deliberate induction of RAS

Before the advent of event monitoring (next section), ocular compression by reproducing RAS precisely was commonly used as a diagnostic test.[5] Diagnostic ocular compression is now confined to three situations: (i) when the parents are extremely keen for the doctor to see one of the RAS; (ii) when the history of the suspected RAS is distinctly unusual (see Automatisms); and (iii) when a history suggesting anoxic-epileptic seizures (see Anoxic-epileptic seizures under Complications) is difficult to confirm.[20]

Head-up tilt is a less worrisome provocation for the older child (over 7 years) and may be required occasionally when syncopes are severe but infrequent.

Event monitoring

Though the diagnosis of RAS is made primarily by the clinical history, it is supported by the demonstration of cardiac asystole during a typical attack. Such confirmation is essential if treatment by a pacemaker is being considered for frequent severe episodes. Cardiac event recorders are available in a number of different forms, including 'credit cards' and 'wrist watches', but we have found the King of Hearts monitor (Scottish Medical) to be particularly robust

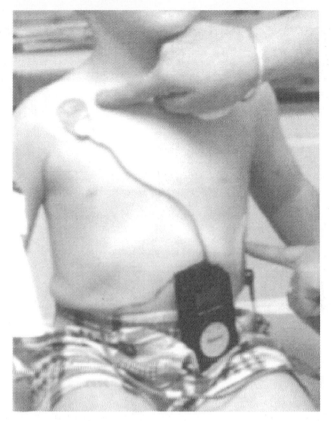

Fig. 1.2 King of Hearts (Scottish Medical) cardiac event monitor with leads and electrodes. This can be worn for several weeks with only the electrodes requiring to be changed.

for toddlers and capable of producing good quality ECGs. The monitor is the shape and size of a standard radiopager (Fig. 1.2) and is attached via two leads to two electrodes on the child's chest. The monitor constantly records the ECG, continually updating and holding in its memory the last 30 s of ECG. Should an event happen, the record button is pressed and the monitor stores the 30 s of ECG prior to and the 60 s can then be sent down the telephone printed out and analysed (Figs 1.1 & 1.2). We have monitored over a 100 children with a clinical diagnosis of RAS and it is a curious observation that many toddlers with reportedly frequent attacks will inexplicably improve as soon as the monitor is fitted. We have observed that the likelihood of obtaining an ECG recording during typical RAS is increased if the child is less than 5-years-old and has attacks at least once a week. On some monitors, the time periods are programmable (Fig. 1.3).

Biochemical studies

Despite earlier studies to the contrary, it seems clear that prolactin is elevated after tilt induced syncope[21] and so not a discriminator against epileptic

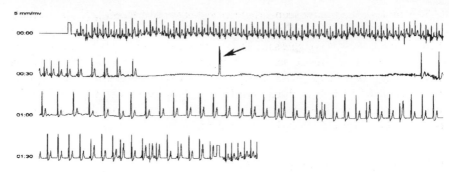

Fig. 1.3 Episode of cardiac asystole on a cardiac event recorder during one episode of RAS. The monitor was programmed to record for 40 s prior to and for 60 s after activation of the record button (arrow). Each strip is 30 s. Initially, there is sinus tachycardia corresponding to the child running, but, in response to a noxious stimulus (in this case a bump on the elbow), the heart slows within a few seconds to complete cardiac asystole lasting over 20 s. On return of cardiac rhythm, there is bradycardia with a nodal rhythm of 55–60 beats/min. This continues beyond the end of the recording. As in Figure 1, the EMG signal of the (non-epileptic) tonic seizure is seen towards the end of the asystole.

seizures. No one has measured prolactin after asystole-confirmed RAS, but one would expect it to increase.

DIFFERENTIAL DIAGNOSIS

The confusion wrought both by the conflicting terminology and by the uncertainties about the biological bases make for some difficulty here.

Cyanotic breath-holding

Many argue that there is nothing fundamentally different between blue breath-holding[7] and RAS. In both there may be rapidly repeated expiratory grunts and in both there may be typical anoxic seizures, albeit with no change in heart rate, tachycardia or bradycardia in cyanotic breath-holding spells. The studies of DiMario[22] suggest that there may be biological differences in autonomic function between children with RAS and those with cyanotic breath-holding, those with RAS having central parasympathetic dysfunction. Investigations in adults are beginning to show varieties of vasovagal reactions.[28] Similar heterogeneity of response detail may well apply to RAS. Meanwhile, the important message to practitioners is not to confuse any of these conditions with temper tantrums!

Imposed upper airways obstruction

This is a differential diagnosis of cyanotic breath-holding rather than of RAS, hence the value of distinguishing clinically between respiratory and cardiac syncopes.

Long QT syndrome

Not surprisingly, the syncopes and anoxic seizures of the long QT syndrome may easily and dangerously be confused with cardio-inhibitory syncopes and

RAS. Although there now seems to be little chance of detecting all individuals carrying a long QT gene mutation unless one has access to molecular biology at the highest level,[18] the message must be that if the history is of a syncope with or without an anoxic seizure then an ECG should be obtained. If the history suggests syncope/RAS precipitated by extremes of emotion, surprise, fright, startle (especially auditory startle[17]), vigorous exercise or sleep, then the paediatrician should not let the cardiologist off the hook until the diagnosis is secure. If one is certain enough, ask for the molecular biology.[18]

Pallid syncope of the limp variety

In the past, authors[3] thought that this was the same thing as RAS. Actually, we do not know the mechanism of such limp attacks, except that there cannot be cardiac standstill for as long as 10 s or else there would be a motor anoxic seizure.[5]

Familial rectal pain

This dominantly inherited disorder (which may also appear sporadically) presents as severe syncopes in the neonatal period.[24] Although cardiac asystole may be very long (up to 45 s, C. Ferrie, personal communication),[25] the syncopes are not prevented by cardiac pacing but seemingly are respiratory as in cyanotic breath holding or neonatal hyperekplexia. Good clinical clues are that the anoxic seizures may be precipitated by the mother wiping the perineal area associated with a harlequin flushing of the face.[24,25]

Epileptic-anoxic seizures

Epileptic apnoea[10] looks somewhat like imposed upper airways obstruction. With no prior provocation, a motionless stare precedes apnoea and cyanosis. Thus, there should not be confusion with RAS.

COMPLICATIONS

Sleep disorders

Anecdotal evidence suggests that sleep disorders, especially night terrors, are common in children with RAS, and add to family distress. This topic needs to be researched.

Psychological co-morbidity

Child psychiatrists in the past (perhaps in the present?) thought that RAS, which they called breath-holding spells, were a sign of underlying social problems. However, such children are not 'difficult' and the frequency of temper tantrums is no different from that in unaffected children.[26] None-theless, families may become dysfunctional because of frequent severe RAS, and this has been one of the factors in the decision to offer pacemaker therapy (see 'Management, Cardiac pacing' below).

Anoxic-epileptic seizures

Although anoxic seizures from cardiac asystole (RAS) or from breath-holding are not in any sense epileptic seizures, true epileptic seizures may occasionally be triggered by a syncope. We call this combination an anoxic-epileptic seizure.[5,10] Status epilepticus, clonic or absence, may supervene,[5,10,20,27,28] but generalised tonic-clonic seizures as a sequel to RAS or other syncope have not been described. The recognition of absence status after RAS may be particularly difficult, and a history of prolonged unconsciousness after RAS is one of the remaining absolute indications for ocular compression under ECG/EEG control.[20]

In the following case the morbidity associated with status epilepticus and the wish to avoid long-term anti-epileptic medication prompted cardiac pacing.

Case 7

A 2-year-old girl had had RAS since age 8 months, 1–4 episodes daily. After a fall or a bump to the head or being knocked or upset she would be 'away' in about 10 s going rigid and twisted blue round the mouth and looking cold and dead. Her legs would jerk but not every time and then the top half of her would jerk and then there would be a funny breathing noise before she went limp. After about 40 s she would open her eyes and scream hysterically. Night terrors (one a night) started after the onset of RAS. At the age of 19 months, she had one of her usual RAS after falling and banging her head but on this occasion she remained unconscious with rhythmic jerking of her limbs for 40 min, only terminating after diazepam, phenobarbitone and paraldehyde. She collapsed her right lung and was unconscious for a day. She was given sodium valproate from then on. Several RAS were recorded by home monitoring, all with asystole of more than 20 s. She was treated by ventricular pacing with hysteresis (VVI – see 'Cardiac pacing' below) and stopped her valproate. Aged 3 years, she has had no further episodes of loss of consciousness (or epileptic seizures) but may have up to 8 or 9 'near-misses' (a gasp, colour draining, eyes starting to roll, after being hurt) daily lasting 2 s.

MANAGEMENT

Appreciation of parents' perceptions

'May be frightening to parents but nothing to worry about' was the subtitle of a review on RAS.[9] Parents do appreciate seeing a paediatrician who knows about RAS and who appreciates that there may be justifiable worries about the effect of RAS on the child, the family, friends, school and so forth. In alleviating anxiety, the parent support group acknowledged at the end of this chapter has proved most valuable. It should be said again that many parents translate the diagnosis of breath-holding spells as temper tantrums, being in control, doing it voluntarily, whereas they know that their child cannot help it, it is a reflex.

Medical therapy

Atropine

Atropine sulphate and atropine methonitrate were shown in an open trial[11] to prevent RAS; more data are included elsewhere.[5] Nowadays most families do not seem to like the atropine side-effects and actually prefer a cardiac pacemaker (see below)!

Iron

A recent double-blind trial[29] showed a beneficial effect of iron in 'breath-holding spells'. In this trial, placebo was given instead of iron to alternate children, without randomisation. Whether iron supplementation would reduce the recurrence of RAS in a developed country is not known.

Piracetam

In a placebo controlled double blind trial piracetam in a dose of 40 mg/kg/day was effective in controlling 'breath-holding spells'.[30] The trial was randomised, but the method of randomisation was not reported. Whether children with RAS and confirmed ictal asystole would respond is not yet known.

Cardiac pacing

As indicated earlier, there is strong evidence to support the view that cardiac asystole secondary to powerful vagal stimulation is the underlying mechanism for RAS.[1,5,11] This has raised the question as to whether cardiac pacing would prevent RAS. Studies in a small number of children have reported apparently striking success with cardiac pacing,[31–33] but the placebo effect of pacing was not tested.

In adults with vasovagal syncope and asystole the therapeutic use of pacemakers has been controversial. Not all patients appear to benefit from pacing[34] and the studies would suggest that dual chamber pacing (pacing both the atria and ventricles to achieve synchronous atrioventricular contraction) is required[35] as pacing only the ventricle can sometimes make symptoms worse.[34] A recently completed multicentre randomised trial[35] showed that the implantation of dual-chamber pacemakers with rate-drop response reduced the likelihood of recurrence of vasovagal syncope. However, a placebo response could not be excluded.[36]

After ethical approval and with informed consent, we conducted, between 1996 and 1998, a double-blind trial to determine whether severe RAS can be prevented by cardiac pacing and, if so, whether dual chamber pacing with rate drop response was superior to single chamber ventricular pacing.[37] Dual chamber pacemakers were implanted into 12 children (8 male) aged 2–14 years (median 2.4 years) with frequent episodes of RAS and a recorded prolonged asystole of over 10 s during an attack. The pacemaker was programmed to sensing only, i.e. no pacing (ODO), single chamber ventricular pacing with hysteresis (VVI), and dual chamber pacing with rate drop response (DDD) for three 4 month periods, with each patient allocated to one of the six possible sequences of these modes, according to chronological order of pacemaker implantation. The parent and patient were blinded to the pacemaker mode and asked to record all episodes of syncope or presyncope ('near-miss' events). The doctor analysing the results was blinded to the patient and pacemaker mode.

One patient was withdrawn from the study after the pacemaker was removed due to infection. In the remaining children, both dual chamber and single chamber pacing significantly reduced the episodes of syncope (RAS) compared with sensing only (both $P = 0.008$). In contrast to studies in adults, single chamber ventricular pacing with hysteresis was found to be as effective as dual chamber pacing with rate drop response for prevention of syncopes and RAS. It may be that blood pressure in children is more dependent upon heart rate than atrioventricular synchrony or indeed that as previously hypothesised[1] RAS represent a pure vagal cardio-inhibitory form of syncope with minimal hypotension from vasodilatation.

Although we found that ventricular pacing with hysteresis was as effective as dual chamber pacing with rate drop response for preventing syncopes with RAS, the latter (DDD) was more effective for reducing overall symptoms including 'near-misses' ($P = 0.016$). As mentioned earlier, in adults dual chamber pacing with rate drop response has been found to be the most effective pacemaker programme for vasovagal syncope currently available.[35]

In terms of symptomatic response to pacemaker implantation, six patients had no loss of consciousness when paced compared with syncopal episodes when the pacemaker was programmed to sensing only, three patients had no further episodes of syncope whether paced or not (suggesting a possible placebo effect from pacemaker implantation itself), and two children continued to have episodes despite being paced. The latter may have had a significant hypotensive or indeed a respiratory component to the syncope as in so-called cyanotic breath-holding spells.[7]

We concluded that permanent cardiac pacing provides an effective treatment for patients with RAS. In view of the potential problems and complications of pacing in young children, we would advise that pacing be limited to those with frequent and severe attacks in whom medical treatment has failed or is declined, bearing in mind that in older children fewer attacks may be tolerated. Prior to pacemaker implantation, prolonged asystole (10 s or more) should be demonstrated during an attack, preferably on more than one occasion. This would normally be done by using a cardiac event monitor (or by head-up tilt testing in older children). A ventricular system is as effective as dual chamber pacing for preventing syncope and RAS, although a dual chamber pacemaker with rate drop function is more effective at reducing overall symptoms. At the present time, we would recommend ventricular pacing with wide hysteresis in younger children and dual chamber pacing with rate drop function in older children.

We should add that this controlled study was UK wide (supported by the Reflex Anoxic Seizure Information and Support Group), and that cardiac pacing for RAS is only rarely required.[37]

Counselling on natural history and genetics

In general, one has optimism that the child will 'grow out of it'. However, the data on which to base such a prognosis are thin. One of the best early studies[4] showed that 17% of prospectively studied children with breath-holding ('cyanotic and pallid infantile syncope') went on to develop 'syncope' later. One has the impression that it is not rare for cardio-inhibitory syncopes beginning as RAS to persist indefinitely, as in cases presented earlier.[10]

Parents are naturally anxious that their child may die in an attack, and a keystone of management is the reassurance that this does not happen (unless the true diagnosis is long QT syndrome or Munchausen by proxy abuse). Such reassurance may be undermined by stories on the Internet of children dying from 'breath-holding spells'. Clear explanation of the mechanism of RAS and how serious brain hypoxia must abolish the vagal inhibition of the heart (negative feed-back)[38] is almost always sufficiently reassuring. The parent support group may be additionally helpful.

Genetic aspects or at any rate family histories have been studied both from the childhood[39] and the adult[40] perspective. Dominant inheritance with incomplete penetrance was suggested in the paediatric study albeit cyanotic breath-holding and RAS were lumped together. Adults with confirmed vasovagal syncope who had a positive family history were likely to have started their attacks before the age of 9 years.

Key points for clinical practice

- Reflex anoxic seizures (RAS) are non-epileptic motor events triggered by bumps and unexpected pain which look like 'breath-holding' but whose mechanism is reflex cardiac standstill.

- A discerning history should make the diagnosis in almost every case.

- Do not forget that children with brain disorders, such as cerebral palsy, may have RAS rather than epilepsy.

- When taking the family history, remember that the diagnosis of epilepsy is often wrong in adults as well as in children.

- Management of RAS includes making the parents aware that one understands what the condition is. It is essential not to give the impression that the child is just having temper tantrums.

- When RAS are accompanied by automatisms or hallucinations or out-of-body experiences it is important to resist the diagnosis of epilepsy.

- When (rarely) epileptic seizures are triggered by RAS they may be treated by anti-epileptic drugs and/or the RAS may themselves be prevented. Such anoxic-epileptic seizures do not imply later epilepsy.

- On rare occasions, RAS may need to be prevented by atropine or cardiac pacing. Other therapies are of uncertain value.

- The RAS patient support group is an invaluable resource which should be made available to families (Co-ordinator Trudie Lobban, PO Box 175, Stratford upon Avon, Warwickshire CV37 8YD, UK, tel/fax +44 1789 450564, E-mail Lobban_Fits_Faints@compuserve. com

CONCLUSION

Reflex anoxic seizures (RAS) are non-epileptic motor events (stiffening, jerks, spasms) triggered by noxious stimuli (head bump, pain, irritation) and mediated by short latency vagal mediated cardiac asystole. Other authors have called these white or pallid breath-holding spells or pallid infantile syncope but affected children need not be pale nor limp nor show 'breath-holding'. RAS are the result of ultra-fast vasovagal or pure vagal neurocardiogenic (neurally mediated) syncopes.

Very similar anoxic seizures (non-epileptic seizures) are caused by the more common so-called blue (cyanotic) breath-holding spells with prolonged expiratory apnoea, of complex and controversial mechanism.

To distinguish RAS from blue breath-holding (BBH) with certainty, it is necessary to record to record the ECG during an attack. In RAS, there is asystole of at least 10 s, whereas in BBH there is either bradycardia or tachycardia or some combination.

Rarely, as when RAS are very frequent and severe or complicated by true epileptic seizures, or persist into later childhood, specific therapy by atropine or cardiac pacing may be necessary, but usually understanding reassurance and support will allow normal development and potential.

References

1 Stephenson JBP. Reflex anoxic seizures ('white breath-holding'): nonepileptic vagal attacks. Arch Dis Child 1978; 53: 193–200
2 Breningstall GN. Breath-holding spells. Pediatr Neurol 1996; 14: 91–97
3 Bower BD. Pallid syncope (reflex anoxic seizures). Arch Dis Child 1984; 59: 1118–1119
4 Lombroso CT, Lerman P. Breath-holding spells (cyanotic and pallid infantile syncope). Pediatrics 1967; 39: 563–581
5 Stephenson JBP. Fits and Faints. London: MacKeith, 1990
6 Hannon DW. Breath-holding spells: waiting to inhale, waiting for systole, or waiting for iron therapy. J Pediatr 1997; 130: 510–512
7 Stephenson JBP. Blue breath holding is benign. Arch Dis Child 1991; 66: 255–257
8 Southall DP, Talbert DG, Johnson P et al. Prolonged expiratory apnoea: a disorder resulting in episodes of severe arterial hypoxaemia in infants and young children. Lancet 1985; 2: 571–577
9 Appleton RE. Reflex anoxic seizures. BMJ 1993; 307: 214–215
10 Stephenson JBP. Nonepileptic seizures, anoxic-epileptic seizures, and epileptic-anoxic seizures. In: Wallace S (ed) Epilepsy in Children. London: Chapman & Hall, 1996; 5–26
11 McWilliam RC, Stephenson JBP. Atropine treatment of reflex anoxic seizures. Arch Dis Child 1984; 59: 473–475
12 Lempert T. Recognising syncopes: pitfalls and surprises. J R Soc Med 1996; 89: 372–375
13 Roddy SM, Ashwal S, Schneider S. Venepuncture fits: a form of reflex anoxic seizure. Pediatrics 1983; 72: 715–718
14 Blackmore S. Experiences of anoxia: do reflex anoxic seizures resemble near-death experiences? J Near-Death Studies 1998; 17: 111–120
15 Smith D, Defalla BA, Chadwick DW. The misdiagnosis of epilepsy and the management of refractory epilepsy in a specialist clinic. Q J Med 1999; 92: 15–23
16 Gibbs J, Appleton RE. False diagnosis of epilepsy in children. Seizure 1992; 1: 15–18
17 Wilde AA, Jongbloedd RJ, Doevendans PA et al. Auditory stimuli as a trigger for arrhythmic events differentiate HERG-related (LQTS2) patients from KVLQT1-related patients. J Am Coll Cardiol 1999; 33: 327–332

18 Priori SG, Napolitano C, Schwartz PJ. Low penetrance in the long QT syndrome: clinical impact. Circulation 1999; 99: 529–523

19 McCrory PR, Berkovic SF. Concussive convulsions. Incidence in sport and treatment recommendations. Sports Med 1998; 25: 131-136

20 Guerrini R, Battaglia A, Gastaut H. Absence status triggered by pallid syncopal spells. Neurology 1991; 41: 1528–1529

21 Oribe E, Amini R, Nissenbaum E, Boal B. Serum prolactin concentrations are elevated after syncope. Neurology 1996; 47: 60–62

22 DiMario FJ, Bauer L, Baxter D. Respiratory sinus arrhythmia in children with severe cyanotic and pallid breath-holding spells. J Child Neurol 1998; 13: 440–442

23 Furlan R, Piazza S, Dell'Orto S et al. Cardiac autonomic patterns preceding occasional vasovagal reactions in healthy humans. Circulation 1998; 98: 1756–1761

24 Schubert R, Cracco JB. Familial rectal pain: a type of reflex epilepsy? Ann Neurol 1992; 32: 824–825

25 Stephenson JBP, Ferrie CD. Syncope and anoxic seizures in familial rectal pain. Brain Dev 1998; 20: 487

26 DiMario FJ, Burleson JA. Behaviour profile of children with severe breath-holding spells. J Pediatr 1993; 122: 488–491

27 Battaglia A, Guerrini R, Gastaut H. Epileptic seizures induced by syncopal attacks. J Epilepsy 1989; 2: 137–146

28 Emery ES. Status epilepticus secondary to breath-holding and pallid syncopal spells. Neurology 1990; 40: 859

29 Daoud AS, Batieha A, Al-Sheyyab M, Abuekteish F, Hijazi S. Effectiveness of iron therapy on breath-holding spells. J Pediatr 1997; 130: 547–550

30 Donma MM. Clinical efficacy of piracetam in treatment of breath-holding spells. Pediatr Neurol 1998; 18: 41–45

31 Sapire DW, Casta A, Satley W, O'Riordan AC, Balsara RK. Vasovagal syncope in children requiring pacemaker implantation. Am Heart J 1983; 106: 1406–1411

32 Porter CJ, McGoon MD, Espinosa RE, Osborn MJ, Hales DL. Apparent breath-holding spells associated with life-threatening bradycardia treated by permanent pacing. Pediatr Cardiol 1994; 15: 260

33 Sreeram N, Whitehouse W. Permanent cardiac pacing for reflex anoxic seizures. Arch Dis Child 1996; 75: 462

34 Petersen MEV, Price D, Williams T, Jensen N, Rift K, Sutton R. Short AV interval VDD pacing does not prevent tilt induced vasovagal syncope in patients with cardioinhibitory vasovagal syndrome. Pacing Clin Electrophysiol 1994; 17: 882–891

35 Connolly SJ, Sheldon R, Roberts RS, Gent M. The North American Pacemaker Study (VPS) a randomized trial of permanent cardiac pacing for the prevention of vasovagal syncope. J Am Coll Cardiol 1999; 33: 16–20

36 Benditt DG. Cardiac pacing for prevention of vasovagal syncope. J Am Coll Cardiol 1999; 33: 21–23

37 McLeod KA, Wilson N, Hewitt J, Norrie J, Stephenson JBP. Cardiac pacing for severe childhood neurally-mediated syncopes with reflex anoxic seizures. Heart 1999; In press

38 Stephenson JBP. Reflex anoxic seizures and ocular compression. Dev Med Child Neurol 1980; 22: 380–386

39 DiMario FJ, Sarfarazi M. Family pedigree analysis of children with severe breath-holding spells. J Pediatr 1997; 130: 647–651

40 Mathias CJ, Deguchi K, Bleasedale-Barr K, Kimber JR. Frequency of family history in vasovagal syncope. Lancet 1998; 352: 33–34

Janet M. Rennie Geraldine B. Boylan

CHAPTER

2

Neonatal seizures

WHAT IS DIFFERENT ABOUT NEONATAL SEIZURES?

Seizures are the most frequent clinical sign of a central nervous system disorder in babies, not least because other clinical signs are often subtle or lacking. A seizure is best defined as any paroxysmal alteration in neurological function, and this definition includes autonomic nervous system change as well as change which is seen only on the EEG. EEG definitions vary, but paroxysms are considered to be seizures if they last more than 5–10 s. Seizures occur more frequently in the neonatal period than at any other time of life. Seizures are a common emergency in neonatal paediatrics and, for this reason alone, it is important to have a clear protocol for investigation and management. Knowledge of the likely prognosis helps in counselling parents who are understandably anxious about any 'brain' problem in their infant. A proportion of surviving children will inevitably be handicapped and, in some, their caregivers will pursue litigation in an attempt to recover the costs of their ongoing care. Detailed recording of prompt and appropriate decision making is particularly important because these notes are closely scrutinized, often many years after the events, by individuals who were not involved at the time. Comments such as 'fitting, BM stix 1' with no elaboration and no further entry in the case notes until 12 h later 'ventilated, low sugars, frequent clonic movements of limbs' are unlikely to assist a defence team.

Dr Janet M Rennie MA MD FRCP FRCPCH DCH, Consultant and Senior Lecturer in Neonatal Medicine, Room 401, 4th Floor Ruskin Wing, King's College Hospital, Denmark Hill, London SE5 9RS, UK (for correspondence)

Ms Geraldine B Boylan MSc, Research Fellow, Neonatal Unit, King's College Hospital, Denmark Hill, London SE5 9RS, UK

CLINICAL PRESENTATION OF NEONATAL SEIZURE

Neonatal seizures are uniquely varied and subtle. Classic 'tonic–clonic' seizures are rarely seen. Typical neonatal seizure manifestations include apnoea; staring; pallor; eye deviation; eye opening; chewing/sucking; limb posturing; change in blood pressure; increased salivation or secretions; swimming/pedalling limb movements. Video-EEG studies have led to the realisation that many (previously ignored) subtle stereotyped repeated movements were in fact seizures. Often it is only in retrospect that a brief stereotyped movement is recognised to have accompanied an electrical seizure discharge. The clinical manifestations may be slight but the EEG changes can be dramatic. The reasons behind the subtle clinical manifestation of seizure probably relate more to the lack of myelination and development of the infant nervous system rather than the 'benign' nature of the seizures themselves. The early clinical studies termed these seizures 'slight' but we now realise that the lack of impressive clinical signs does not mean that the seizures are unimportant. Volpe's (1992) classification of neonatal seizures has become widely adopted and has the merit of simplicity (Table 2.1).[1] Video-EEG studies have also led to the realisation that neonatal seizures exhibit 'electroclinical dissociation'; that is, that a clinical seizure can occur without a characteristic electrical signature and vice-versa. Only very rarely is a stereotyped, repetitive clinical paroxysm accompanied by a sharp wave or polyspike electrical discharge which begins and ends at the same time as the clinical seizure. This makes the study of neonatal seizures uniquely difficult.

INCIDENCE

A true prospective study using video-EEG monitoring of all births in a defined geographical population will never be done. Studies reporting only clinically diagnosed seizures inevitably represent an underestimate, but this incidence varies between 10–13% in preterm infants and 0.1–0.5% in those born at term.[2] The vast majority of neonatal seizures occur on the first day, and 70% of all cases eventually recognised have been diagnosed by the fourth day.

MECHANISMS

The particular susceptibility which babies undoubtedly have to develop seizures is due to the following:[3,4]

1. There is a relative excess of glutamate, the excitatory neurotransmitter, in the neonatal brain.
2. There is a reduced number of receptors for inhibitory neurotransmitters and a high density of excitatory receptors in the neonatal brain.
3. Gamma-amino butyric acid (GABA) is the main inhibitory neurotransmitter in the brain. The nature of $GABA_A$ receptors in babies can make GABA excitatory. Brain GABA levels are low in the neonatal period.
4. NMDA (excitatory) receptors are abundant, more easily triggered by glutamate, and less easily inhibited by magnesium in the neonatal brain

Table 2.1 Types of seizure in the newborn. Adapted from Volpe (1992)[1]

Type	Clinical signs	EEG
Subtle	Eye signs – eyelid fluttering, eye deviation, fixed open stare, blinking. Apnoea. Cycling, boxing, stepping, swimming movements of limbs. Mouthing, chewing, lip smacking, smiling. 'motor automatisms'	Often no EEG changes – EEG change is most likely with ocular manifestations. Focal abnormalities
Tonic	Stiffening. Decerebrate posturing. Includes conjugate deviation of the eyes.	EEG variable; often EEG change if focal posturing
Clonic	Repetitive jerking, distinct from jittering. Can still be felt in the restrained limb. Clonic seizures can be unifocal or migrate	Usually has EEG change
Myoclonic	Rapid isolated jerks, usually bilateral but can be unilateral or focal. Sleep myoclonus is benign	EEG often normal, although background EEG can be abnormal

compared to the adult. NMDA receptors are largely calcium dependent in the newborn.

5. Na/K-ATPase, the energy dependent cellular ion pump, is often deprived of glucose and/or oxygen in the neonatal period and then admits sodium to the cell which leaks potassium. Accumulated extracellular potassium contributes to a hyperexcitability state.

6. There is an increased density of synapses in the normal neonatal brain (many will drop out) and this supports 'hypersynchrony', 'recurrent excitation' or 'kindling', the phenomenon whereby an electrical seizure is propagated around the brain.

7. 'Surround inhibition', the response of neurons around an area of excitability which contains a seizure, is less effective in the immature brain.

DIAGNOSIS

The key feature which differentiates neonatal seizures from those in older children and adults is the extremely subtle nature of the clinical manifestations. Paradoxically, this leads to both under- and over-diagnosis. Not only are the clinical manifestations subtle, but newborn infants often have electroclinical dissociation; that is, babies can have typical seizure manifestations without a characteristic electrical signature and vice-versa. Only rarely do clinical and electrographic seizures occur simultaneously. Movements which can represent seizure activity include jaw trembling, eye opening, eye deviation, blinking, lip-smacking, and bicycling/swimming/boxing movements of the limbs. Heart rate or blood pressure changes are detected in infants undergoing intensive care, and apnoea can be a seizure manifestation. Myoclonic jerking can be seen, sometimes due to benign neonatal sleep myoclonus. Clonic jerking is more often accompanied by an electrographic discharge than subtle seizures. Tonic seizures involve opisthotonic posturing, or tonic extension of the limbs.

The message from video-EEG studies is that it can be very difficult to detect seizures using clinical observation alone.[5,6] Any stereotyped movement or unusual behaviour in a high risk infant should arouse suspicion. Although, as already mentioned, 'subtle' seizures were at first characterized as 'slight',[7] study over time has confirmed that subtle seizures are often a manifestation of serious underlying central nervous system disorder. The only way to confirm whether or not an abnormal motor pattern truly represents a seizure is to carry out an EEG, ideally with simultaneous video monitoring. Even then the clinical manifestation of the seizure does not usually correlate with the anatomic site of the paroxysmal electrical discharge. Interpreting the neonatal EEG is a specialized skill. Digitization already allows the rapid transmission of large EEG data files for expert interpretation, and the use of this method will enable this valuable investigation to become more widely available than at present.

INVESTIGATION

General

Investigations are required, aimed at determining the cause of the seizure. A lumbar puncture is mandatory. Serum electrolytes including glucose, calcium and magnesium; an infection screen including a lumbar puncture and cranial ultrasound imaging are a minimum. Cranial ultrasound scanning represents the minimum neuro-imaging and, if the results are normal, an MRI scan should be done. CT is superior to MRI for the detection of calcification and haemorrhage, but ultrasound will usually detect these reliably and CT involves a large X-ray exposure. Glucose and electrolytes should be measured to exclude hypoglycaemia and hypocalcaemia. Pyridoxine dependency cannot be diagnosed in the laboratory and if this diagnosis is suspected a trial of pyridoxine therapy is the only option.

EEG

The EEG was discovered in Liverpool in 1875. Caton's original description was of 'feeble currents of varying direction pass through the multiplier when the electrodes are placed on two points of the external surface, or on the surface of the skull'. Epileptiform discharges are sharp waves or spikes with or without slow waves which are clearly distinguishable from background EEG activity. Neonatal electrographic seizures often begin in a focal area but often spread to involve most of the cortex. Neonatal seizures may be unifocal, that is they arise from one discrete area or focus, or they may be multifocal, that is seizures arise from a number of different independent foci. Most often, neonatal seizures are unifocal or arise in two areas of the brain. Temporal seizures frequently correlate with clinical apnoea.[20]

Neonatal electrographic seizures are not usually sustained, with 97% lasting less than 9 min.[8] In preterm infants seizure duration is shorter than at term.[9,10] In spite of this, the total seizure burden can be very significant. Neonatal status is currently defined as a total seizure time occupying 50% of a recording or 30 min (a routine adult EEG lasts 20-30 minutes). This is a rather arbitrary definition which needs revision for prolonged neonatal recordings. To the uninitiated, repeated stereotyped electrical discharges which resemble an ECG are not a normal feature of the EEG and are probably seizures (Fig. 2.1B).

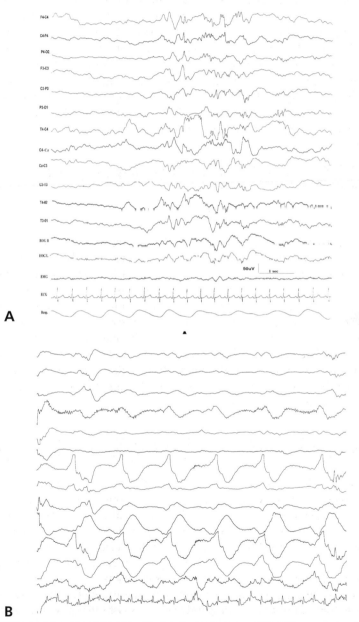

Fig. 2.1 (**A**) Normal trace alternant pattern in a full term infant; (**B**) seizure in a full term infant.

The interictal (between seizure) EEG, or the background activity of the EEG when seizures are not present, can give very helpful information about prognosis.[11] The number and type of seizures is not helpful in this regard, although few authors have examined the prognosis for the subgroup of infants with very prolonged electrographic seizures. The background EEG needs to be interpreted with knowledge of the normal background appearance for the gestational age. Generalised burst-suppression is an ominous pattern at any gestation. At term it must be correctly distinguished from the trace alternant pattern of quiet sleep (Fig. 2.1A). In very preterm infants of 26–32 weeks gestation, the EEG is normally discontinuous, 'trace discontinu'. At less than 26 weeks gestation, the periods of discontinuity can last for several minutes, although above this gestation suppressed periods (even in trace discontinu) do not on average last for more than 20–30 s. This means that a continuously low voltage ('depressed'; 'flat'; 'attenuated') EEG with or without bursts is abnormal even for very immature babies. A low voltage EEG is one where the background activity is generally less than 15 µV (25 µV in wakefulness); in an isoelectric EEG it is less than 5–10 µV. A misleading trace can be excluded by confirmation that there is an ECG artefact visible on the EEG: this ensures that the impedance of the electrodes is sufficiently low to exclude inadequate recording quality as a reason for electrical silence. This is particularly important in babies who often have scalp caput or cephalhaematomas which can affect the amplitude of the EEG. Sensory and auditory stimulation should be tried to ensure that the EEG is truly non-reactive, and recordings made using high sensitivity, gain settings and with meticulous care.

EEG evidence of diffuse cerebral injury (burst-suppression; multifocal sharp waves; dysmaturity; attenuation; electrical silence) is not specific for the pathological process and may be the result of hypoxia–ischaemia, infarction, infection, metabolic disorder or a structural abnormality.[12] A persistently focal abnormality on the EEG should lead to a search for a focal pathology with careful imaging. The role of the EEG in the prognosis of hypoxic ischaemic encephalopathy is discussed later in a specific section in view of its importance.

Cerebral function monitoring

The cerebral function monitor (CFM) is a device which presents a compressed, rectified and filtered signal from one channel of EEG on a paper trace at the cotside. In neonates a CFM trace is usually obtained via a pair of electrodes applied over the parietal lobes with a reference electrode over the frontal lobe.[13] The display is written out at 6–30 cm/h. The amplitude scale is semi-logarithmic. A generally low voltage trace can be distinguished from one with a normal voltage, and prolonged seizures cause a spiky pattern. Whilst the method has the merit of simplicity, and interpretation using pattern recognition can be taught to residents and nurses, CFM will inevitably be less sensitive that EEG as a 'seizure detection' monitor. Seizures which are short-lived (5–30 s) or do not generalise cannot be detected.[14,15] The very compressed nature of the trace makes it difficult to exclude movement artefact. Deterioration of the electrode impedance over time can make the background voltage unreliable and it is more difficult to be sure that scalp swelling is not artificially reducing the amplitude. However, useful results have been obtained when the CFM has been used with care.[16,17]

'CLINICAL ONLY' SEIZURES

A small group of babies have repetitive stereotyped movements which are thought to be abnormal but never develop an electrographic seizure manifestation. Using prolonged EEG monitoring, we have found that, when the background EEG is abnormal, then continued monitoring in this group eventually reveals an electroclinical seizure. The original descriptions of 'non-epileptic' or 'clinical only' seizures were in babies who were clearly neuro-logically sick, obtunded and with a paucity of normal spontaneous movements.[18] All the infants with clinical only seizure described by Mizrahi and Kellaway[6] had abnormal background EEGs. In these babies, the tonic posturing and motor automatisms could be induced by sensory stimulation, and was inhibited by stilling the limb.

In our experience, there is a further group of infants in whom the background EEG remains normal, who have normal neuro-imaging and who appear entirely well between attacks. These babies appear to have repetitive, stereotyped motor automatisms as a benign phenomenon. The movements do not still on holding the limb. Autonomic changes do not occur. Thus, these infants appear to be a different population from those with clinical only seizures originally described by Mizrahi and Kellaway.[19] Treatment should be avoided in this group because the prognosis is excellent without it.[20] Some of the mothers of our babies were known to be using psychometric drugs either on prescription, or off it. This group can be rapidly distinguished from the group in whom the clinical automatisms are not a benign phenomenon. The non-benign group are obtunded; the background EEG is abnormal; and if monitoring is continued long enough these babies will eventually display an electroclinical seizure.

PATHOPHYSIOLOGY/CEREBRAL BLOOD FLOW CHANGES

The most important question is whether or not it is necessary to treat all neonatal seizures to electrical quiescence. This question arises in part because the most frequently used anticonvulsant, phenobarbitone, is known to increase electroclinical dissociation.[21] Clinically, things may look better because the infant is quieter, but electrographic seizures continue unabated. If EEG monitoring is in place, there may be just as many electrical seizures as before. Both electroclinical and electrographic seizures are accompanied by physiological changes, including a rise in blood pressure and a rise in cerebral blood flow.[22] We used Doppler estimation of cerebral blood flow velocity to measure blood pressure, respiration, heart rate and cerebral blood flow velocity during different types of neonatal seizure. Changes in cerebral blood flow velocity and blood pressure were seen, and were of similar magnitude in both electroclinical and electrographic seizure.[23] These results can be interpreted to mean that it is necessary to treat neonatal seizures to electrical quiescence if the outcome is to be improved. The seizure burden which is currently tolerated in the newborn would not be considered reasonable in adults or older children. Neonatal rats subjected to recurrent brief seizures have long-term changes in behaviour and permanent changes in brain development with 'mossy fibre' sprouting in the hippocampus.[24] At present, the therapeutic options do not allow neonatal seizure control to be achieved with any degree of certainty and more work is needed to establish effective regimens before large scale clinical trials can be done.

AETIOLOGY

Seizures are a non-specific manifestation of disorders of the central nervous system and metabolic disruption. At term, hypoxic ischaemic encephalopathy remains the most common underlying factor. In preterm infants, intracranial haemorrhage is the most common cause. Meningitis, focal cerebral infarction, metabolic disorders and congenital abnormalities of the brain can cause seizures at any gestation. Some authors have suggested that there is a relationship between the type of seizure and the aetiology. Table 2.2 shows the relative frequency in some recent studies.

TREATMENT

Treatment of neonatal seizures has changed little in the last 30 years. Intensive care support may be required for infants who have apnoea as a major manifestation, or for the underlying disease. Seizures due to metabolic disturbance such as hypoglycaemia or hypocalcaemia may respond to correction of the underlying metabolic defect, although it may accompany another condition such as hypoxic ischaemic encephalopathy.

Table 2.2 Causes of neonatal seizure

	1	2	3	4	5*	6**	7
Number of cases			71	131	100	40	100
Hypoxic–ischaemic encephalopathy	53%	16%	49%	30%	49%	37%	32%
Intracranial haemorrhage	17%		14%		7%	12%	16%
Cerebral infarction (stroke)					12%	17%	7%
Meningitis	8%	3%	2%	7%	5%	5%	14%
Maternal drug withdrawal			4%				
Hypoglycaemia	3%	2%	0.1%	5%	3%		2%
Hypocalcaemia, hypomagnasaemia				22%			4%
Rapidly changing serum sodium							
Congenitally abnormal brain			8%	4%	3%	17%	3%
Fifth day fits			52%				
Benign familial neonatal seizures							1%
Benign neonatal sleep myoclonus							1%
Pyridoxine dependent seizures							
Hypertensive encephalopathy			1.4%				
Kernicterus					1%		
Inborn errors of metabolism					3%		3%

*This series included > 31 week gestation infants only.
**This series was limited to cases presenting in the first 48 h of life. Blanks occur where no cases were recorded in a particular study. Data in column 1 are from Levene and Trounce (1986),[25] column 2 from Goldberg (1983);[26] column 3 from Andre et al. (1988);[27] column 4 from Bergman et al. (1983);[28] column 5 from Estan and Hope (1997);[29] column 6 from Lien et al. (1995);[30] and column 7 from Mizrahi and Kellaway (1998).[19]

Phenobarbitone remains the mainstay of therapy; the initial dose is 20 mg/kg in unventilated babies and 30 mg/kg in those who are already ventilator dependent (Table 2.3), aiming to achieve a serum level of 20–40 mg/l (88–176 µmol/l). Phenobarbitone achieves clinical control in about 30% of cases; some claim better clinical control (70%) with doses of up to 40 mg/kg and serum levels above 40 mg/l.[31]

Babies with seizures which do not respond to phenobarbitone in adequate dose must be treated with an additional anticonvulsant. Phenytoin 20 mg/kg over 20 min has been a popular option, but this agent can cause significant myocardial depression and should be avoided in babies requiring inotropic support. Midazolam and clonazepam, anecdotally, achieve better EEG control although a formal evaluation is required. Of the two, midazolam has a shorter half-life, does not accumulate, avoids the side effect of increased oropharyngeal secretions and is our current second line. Others have reported success with lignocaine. The published neonatal experience with any of the third line

Table 2.3 Anticonvulsant drug dose in the newborn

Drug	Initial dose	Route	Maintenance dose	Route	Half-life	Therapeutic level
Pheno-barbitone	15–30 mg/kg	IV	4–5 mg/kg/24 h	O	100–200 h	20–40 mg/l 90–180 µmol/l
Phenytoin	20 mg/kg in 2 doses	IV	5 mg/kg/24 h in 2 doses	IV/O	20 h (75 in prems)	10–20 mg/l 40–80 µmol/l
Paralde-hyde	0.2 ml/kg IM or 0.3 ml/kg (0.6 ml/kg of mixture) PR	deep IM or rectal	For rectal use dilute 1:1 with arachis oil, give no more than t.d.s.		10 h	
Diazepam	0.2 mg/kg	IV	0.2 mg/kg	IV	20–60 h	
Clonazepam	100 µg/kg	IV	4 µg/kg/h	IV	30 h	30–100 mg/l
Carbam-azepine	5 mg/kg	O	5–15 mg/kg/12 hourly	O	3–15 h	4–12 mg/l (17–50 µg/l)
Valproate	20 mg/kg	IV	10 mg/kg/12 hourly	O	26–47 h	40–50 mg/l 275–350 µmol/l
Lignocaine	2 mg/kg	IV	2 mg/kg/h maximum 6 mg/kg/h	IV	200 min	2.4–6 mg/l in adults ? little value in infants
Midazolam	0.15 mg/kg	IV	0.1–0.4 mg/kg/h	IV	0.8 h	?
Valproate	20–26 mg/kg	O	5–10 mg/kg/12 hourly	O		40–50 µg/l
Vigabatrin	50 mg/kg	O	50 mg/kg/day	O	?	? — little neonatal experience

Note: although technically correct, abbreviations like g (1000 milligrams), mg (1000 micrograms), µg (1000 nanograms) and ng (1000 picograms) should be avoided when prescribing as they can easily be misread when written by hand.

anticonvulsants (Table 2.3) is very limited. There is a single publication reporting the use of Vigabatrin in the newborn.[32] This drug is a GABA analogue and has been used with some success in infantile spasms in a dose of 60–100 mg/kg/day. Visual field defects have been described in older children and adults treated with Vigabatrin and, in view of the difficulty in assessing visual field defects in infants, neonatal use may be limited. Lamotrigine is believed to stabilise neuronal membranes and inhibit excitatory neurotransmitters, but has not so far been used in the newborn.

Pyridoxine dependency

Pyridoxine dependent seizures are a rare but treatable subgroup of neonatal seizures, which can begin in intra-uterine life. The condition results from an autosomal recessive disorder in which there is a reduction in brain and CSF levels of gamma amino butyric acid (GABA). The diagnosis is difficult because it is one of exclusion. A trial of pyridoxine under EEG control is recommended when all else fails. The trial should be carried out in an intensive care environment in case of severe hypotonia. Some previous advice about this disorder suggested too low a dose of pyridoxine, and a subgroup of affected babies respond only to very high doses given for 2 weeks. This information has served only to make this diagnosis even more difficult. If a baby responds to an intravenous injection of pyridoxine (100 mg intravenously) with abolition of clinical and electrographic seizures then pyridoxine treatment (50–100 mg/day orally with 5 mg folate) should be continued for 6 months before a trial of withdrawal in hospital with frequent EEG monitoring. The issue has been clouded further by reports of babies who responded only after days of massive doses of pyridoxine. If seizures recur when treatment is withdrawn then it should be continued for life.

Seizures in hypoxic–ischaemic encephalopathy

Hypoxic ischaemic encephalopathy (HIE) deserves special mention because this disorder is a common and important cause of seizure. The diagnosis of HIE is supported by an abnormal antenatal history, birth depression, perhaps a low cord pH, need for resuscitation and an abnormal neurological state between seizures. The characteristic time of onset of seizure in HIE is 8–36 h after birth. Frequently, it is reported that infants who suffered from fetal distress and required resuscitation at birth are 'fitting in the delivery room'. Our video-EEG studies reveal that these seizures are usually 'clinical only' at this stage, and are due to an abnormal increase in tone. The background EEG in cases of intrapartum acquired seizure is depressed at this time, and electrical seizures reliably emerge after 8–36 h. At this time, the activity of the EEG increases. Babies appear to be rather like lambs, in that if there is an intrapartum insult the EEG is at first depressed, and then evolves to show seizure activity about 8 h after birth.[33,34] An EEG obtained shortly after birth in which electrical seizure activity was already manifest would strongly suggest an insult over 8 h before delivery, although further studies are clearly needed to establish this important point.

Encephalopathy can develop in the neonatal period even when the insult was established several days or weeks before birth, but in these cases the EEG does not follow the typical sequence seen after an intrapartum acquired insult.

Background EEG is of most value in prognosis of HIE when recorded early, within 24–48 h of birth.[35] Recently reliable prognosis has been claimed with depressed CFM or clinical seizure recognition at 3–6 h, at a time when intervention might be effective.[17,36,37] However, we have found that a full EEG obtained as early as this can normalise and the prognosis is then good. A normal background EEG at any time within the first 24 h suggests a good prognosis, even if there are multiple seizures present. An abnormal background EEG may normalise, or deteriorate. A persistently depressed background is an ominous prognostic feature.[38,39] Infants with a persistently isoelectric EEG usually die or develop multicystic encephalomalacia. Burst-suppression is equally serious. In our recent experience of term babies with HIE, all 7 babies with a clinical grade III encephalopathy also had marked EEG changes, including prolonged discontinuity (more than 20 s) which took a week to normalise. Three of the babies died, two have hypsarrythmia and two are quadriplegic requiring tube feeding. The EEG grading of severity was in good agreement with the clinical grading, and EEG is useful when clinical signs are obscured by therapeutic paralysis or drug treatment. Early dyschronism (dysmaturity) of the EEG with moderate discontinuity is thought by some to indicate that the insult was prenatal rather than intrapartum. Others have found that moderate discontinuity can occur after intrapartum acquired hypoxia, and we would agree with them. The prognosis in term infants with hypoxic ischaemic encephalopathy who have dysmature EEG patterns is usually good,[39,40] although the same may not be true for preterm infants with other diagnoses.

PROGNOSIS

This is mainly related to the cause of the seizures. Following hypoxic–ischaemic encephalopathy at term, 25% of those who develop grade II Sarnat and Sarnat encephalopathy will suffer sequelae. The combination of a 5 min Apgar score < 5, fits and signs of encephalopathy was a poor one with 33% dead and 55% with handicap.[41] Of 70 cases of clinical seizure in very low birthweight infants followed in Cambridge, 43 (59%) died, 16 (22%) had a major handicap and 11 (15%) were normal at 18 months (personal observations). These data are remarkably similar to those of Watkins et al. ($n = 65$),[42] Van Zeben et al. ($n = 72$),[43] and Scher et al. ($n = 62$),[9] although as many as 90% of the preterm infants in some series died.[28] The prognosis after hypocalcaemic seizure and in familial neonatal seizure is excellent. Symptomatic hypoglycaemia and meningitis have a 50% chance of sequelae in the survivors.[7,28] The value of a normal neurological examination at discharge in providing early reassurance should not be underestimated; 11 of 14 infants with seizures who were normal at 4 years were assessed as normal at this stage.[44] However this initially normal group of Oxford children then had problems with spelling and memory in adolescence.[45]

Key points for clinical practice

- Seizures are more common in the neonatal period than at any other time of life; they are particularly frequent on the first day. The incidence is about 10% in preterm infants and about 0.1–0.5% at term.

- Subtle seizures are the usual neonatal seizure type. Manifestations of subtle seizures include apnoea; staring or deviation of the eyes; chewing, blinking or cycling movements.

- Neonatal seizures exhibit electroclinical dissociation; that is there is poor agreement between the clinical and electrical paroxysms. Clinical manifestations can occur without a characteristic electrographic signature and vice-versa.

- Investigation of seizures should include a search for metabolic disorder and infection. A cranial ultrasound scan is the minimum neuro-imaging, and if this result is normal an MRI is strongly recommended.

- Although electrographic seizures are not usually sustained in the neonate, the total electrical seizure burden is often great, the clinical manifestations being the 'tip of the iceberg'.

- Phenobarbitone increases electroclinical dissociation, and at present no drug regimen reliably achieves electrical quiescence of seizures in babies.

- The cerebral haemodynamic response to seizure — raised cerebral blood flow — is seen whether the seizures are electroclinical or electrographic. The rise in cerebral blood flow is not due solely to a rise in blood pressure, which tends to be seen when there are marked motor automatisms.

- The interictal EEG is a good guide to prognosis, especially when performed at 12–48 h. A very depressed background or burst suppression at this time indicates a poor prognosis: a depressed background at < 12 h may normalise. Drugs such as morphine and phenobarbitone can depress the neonatal EEG.

- There appears to be a group of infants who only ever have clinical seizure manifestations, who have a normal EEG, normal neuro-imaging and who remain entirely well. Treatment with anti-epileptic drugs can be avoided in this small group whose prognosis is good.

References

1 Volpe JJ. Neonatal seizures. In: Volpe JJ, ed. Neurology of the Newborn, 3rd edn. Philadelphia, PA: Saunders; 1995; 172–207
2 Rennie JM. Neonatal seizures. Eur J Pediatr 1997; 156: 83–87
3 Moshe SL. Seizures in the developing brain. Neurology 1993; 43: S3–S7
4 Moshe SL, Albala BJ, Ackerman RF et al . Increased seizure susceptibility in the neonatal brain. Dev Brain Res 1983; 7: 81–85
5 Weiner SP, Painter MJ, Geva Guthrie RP, Scher MS. Neonatal seizures electroclinical dissociation. Pediatr Neurol 1991; 7: 363–368

6 Mizrahi EM, Kellaway P. Characterization and classification of neonatal seizures. Neurology 1987; 37: 1837–1844

7 Rose A, Lombroso CT. Neonatal seizure states: a study of clinical, pathological, and electroencephalographic features in 137 full-term babies with a long-term follow-up. Pediatrics 1970; 45: 404–425

8 Clancy RR, Ledigo A. The exact ictal and interictal duration of electroencephalographic neonatal seizures. Epilepsia 1987; 28: 537–541

9 Scher MS, Aso K, Beggarly ME et al . Electrographic seizures in preterm and full-term neonates: clinical correlates, associated brain lesions, and risk for neurologic sequelae. Pediatrics 1993; 91: 128–134

10 Scher MS, Hamid MY, Steppe DA et al. Ictal and interictal electrographic seizure durations in preterm and term neonates. Epilepsia 1993; 34: 284–288

11 Laroia N, Guillet R, Burchfield J et al . EEG Background as predictor of electrographic seizures in high-risk neonates. Epilepsia 1998; 39: 545–551

12 Aso K, Scher MS, Barmada MA. Neonatal electroencephalography and neuropathology. J Clin Neurophysiol 1998; 6: 103–123

13 Viniker DA, Maynard DE, Scott DF. Cerebral function monitor studies in neonates. Clin Electroencephalogr 1984; 15: 185–192

14 Hellstrom-Westas L. Comparison between tape recorded and amplitude integrated EEG monitoring in sick newborn infants. Acta Paediatr 1992; 81: 812–819

15 Murdoch-Eaton D, Toet M, Livingston J et al . Evaluation of the Cerebro-trac 2500 for monitoring of cerebral function in the neonatal intensive care. Neuropaediatrics 1984; 25: 122–128

16 Archbald F, Verma UL, Tejani NA et al. Cerebral function monitor in the neonate. II. Birth asphyxia. Dev Med Child Neurol 1984; 26: 162–168

17 Hellstrom-Westas L, Rosen I, Svenningsen NW. Predictive value of early continuous amplitude integrated EEG recordings on outcome after severe birth asphyxia in full term infants. Arch Dis Child 1995; 72: F34–F38

18 Kellaway P, Mizrahi EM. Clinical, electroencephalographic, therapeutic and pathophysiologic studies of neonatal seizures. Neonatal Seizures Book 1990; 1–14

19 Mizrahi EM, Kellaway P. Diagnosis and Management of Neonatal Seizures, 1st edn. Philadelphia, PA: Lippincott-Raven; 1998

20 Boylan GB, Pressler RM, Rennie JM et al. Outcome of electroclinical, electrographic and clinical seizures in the newborn infant. Dev Med Clin Neurol; In press

21 Connell JA, Oozeer R, de Vries LS et al . Clinical and EEG response to anticonvulsants in seizures. Arch Dis Child 1989; 64: 459–464

22 Borch K, Pryds O, Holm S et al. Regional cerebral blood flow during seizures in neonates. J Paediatr 1998; 132: 431–435

23 Boylan GB, Pressler R, Rennie JM et al. Cerebral blood flow velocity during neonatal seizures. Arch Dis Child 1999; 80: F105-F110

24 Holmes GL, Gairsa J-L, Chevassus-Au-Louis N et al. Consequences of neonatal seizures in the rat: morphological and behavioral effects. Ann Neurol 1998; 44: 845–857

25 Levene MI, Trounce JQ. Causes of neonatal convulsions. Arch Dis Child 1986; 61: 78–79

26 Goldberg HJ. Neonatal convulsions – a ten year review. Arch Dis Child 1983; 57: 633–635

27 Andre M, Matisse M, Vert P et al. Neonatal seizures – recent aspects. Neuropaediatrics 1988; 19: 201–207

28 Bergman I, Painter MJ, Hirsch RP et al. Outcome in neonates with convulsions treated in ICU. Ann Neurol 1983; 14: 642–647

29. Estan J, Hope PL. Unilateral neonatal cerebral infarction in full term infants. Arch Dis Child 1997; 76: F88–F93

30 Lien JM, Towers CV, Quilligan EJ et al. Term early-onset neonatal seizures: obstetric characteristics, etiologic classifications and perinatal care. Obstet Gynaecol 1995; 85: 163–169

31 Gilman, JT. Rapid sequential phenobarbitone therapy of neonatal seizures. Pediatrics 1989; 83: 674–678

32 Baxter PS. Vigabatrin monotherapy in resistant neonatal seizures. Seizure 1995; 4: 57–59

33 Williams CE, Gunn A, Gluckman PD. Time course of intracellular oedema and epileptiform activity following prenatal cerebral ischaemia in sheep. Stroke 1991; 22: 516–21

34 Barabas, RE. Timing of brain insults in severe neonatal encephalopathies with isoelectric EEG. Pediatr Neurol 1993; 9: 39–44

35 Pezzani C, Radvani-Bouvet MF, Relier JP, Monod N. Neonatal electroencephalography during the first 24 hours of life in full term newborn infants. Neuropaediatrics 1986; 17: 11–18

36 Ekert P, Perlman M, Steinlin M, Hao Y. Predicting the outcome of postasphyxial hypoxic-ischemic encephalopathy within 4 hours of birth. J Paediatr 1997; 131: 613–617

37 Eken P, Toet MC, Groenendaal F, de Vries LS. Predictive value of early neuroimaging, pulsed Doppler and neurophysiology in full term infants with hypoxic ischaemic encephalopathy. Arch Dis Child 1995; 73: f75–f81

38 Watanabe K, Miyazaki S, Hara K et al. Behavioral state cycles, background EEGs and prognosis of newborn with perinatal hypoxia. Electroencephalog Clin Neurophysiol 1980; 49: 618–625.

39 Holmes G, Rowe J, Schmidt R et al. Prognostic value of the electroencephalogram in neonatal seizures. Electroencephalogr Clinic Neurophysiol 1982; 53: 60–72

40 Rowe JC, Holmes GL, Hafford J. Prognostic value of the EEG in term and preterm infant following neonatal seizures. Electroencephalog Clin Neurophysiol 1985; 60: 183–192

41 Ellenberg JH, Nelson KB. Cluster of perinatal events identifying children at high risk for death and disability. J Pediatr 1988; 113: 546–552

42 Watkins A, Szymonowicz W, Jin X et al. Significance of seizures in very low birthweight infants. Dev Med Child Neurol 1988; 30: 162–169

43 van Zeben-van der Aa DM, Veerlove-Vanhorick SP, den Ouden AL et al. Neonatal seizures in very preterm and low birthweight infants: mortality and handicaps at two years in a nationwide cohort. Neuropaediatrics 1990; 21: 62–65

44 Dennis J. Neonatal convulsions: aetiology, late neonatal status and long term outcome. Dev Med Child Neurol 1978; 20: 143–158

45 Temple CM, Dennis J, Crney R et al. Neonatal seizures: long term outcome and cognitive development among 'normal' survivors. Dev Med Child Neurol 1995; 37: 108–118

Sangkae Chamnanavanakij Jeffrey M. Perlman

Management of perinatal hypoxic–ischaemic encephalopathy

INTRODUCTION

Brain injury that occurs during the perinatal period is one of the most commonly recognized causes of severe, long-term neurological deficits in children, often referred to as cerebral palsy (CP). It is estimated that CP affects approximately 2–3 per 1000 school-aged children.[1] The overwhelming evidence suggests that the proportion of CP attributed to perinatal events, i.e. 'birth asphyxia', is small and representing approximately 10–20% of all cases.[1,2] However, this is the most relevant and important group of infants with CP because therapeutic strategies aimed to minimize or prevent cerebral injury are feasible.

Hypoxic–ischaemic brain injury is an evolving process initiated during an insult and extending into the recovery period, the latter referred to as the 'reperfusion phase' of injury. Clinically, it is the latter phase that is amenable to potential intervention(s). Current management strategies continue to remain largely supportive and are not targeted toward the processes of ongoing injury.[3] Thus, it is not surprising that, despite the improvement in perinatal practice during the past several decades, the incidence of CP attributed to intrapartum asphyxia remains essentially unchanged.[1] However, novel exciting strategies aimed at preventing ongoing injury are being evaluated and may, in the near future, offer an opportunity for neuroprotection. In this chapter, we briefly review the cellular characteristics of hypoxic–ischaemic cerebral injury and the current and future therapeutic strategies aimed at ameliorating ongoing brain injury following intrapartum hypoxia–ischaemia.

Sangkae Chamnanavanakij MD, Department of Pediatrics, Division of Neonatal-Perinatal Medicine, University of Texas Southwestern Medical Center, 5323 Harry Hines Blvd, Dallas, TX 75235-9063, USA

Jeffrey M. Perlman MB, Department of Pediatrics, Division of Neonatal-Perinatal Medicine, University of Texas Southwestern Medical Center, 5323 Harry Hines Blvd, Dallas, TX 75235-9063, USA (for correspondence)

The principal pathogenetic mechanism underlying most of the neuropathology attributed to intrapartum hypoxia–ischaemia is impaired cerebral blood flow (CBF). This is most likely to occur as a consequence of interruption in placental blood flow and gas exchange, often referred to as 'asphyxia'.

At the cellular level, the reduction in cerebral blood flow and oxygen delivery initiates a cascade of deleterious biochemical events. Depletion of oxygen precludes oxidative phosphorylation, and a switch to anaerobic metabolism. This is an energy inefficient state resulting in rapid depletion of high-energy phosphate reserves including ATP, accumulation of lactic acid and the inability to maintain cellular functions.[4] Transcellular ion pump failure results in the intracellular accumulation of Na^+, Ca^{2+} and water (cytotoxic oedema). The membrane depolarization results in a release of excitatory neurotransmitters (i.e. glutamate) from axon terminals. The glutamate then activates specific cell surface receptors resulting in an influx of Na^+ and Ca^{2+} into postsynaptic neurons. Within the cytoplasm, there is an accumulation of free fatty acids secondary to increased membrane phospholipid turnover. The fatty acids undergo peroxidation by oxygen free radicals that arise from reductive processes within mitochondria and as byproducts in the synthesis of prostaglandins, xanthine and uric acid (see Fig 3.1). Ca^{2+} ions accumulate within the cytoplasm as a consequence of increased cellular influx as well as decreased efflux across the plasma membrane combined with release from mitochondria and endoplasmic reticulum. In selected neurons, the intracellular calcium induces the production of nitric oxide, a free radical, diffusing to adjacent cells susceptible to nitric oxide toxicity. The combined effects of cellular energy failure, acidosis, glutamate release, intracellular Ca^{2+} accumulation, lipid

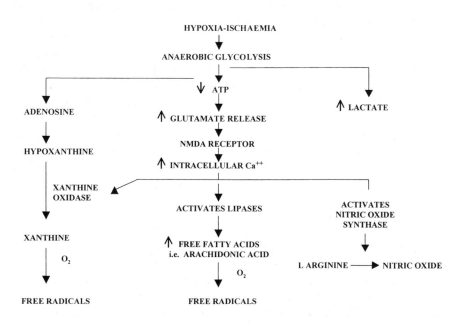

Fig. 3.1 Potential biochemical mechanisms of hypoxic–ischaemic cerebral injury.

peroxidation and nitric oxide neurotoxicity serve to disrupt essential components of the cell with its ultimate death.[2,5] Many factors, i.e. the duration or severity of the insult, will influence the progression of cellular injury following hypoxia–ischaemia.

Delayed (secondary) brain damage

Following resuscitation, which may occur *in utero* or postnatally in the delivery room, cerebral oxygenation and perfusion is restored. During this recovery phase, the concentration of phosphorus metabolites and the intracellular pH returns to baseline. However, the process of cerebral energy failure recurs 6–48 h later in a second phase of injury. This phase is characterized by a decrease in the ratio of phosphocreatine/inorganic phosphate, although the intracellular pH remains unchanged. This contributes to further brain injury,[4,6] despite the stable cardio-respiratory status. In the human infant, the severity of the second energy failure is correlated with adverse neurodevelopmental outcome at 1–4 years.[7] The mechanisms of secondary energy failure may involve mitochondrial dysfunction secondary to extended reactions from primary insults (e.g. calcium influx, excitatory neurotoxicity, oxygen free radicals or nitric oxide formation). Recent evidence also suggests that circulatory and endogenous inflammatory cells/mediators also contribute to ongoing brain injury.[8]

To discuss this process further, three principal mechanisms of ongoing injury are outlined below.

Accumulation of cytosolic calcium

Calcium is an intracellular second messenger necessarily for numerous cellular reactions. Under physiological condition, cytosolic Ca^{2+} concentration is strictly regulated at a very low intracellular concentration. During hypoxia–ischaemia, there is an increase in Ca^{2+} influx into neuronal cells in part by stimulation of the NMDA receptors of the agonist-operated Ca^{2+} channel by glutamate. In an opposite direction, Ca^{2+} efflux across the plasma membrane is interrupted by energy failure. Moreover, Ca^{2+} is also released into cytoplasm from the mitochondria by the Na^+/H^+-dependent antiport system and from the endoplasmic reticulum by inositol trisphosphate (IP_3) derived from the plasma membrane. These alterations of Ca^{2+} balance result in increased intracellular Ca^{2+}, which interferes with many enzymatic reactions including the activation of lipases, proteases, endonucleases and phospholipases and the formation of oxygen free radicals as byproducts of xanthine and prostaglandin synthesis. Overall, the accumulation of cytosolic Ca^{2+} after hypoxia–ischaemia has detrimental effects on neuronal cells leading to irreversible brain damage.[2,5]

Excitatory neurotransmitter release

Glutamic acid is a major excitatory amino acid within brain. The action of glutamate is mediated by a number of receptor subtypes including the NMDA receptors regulating Ca^{2+} influx through an ion channel, the AMPA (kainate/quisqualate) receptors mediating Na^+ influx and metabotropic receptors activating IP_3 generation for intracellular Ca^{2+} release. In the developing brain, the density of glutamate receptors, particularly of the NMDA subtype, is increased in areas of active development, e.g. striatum or hippocampus.

Within the NMDA receptor site, there are regions of agonist activity, i.e. glutamate, glycine as well as regions of antagonist activity, i.e. Mg^{2+}, phencyclidine or PCP.[2,5]

During hypoxia–ischaemia, glutamate accumulates in the synaptic cleft secondary to increased release from axon terminals as well as impaired re-uptake at presynaptic nerve endings. The excessive glutamate acting on the receptor sites facilitates the intracellular entry of Ca^{2+} via the NMDA receptor-mediated channel and promotes the biochemical cascade mentioned above leading to ultimate neuronal death.[2,5]

Formation of free radicals

Oxygen free radicals. In aerobic cells, oxygen free radicals (i.e. O_2^-, H_2O_2, OH^-) are produced within the cytoplasm and mitochondria. Under physiological condition, the oxygen free radicals are rapidly destroyed by endogenous antioxidants (i.e. superoxide dismutase, endoperoxidase, catalase) and scavengers (i.e. cholesterol, α-tocopherol, ascorbic acid, glutathione).[5,8] During and following hypoxia–ischaemia, the generation of oxygen free radicals is increased in excess of the protective capability. Two major sources of oxygen free radicals are the byproducts of xanthine (derived from the breakdown of ATP) and prostaglandin synthesis (derived from the breakdown of free fatty acids; see Fig. 3.1). Oxygen free radicals contribute to tissue injury by attacking the polyunsaturated fatty acid component of the cellular membrane resulting in membrane fragmentation and cell death.[5,8]

Nitric oxide. Nitric oxide (NO) is a weak free radical formed during the conversion of L-arginine to L-citrulline by nitric oxide synthase (NOS). NOS is strongly activated during hypoxia–ischaemia as well as during reperfusion and a large amount of NO is produced for extended periods. NO when combined with superoxide generates a potent radical, peroxynitrite, which activates lipid peroxidation. In addition, NO also enhances glutamate release.[8]

Iron. Physiologically, iron (Fe) is maintained in the non-toxic ferric state and bound to proteins (i.e. ferritin, transferrin). During hypoxia–ischaemia, free ferric iron is released from these proteins and reacts with peroxide to generate potent hydroxyl radicals. In addition, free ferric iron is reduced to a ferrous form, which further contributes to free radical injury.[8]

Mechanisms of neuronal cell death following hypoxia–ischaemia

The mechanism of neuronal cell death in animals and human following hypoxia–ischaemia includes neuronal necrosis and apoptosis. The intensity of the initial insult may determine the mode of death with severe injury resulting in necrosis, while milder insults result in apoptosis.[9] Necrosis is a passive process of cell swelling, disrupted cytoplasmic organelles, loss of membrane integrity and eventual lysis of neuronal cells and activation of an inflammatory process. By contrast, apoptosis is an active process distinguished from necrosis by the presence of cell shrinkage, nuclear pyknosis, chromatin condensation and genomic fragmentation, events that occur in the absence of an inflammatory response.[10] These two processes of neuronal death can be demonstrated following hypoxia–ischaemia in both animals and humans.[10] Since the mechanisms of neuronal necrosis versus apoptosis are likely to differ, strategies to minimize brain damage in an affected infant following hypoxia–ischaemia will have to include interventions that target both processes.

MANAGEMENT

The goals of management of a newborn infant who has sustained an hypoxic-ischemic insult should include: (i) supportive care to facilitate adequate perfusion and nutrients to the brain; and (ii) interventions to ameliorate the processes of ongoing brain injury. Each of these approaches is discussed next.

Identification of high risk infants

The initial step in management is early identification of those infants at greatest risk for evolving to the syndrome of hypoxic–ischaemic encephalopathy (HIE). This is a highly relevant issue because the therapeutic window, i.e. the time interval following hypoxia–ischaemia during which interventions might be efficacious in reducing the severity of ultimate brain injury, is likely to be short, i.e. estimated to vary from 2–6 h. Given this presumed short window of opportunity, infants must be identified as soon as possible following delivery so that early interventions can be implemented. Clinical investigations suggest that infants at highest risk for hypoxic–ischaemic brain damage include those who are severely depressed at birth (low extended Apgar score), exhibit fetal acidemia (cord umbilical artery pH < 7.00 and/or base > –14 mEq/l), require intensive delivery room resuscitation (i.e. intubation, chest compression ± epinephrine administration),[11] and exhibit an early abnormal neurological examination and/or abnormal assessment of cerebral function, i.e. integrated EEG.[12]

Supportive care

The various aspects of the supportive management of an infant at risk for hypoxic–ischaemic cerebral injury are summarised below and in Table 3.1.

Table 3.1 A guide to the supportive management of an infant at risk for hypoxic–ischaemic cerebral injury

Ventilation	Maintain pCO_2 within a normal range
Perfusion	Promptly treat hypotension Avoid hypertension
Fluid status	Initial fluid restriction Follow serum sodium and daily weights
Blood glucose	Maintain blood glucose within a normal range
Seizures	Treat clinical seizures, particularly with an electrographic correlate
Electrolyte imbalance	Monitor serum electrolytes, calcium and magnesium
Infection	Lumbar puncture in suspected cases of CNS infection

Ventilation

Assessment of adequate respiratory function is critical in the infant with HIE. Inadequate ventilation and frequent apnoea episodes are not uncommon in severely affected infants necessitating assisted ventilation. In mechanically ventilated infants, careful monitoring of the arterial blood gases and level of $PaCO_2$ is of particular importance. Thus, changes in $PaCO_2$ affect CBF with hypercarbia resulting in increases and hypocarbia in decreases in CBF.[13] The increase in CBF with hypercarbia increases the risk of hemorrhage in vulnerable capillary bed, e.g. germinal matrix in premature infants. Despite this potential adverse effect, immature rats subjected to cerebral hypoxia–ischaemia with CO_2 added to the hypoxic gas mixture had less severe brain injury than hypocapnic or normocapnic animals.[14] In contrast, the decrease in CBF associated with hypocarbia may be deleterious to developing brain. Thus, poorer neuro-developmental outcome has been noted in hyperventilated term infants with persistent pulmonary hypertension.[15] as well as an association between the development of periventicular leukomalacia and low $PaCO_2$ levels in preterm infants.[16] Until a cause and effect relationship can be clearly demonstrated, we recommend maintaining the $PaCO_2$ within a normal range.

Maintenance of adequate perfusion

One of the consequences of hypoxia–ischaemia is a disturbance of vascular autoregulation resulting in pressure-passive circulation.[17] In this state, changes in mean arterial blood pressure even if modest may significantly influence CBF. In this regard, it is not uncommon for infants with hypoxia–ischaemia to exhibit hypotension. This may be related to superimposed hypoxic–ischaemic myocardial injury, peripheral vasodilation, a central mechanism or rarely hypovolemia. Irrespective of the mechanism given a pressure-passive circulation, a decrease in blood pressure will result in a decrease in CBF potentially resulting in further ischemic injury within vulnerable regions, i.e. parasagittal cerebral convexities in term and periventricular white matter in preterm infants. Thus, the management strategy should be to maintain the arterial blood pressure within a normal range for age and gestation. For those hypotensive infants, the treatment will depend on the cause, i.e. inotropic support for myocardial dysfunction or volume replacement for intravascular depletion, etc.

In contrast to hypotension, an increase in arterial blood pressure is much less common in asphyxiated infants. Transient hypertension is occasionally seen shortly after birth, presumably as an adaptive mechanism to maintain cerebral perfusion. More prolonged hypertension, when it occurs, is often centrally mediated as a consequence of neonatal seizures. The hypertension is often accompanied by bradycardia and desaturation episodes. These episodes may be observed in the non- and paralyzed infant and are presumed to be secondary to sympathetic release since they can be eliminated by cord transection.[2] Controlling the epileptic activity may correct the hypertension.

Fluid status

Hypoxic–ischaemic infants often progress to a fluid overload state. This may be related to renal failure secondary to acute tubular necrosis or to inappropriate antidiuretic hormone release (SIADH). Clinically, infants present with an increase in weight, low urine output and hyponatremia. The management is fluid restriction. In some infants with concomitant hypotension, fluid management may become extremely complicated.

Control of blood glucose concentrations

In the context of cerebral hypoxia–ischaemia, experimental studies suggest that both hyperglycemia and hypoglycemia may accentuate brain damage. Regarding hyperglycemia in adult experimental models as well as in humans, brain damage is accentuated.[3] However, in immature animals subjected to cerebral hypoxia–ischaemia, hyperglycemia to blood glucose concentration of 600 mg/dl entirely prevents the occurrence of brain damage.[18] Regarding hypoglycemia, perhaps a more common finding in infants with hypoxia–ischaemia, the effects in experimental animals vary and are related to the mechanisms of the hypoglycemia. Thus, insulin-induced hypoglycemia is detrimental to immature rat brain subjected to hypoxia–ischaemia. However, if hypoglycemia is induced by fasting, a high degree of protection is noted.[19] This protective effect is presumed to be secondary to the increased concentrations of ketone bodies, which presumably serve as alternative substrates to the immature brain.

In the management of hypoxia–ischaemia, glucose level should be screened shortly after birth and monitored closely. Based on the divergent effects of glucose levels in experimental studies, the blood glucose should be maintained within the physiologic range. To prevent hypoglycemia, a continuous infusion of glucose at the rate of 4–6 mg/kg body weight/min should be started in affected infants and continued until enteral feedings are well tolerated.

Seizures

Hypoxic–ischaemic cerebral injury is the most common cause of early onset neonatal seizures.[2] Although seizures are a consequence of the underlying brain injury, seizures activity in itself may contribute to ongoing injury. Experimental evidence strongly suggests that repetitive seizures disturb brain growth and development as well as increase the risk for subsequent epilepsy.[20,21] Despite the potential adverse effects of seizures, the question of which infants should be treated remains controversial.[22] This is in part related to the observation that not all clinical seizures have an electrographic correlation.[22] Practically, we initially treat all clinical seizures with an anticonvulsant, usually phenobarbital and continue to treat clinical seizures until we have maximized the anticonvulsant therapy (e.g. phenobarbital, phenytoin or lorazepam) particularly when the seizures are associated with systemic signs, i.e. hypertension, bradycardia and/or desaturations. Electrographic seizures in the absence of clinical seizures in the non-paralyzed infant are not treated because they are generally brief in nature and require excessive anticonvulsants for controlling the seizure activity.

Prophylactic phenobarbital

Experimental data indicate that barbiturate pretreatment and even early post-treatment in adult animals subjected to cerebral hypoxia–ischaemia reduces the severity of ultimate brain damage. The prophylactic administration of 'high dose' barbiturates to infants at highest risk for evolving to HIE has been evaluated in two small studies with conflicting results.[23,24] In the first randomized study, the administration of thiopental initiated within 2 h and infused for 24 h did not alter the frequency of seizures, intracranial pressure or short-term neurodevelopmental outcome at 12 months.[23] Of importance was the observation that systemic hypotension occurred significantly more often in the treated group. In the second randomized study, phenobarbital 40 mg/kg body weight administered intravenously between 1–6 h to asphyxiated infants was associated with subsequent neuroprotection.[24] Although there was no difference in the frequency of seizures between the two groups in the neonatal period, 73% of the pretreated infants compared to 18% of the control group (P < 0.05) revealed normal neurodevelopmental outcome at 3 year follow-up. No adverse effect of phenobarbital administration was observed in this study. Thus, the role of prophylactic barbiturates in high-risk infants remains unclear at this current time and may be worthy of further investigation.

Cerebral oedema and increased intracranial pressure

Based on an understanding on the mechanisms of brain injury, it is not surprising that cytotoxic oedema complicates the clinical course of infants with HIE. In severe cases, cerebral edema is accompanied by the elevation of intracranial pressure which impairs tissue perfusion. Strategies that have been considered in the treatment of this complication include hyperventilation, glucocorticosteroids and mannitol. Indeed, mannitol was evaluated in a limited uncontrolled study in term infants with severe perinatal asphyxia.[25] Although a temporary effect on reduction of intracranial pressure was observed, the outcome was dismal in all cases. At the current time, there is no known strategy available for clinicians to lower intracranial pressure following hypoxia–ischaemia in neonates.

Electrolyte imbalance

Infants with HIE frequently develop electrolyte abnormalities, e.g. hypo-natremia, hypocalcemia or hypomagnesemia. Hyponatremia as mentioned above is likely due to impaired renal function and/or inappropriate anti-diuretic hormone release. The treatment of hyponatremia is fluid restriction until an improvement of urine output and a decrease in weight is noted. Hypocalcemia and hypomagnesemia are also commonly noted in infants with HIE. These abnormalities in a symptomatic infant should be appropriately treated with a slow infusion of calcium gluconate or magnesium sulphate.

Infection

Clinical manifestations of hypoxic–ischaemic encephalopathy (e.g. irritability, lethargy, and coma) may mimic other diseases including sepsis and infections of the central nervous system. Therefore, in some suspected cases, a lumbar puncture should be performed to exclude meningitis.

Supportive care as outlined above, while important in the overall management of infants with HIE, is clearly not focussed on the more relevant and specific issue, i.e. the prevention of the secondary phase of brain injury. Interventions currently under intense study especially in experimental animals include the use of hypothermia, free radical scavengers, excitatory amino acid antagonists, calcium channel blockers and nitric oxide synthase inhibitors. These interventions are briefly discussed next.

Potential neuroprotective strategies aimed at ameliorating secondary brain injury

Hypothermia

Modest systemic or selective cooling of the brain by as little as 2–4°C has been shown to reduce the extent of tissue injury in experimental studies as well as human following events such as stroke or trauma.[26,27] Potential mechanisms of neuroprotection with hypothermia include inhibition of glutamate release, reduction of cerebral metabolism which in turn preserves high energy phosphates, decrease in intracellular acidosis and lactic acid accumulation, preservation of endogenous anti-oxidants, reduction of nitric oxide production, prevention of protein kinase inhibition, improvement of protein synthesis, reduction of leukotriene production, prevention of blood brain barrier disruption and brain oedema and inhibition of apoptosis.[28–30] Although neuroprotection following intra-ischaemic hypothermia is well established, the effects of post-ischaemic hypothermia are less certain. The latter is the usual scenario in the human newborn. Before initiating hypothermia as a strategy, several factors need to be considered. The first relates to duration of therapy. Thus, brief post-ischaemic hypothermia, i.e. less than 6 h, results in only partial or temporary neuroprotection in most experimental animals. Prolonging post-ischaemic hypothermia from 24 h to 72 h attenuates brain damage and improves behavioural performance.[28–30] The second factor relates to the degree of hypothermia. Accordingly, moderate hypothermia at brain temperatures of 32–34°C initiated immediately or within a few hours after reperfusion and continued for 24–72 h has been shown to favourably affect outcome in adult and newborn animals.[28–30] The third factor relates to the delay in initiation of therapy. Clearly, the sooner hypothermia can be initiated, the more likely it is to be successful.[28–30] The fourth factor relates to the method of achieving hypothermia. Selective head cooling is attractive because it reduces potential side effects (see below) but is associated with differential gradients within the brain.[31] Total body cooling is more likely to be associated with side effects but less temperature gradient within the brain. A major concern of hypothermia in newborn infants relates to adverse effects including hypoglycemia, reduction of myocardial contractility and ventilation-perfusion mismatch, increased blood viscosity, acid-base and electrolyte imbalance and an increased risk of infection.[28–30]

To address the practicality and safety of selective head cooling with mild or minimal systemic hypothermia, a pilot study was recently conducted in term neonates with moderate to severe encephalopathy.[32] The study group comprised term infants with an Apgar score ≤ 6 at 5 min or an umbilical artery pH ≤ 7.09 plus evidence of encephalopathy who were randomized to no cooling (rectal temperature 37.0 ± 0.2°C; n = 10), minimal systemic cooling (rectal temperature 36.3 ± 0.2°C; n = 6) or mild systemic cooling (rectal temperature 35.7 ± 0.2°C; n = 6). Head cooling was achieved by circulating water at 10°C through a coil of tubing wrapped around the head for up to 72 h. With mild cooling, the nasopharyngeal temperature was 34.5°C during cooling, 1.2°C lower than the rectal temperature. No adverse effects of the cooling were noted. From the pilot data presented, it appears that mild selective head cooling is a safe and convenient method of rapid reduction of cerebral temperature. These observations should serve as a springboard for the development of multi-centre studies to evaluate the role of hypothermia as a neuroprotective strategy. However, several critical questions need to be addressed prior to the implementation of this intervention in multi-centre studies: (i) what is the ideal temperature for selective head cooling?; (ii) which is the best mode of administration, i.e., selective head versus total body cooling?; and (iii) how long should hypothermia be maintained?

Oxygen free radical inhibitors and scavengers

One therapeutic approach for the destruction of oxygen free radicals generated during and following hypoxia–ischaemia is the administration of specific enzymes known to degrade highly reactive radicals to a non-reactive component. Superoxide dismutase and catalase are antioxidant enzymes conjugated to polyethylene glycol which prolongs their circulatory half-life and facilitates penetration across the blood brain barrier.[8] Because of their large molecular sizes, they are restricted to the vascular space. Thus, the positive effects of these conjugated compounds are presumably from within cerebral vasculature by improving cerebral blood flow.[8] In newborn animals, neuroprotection has only been shown when these agents have been administered several hours prior to the hypoxic–ischaemic insult.[3]

A second group of free radical inhibitors that have been shown to be effective in experimental animals are agents that inhibit specific reactions in the production of xanthines. Thus, both allopurinol and oxypurinol, xanthine oxidase inhibitors, protected the immature rat from hypoxic–ischaemic brain damage when the drugs were administered early during the recovery phase following resuscitation.[3] In a recent clinical study, allopurinol administered to asphyxiated infants reduced blood concentrations of oxygen free radicals when compared to control infants.[33]

A third group of free radical inhibitors has targeted the formation of free radicals specifically hydroxyl radical from free iron during reperfusion.[8] Thus, deferoxamine, a chelating agent, prevents the formation of free radical from iron, reduces the severity of brain injury and improves cerebral metabolism in animal models of hypoxia–ischaemia when given during reperfusion.[8]

Finally, lazeroids which are nonglucocorticoid, 21-aminosteroids, preventing iron-dependent lipid peroxidation by scavenging peroxyl radicals have been shown to be neuroprotective in both adult and immature models of hypoxic–ischaemic brain damage.[3]

Excitatory amino acid antagonists

Given the important role of excessive stimulation of neuronal surface receptors by glutamate in promoting a cascade of events leading to cellular death,[2,5] it has been logical to identify pharmacological agents that would either inhibit glutamate release or block its postsynaptic action.

Glutamate receptor antagonists (i.e. NMDA, AMPA subtypes) have been extensively investigated in experimental animals. Non-competitive antagonists provided a reduction in brain damage in adult animals even when administered up to 24 h after the insult. The available NMDA antagonists include dizocilpine (MK-801), magnesium, phencyclidine (PCP), dextrometrophan and ketamine.[3]

MK-801 has been shown to be an efficacious agent in reducing the extent of hypoxic–ischaemic brain damage in both adult and neonatal animal models.[3]

This neuroprotective effect appears to be greater in immature compared to the adult model. This age-related neuroprotective effect may reflect the alterations of density and distribution of glutamate receptor subtypes during development of the brain.

Magnesium is an NMDA antagonist blocking neuronal influx of Ca^{2+} within the ion channel. The effect of magnesium also appears to be dependent on the maturation of the glutamate receptor system. Thus, in a developmental study in mice, excitotoxic neuronal death was limited by magnesium which was effective only after development of several aspects of the excitotoxic cascade, including the coupling of the calcium influx following NMDA overstimulation, and the presence of magnesium-dependent calcium channels.[34]

The potential neuroprotective effect of magnesium has revealed conflicting data in experimental neonatal studies. Thus, when administered shortly following an intracerebral injection of NMDA, magnesium sulphate reduced brain injury in the newborn rat. However, other neonatal studies have failed to demonstrate neuroprotection. Thus, in a piglet model of asphyxia, magnesium sulphate administered 1 h following resuscitation failed to decrease the severity of delayed energy failure. In addition, in a near-term fetal lamb model, magnesium sulphate administered before and during umbilical cord occlusion did not influence the electrophysiological responses or neuronal loss.[3,35,36]

Magnesium sulphate is an attractive agent because of its frequent use in the US. It is often administered to mothers as a tocolytic agent or to prevent seizures in mothers with pregnancy-induced hypertension. Preliminary retrospective observation in premature infants noted a reduced incidence of CP at 3 years in those exposed to antenatal magnesium sulphate.[37] Clearly, future research is necessary in order to determine the potential neuroprotective role of magnesium.

Prevention of nitric oxide formation

The inhibition of NOS is another potential treatment modality to decrease brain injury. The experimental effects of NOS inhibitors vary and are animal species specific and influenced by the pharmacological agent used, the dose and timing of therapy. Thus, in adult experiments, the severity of neuronal loss can be reduced by the prior administration of inhibitors of NOS activity. A similar protective effect has been observed in the immature rat, whereas in fetal sheep, neuronal injury appears to be accentuated following hypoxia–ischaemia.[3] Further studies are clearly necessary.

Calcium channel blockers

The elevation of cytosolic calcium during hypoxic–ischaemic injury makes the reduction of intracellular accumulation a highly desirable therapy. One strategy of preventing calcium toxicity is to inhibit Ca^{2+} influx into neurons by using calcium channel blockers (e.g. flunarizine, nimodipine, nicardipine). Flunarizine has been studied in the fetus and newborn animals and the neuroprotective effect has only been demonstrated when given prophylactically but not following hypoxic–ischaemic insults.[3] Nicardipine was tested in four severely asphyxiated infants but the positive effect was counteracted by the adverse effects of significant haemodynamic disturbance.[38] Indeed, current calcium channel blockers are in general contra-indicated in the neonate and young infant in the US because of significant adverse cardiovascular effects.

Other studied therapies in immature animals

Other avenues of potential neuroprotection include platelet-activating factor antagonists,[39] adenosinergic agents,[40] monosialoganglioside GM_1,[41] and growth factors, e.g. nerve growth factor (NGF),[42] and insulin growth factor-1.[43]

CONCLUSIONS

Much progress has been made toward understanding the mechanisms contributing to ongoing brain injury following hypoxia–ischaemia. This should facilitate more specific pharmacological intervention strategies that might provide neuroprotection during the reperfusion phase of injury. Early identification of infants at highest risk for brain injury is critical if such interventions are to be successful. Moreover, given the small number of asphyxiated full-term infants that are likely to be admitted to any one neonatal intensive care unit over an extended time period implores a multi-centre treatment approach to allow inclusion of an adequate number of infants to achieve statistical validity.

Key points for clinical practice

- The initial step in management is early identification of those infants at greatest risk for evolving to the syndrome of hypoxic ischaemic encephalopathy.

- Current management strategies are largely supportive and unlikely to directly affect outcome. Future strategies, i.e. hypothermia, may provide an opportunity for preventing ongoing injury following hypoxia-ischaemia.

References

1 Perlman JM. Intrapartum hypoxic-ischemic cerebral injury and subsequent cerebral palsy: medico-legal issues. Pediatrics 1997; 99: 851–859

2 Volpe JJ. Hypoxic-ischemic encephalopathy. In: Volpe JJ, ed. Neurology of the Newborn. Philadelphia, PA: Saunders, 1995

3 Vannucci RC, Perlman JM. Interventions for perinatal hypoxic-ischemic encephalopathy. Pediatrics 1997; 100: 1004–1014

4 Wyatt JS, Edwards AD, Azzopardi D, Reynolds EOR. Magnetic resonance and near infrared spectroscopy for investigation of perinatal hypoxic-ischemic brain injury. Arch Dis Child 1989; 64: 953–963

5 Vannucci RC. Experimental biology of cerebral hypoxia-ischemia: relation to perinatal brain damage. Pediatr Res 1990; 27: 317–326

6 Lorek A, Takei Y, Cady EB et al. Delayed ('secondary') cerebral energy failure after acute hypoxia-ischemia in the newborn piglet: continuous 48-hour studies by phosphorus magnetic resonance spectroscopy. Pediatr Res 1994; 36: 699–706

7 Roth SC, Baudin J, Cady E et al. Relation of deranged neonatal cerebral oxidative metabolism with neurodevelopmental outcome and head circumference at four years. Dev Med Child Neurol 1997; 39: 718–725

8 Palmer C. Hypoxic-ischemic encephalopathy. Therapeutic approaches against microvascular injury, and role of neutrophils, PAF, and free radicals. Clin Perinatol 1995; 22: 481–517

9 Bonfold E, Krainc D, Ankarcrona M, Nicotera P, Lipton SA. Apoptosis and necrosis: two distinct events, induced respectively by mild and intense insults with N methyl–aspartate or nitric oxide/superoxide in cortical cell cultures. Proc Natl Acad Sci USA 1995; 92: 7162–7166

10 Edwards AD, Mehmet H. Apoptosis in perinatal hypoxic-ischemic cerebral damage. Neuropathol Appl Neurobiol 1996; 22: 494–498

11 Perlman JM, Risser R. Severe fetal acidemia: neonatal neurologic features and short-term outcome. Pediatr Neurol 1993; 9: 277–282

12 Hellstrom-Westas L, Rosen I, Svenningsen NW. Predictive value of early continuous amplitude integrated EEG recordings on outcome after severe birth asphyxia in full term infants. Arch Dis Child 1995; 72: F34–F38

13 Hansen NB, Brubakk AM, Bratlid D, Oh W, Stonestreet BS. The effects of variations in $PaCO_2$ on brain blood flow and cardiac output in the newborn piglet. Pediatr Res 1984; 18: 1132-01136

14 Vannucci RC, Brucklacher RM, Vannucci SJ. Effect of carbon dioxide on cerebral metabolism during hypoxia-ischemia in the immature rat. Pediatr Res 1997; 42: 24–29

15 Bifano EM, Pfannenstiel A. Duration of hyperventilation and outcome in infants with persistent pulmonary hypertension. Pediatrics 1988; 81: 657–661

16 Graziani LJ, Spitzer AR, Mitchell DG et al. Mechanical ventilation in preterm infants: neurosonographic and developmental studies. Pediatrics 1992; 90: 515–522

17 Pryds O, Greisen G, Lou H, Friis-Hansen B. Vasoparalysis associated with brain damage in asphyxiated term infants. J Pediatr 1990; 117: 119–125

18 Vannucci RC, Mujsce DJ. Effect of glucose on perinatal hypoxic-ischemic brain damage. Biol Neonate 1992; 62: 215–224

19 Yager JY, Heitjan DF, Towfighi J, Vannucci RC. Effect of insulin-induced and fasting hypoglycemia on perinatal hypoxic-ischemic brain damage. Pediatr Res 1992; 31: 138–142

20 Wasterlain CG. Effects of neonatal status epilepticus on rat brain development. Neurology 1976; 26: 975–986

21 Holmes GL, Gairsa JL, Chevassus Au Louis, Ben-Ari Y. Consequences of neonatal seizures in the rat: morphological and behavioral effects. Ann Neurol 1998; 44: 845–857

22 Mizrahi EM. Consensus and controversy in the clinical management of neonatal seizures. Clin Perinatol 1989; 16: 485–500

23 Goldberg RN, Moscoso P, Bauer CR et al. Use of barbiturate therapy in severe perinatal asphyxia: a randomized controlled trial. J Pediatr 1986; 109: 851–856

24 Hall RT, Hall FK, Daily DK. High-dose phenobarbital therapy in term newborn infants with severe perinatal asphyxia: a randomized prospective study with three-year follow-up. J Pediatr 1998; 132: 345–348

25 Levene MI, Evans DH. Medical management of raised intracranial pressure after severe birth asphyxia. Arch Dis Child 1985; 60: 12–16

26 Reith J, Jorgensen HS, Pedersen PM et al. Body temperature in acute stroke; relation to stroke severity, infarct size, mortality, and outcome. Lancet 1996; 347: 422–425

27 Marion DW, Penrod LE, Kelsey SF et al. Treatment of traumatic brain injury with moderate hypothermia. N Engl J Med 1997; 336: 540–546

28 Colbourne F, Sutherland G, Corbett D. Postischemic hypothermia: a critical appraisal with implications for clinical treatment. Mol Neurobiol 1997; 14: 171–201

29 Edwards AD, Wyatt JS, Thoresen M. Treatment of hypoxic-ischaemic brain damage by moderate hypothermia. Arch Dis Child Fetal Neonatal Ed 1998; 78: F85–F91

30 Laptook AR, Corbett RJT. Therapeutic hypothermia: a potential neuroprotective and resuscitative strategy for neonatal hypoxia-ischemia. Prenat Neonat Med 1996; 1: 199–212

31 Towfighi J, Housman C, Heitjan DF, Vannucci RC, Yager JY. The effect of focal cerebral cooling on perinatal hypoxic-ischemic brain damage. Acta Neuropathol 1994; 87: 598–604

32 Gunn AJ, Gluckman PD, Gunn TR. Selective head cooling in newborn infants after perinatal asphyxia. A safety study. Pediatrics 1998; 102: 885–892

33 Van Bel F, Shadid M, Moison RM et al. Effect of allopurinol on postasphyxial free radical formation, cerebral hemodynamics and electrical brain activity. Pediatrics 1998; 101: 185–193

34 Marret S, Gressens P, Gadisseux JF, Evrard P. Prevention by magnesium of excitotoxic neuronal death in the developing brain: an animal model of clinical intervention studies. Dev Med Child Neurol 1995; 37: 473–484

35 Penrice J, Amess PN, Punwani S et al. Magnesium sulfate after transient hypoxia-ischemia fails to prevent delayed cerebral energy failure in the newborn piglet. Pediatr Res 1997; 41: 443–447

36 de Haan HH, Gunn AJ, Williams CE, Heymann MA, Gluckman PD. Magnesium sulfate therapy during asphyxia in near-term fetal lambs does not compromise the fetus but does not reduce cerebral injury. Am J Obstet Gynecol 1997; 176: 18–27

37 Nelson KB, Grether JK. Can magnesium sulfate reduce the risk of cerebral palsy in very low birthweight infants? Pediatrics 1995; 95: 263–269

38 Levene MI, Gibson NA, Fenton AC, Papathoma E, Barnett D. The use of a calcium-channel blocker, nicardipine, for severely asphyxiated newborn infants. Dev Med Child Neurol 1990, 32: 567–574

39 Liu XH, Eun BL, Silverstein FS, Barks JD. The platelet-activating factor antagonist BN 52021 attenuates hypoxic-ischemic brain injury in the immature rat. Pediatr Res 1996; 40: 797–803

40 Halle JN, Kasper CE, Gidday JM, Koos BJ. Enhancing adenosine A1 receptor binding reduces hypoxic-ischemic brain injury in newborn rats. Brain Res 1997; 759: 309–312

41 Tan WK, Williams CE, Mallard CE, Gluckman PD. Monosialoganglioside GM1 treatment after a hypoxic-ischemic episode reduces the vulnerability of the fetal sheep brain to subsequent injuries. Am J Obstet Gynecol 1994; 170: 663–669

42 Holtzman DM, Sheldon RA, Jaffe W, Cheng Y, Ferriero DM. Nerve growth factor protects the neonatal brain against hypoxic-ischemic injury. Ann Neurol 1996; 39: 114-122

43 Johnston BM, Mallard EC, Williams CE, Gluckman PD. Insulin-like growth factor-1 is a potent neuronal rescue agent after hypoxic-ischemic injury in fetal lambs. J Clin Invest 1996; 97: 300–308

Hiran C. Selvadurai   Dominic A. Fitzgerald

Monitoring oxygen in the blood

Blood gases may be arterial, 'arterialised' capillary or venous samples. The situations in which blood gases are used vary greatly and the information provided must be interpreted in relation to the clinical scenario. The various terms used in this article are defined in Table 4.1

DIFFERENTIAL DIAGNOSIS OF HYPOXIA

The causes of hypoxia can be broadly classified into three groups:

Hypoxic hypoxia includes conditions in which the arterial PaO_2 is low. This incorporates conditions with low alveolar PO_2, diffusion impairment, right to left cardiac shunts and ventilation/perfusion (V_A/Q_C) mismatch.

Anaemic hypoxia is caused by a net decrease in the level of normally functioning haemoglobin. This incorporates states with decreased haemoglobin production (red cell aplasia), increased destruction of erythrocytes (haemolysis) or interference with oxygen combining with haemoglobin (carbon monoxide poisoning or methaemoglobinemia).

Hypoperfusion hypoxia may be a localised phenomena (vasculitic states such as Kawasaki's syndrome) or a generalised phenomenon (low cardiac output states). The PAO_2 and the PaO_2 may both be normal, but the reduced oxygen delivery to the tissues may result in tissue hypoxia. In this setting, increasing the FiO_2 is unlikely to improve the situation unless it improves perfusion.

Hiran C. Selvadurai MBBS, Fellow in Paediatric Respiratory Medicine, The Royal Alexandra Hospital for Children, PO Box 3515, Parramatta, Sydney, New South Wales, Australia 2124.

Dominic A. Fitzgerald MBBS PhD FRACP, Paediatric Respiratory Physician, The Royal Alexandra Hospital for Children, PO Box 3515, Parramatta, Sydney, New South Wales, Australia 2124 (for correspondence).

Table 1.1 Abbreviations and definitions

Abbreviation	Definition
PaO_2	Partial pressure of oxygen in arterial blood
PAO_2	Partial pressure of oxygen in alveolar air
$PaCO_2$	Partial pressure of carbon dioxide in arterial blood
$PACO_2$	Partial pressure of carbon dioxide in alveolar air
$TcCO_2$	Transcutaneous measurement of carbon dioxide
V_A	Alveolar ventilation/minute
Q_C	Pulmonary capillary flow/minute
FiO_2	Fractional inspired oxygen concentration
pH	Negative log (to base 10) of the concentration of free hydrogen ions
BE	Base excess
HbF	Fetal haemoglobin ($\alpha_2\beta_2$ polypeptide chains)
HbA	Adult ($\alpha_2\beta_2$) haemoglobin
HbS	Sickle haemoglobin ($\alpha_2\beta'_2$)
SaO_2	Oxygen saturation in arterial blood

Blood gases are the 'gold standard' to which non-invasive modalities such as pulse oximetry and transcutaneous gas monitoring strive to reflect. Monitoring blood gases is an essential aspect of managing the sick child. As all organ systems are affected by acid/base disturbances, blood gas assessment facilitates the diagnosis and management of a wide range of paediatric medical conditions.

Arterial blood gases are useful in a child with asthma who is clinically tiring and not responding to therapy. In such a case, if the arterial blood gas demonstrated a respiratory acidosis, the next level of management with assisted ventilatory support may have to be undertaken. Carruthers et al.[1] have demonstrated that arterial blood gases are unnecessary if the pulse oximetry reading is greater than 92% in room air, in a child whose clinical state is accordingly mild. One must be cautious in giving guidelines based purely on pulse oximetry, as discussed earlier; it does have its limitations and one must use all the available clinical parameters when assessing children in respiratory distress.

Nevertheless, the collection of an arterial blood gas may cause discomfort to a child and the potentially useful information one can obtain from the test needs to be balanced with the potentially negative effects it can have on the child. For example, the child with severe upper airway obstruction due to laryngotracheobronchitis (croup) or acute epiglottitis should be kept as calm as possible. An arterial puncture performed in a chaotic emergency room may well worsen the situation.

The interpretation of arterial blood gases in the newborn period warrants special consideration. The determination of arterial oxygen and carbon dioxide tensions is an important part of the assessment of neonates with tachypnoea and evolving respiratory distress. The interpretations of the results will influence the need for further investigation and/or treatment and the location of further monitoring (neonatal intensive care unit versus in the ward with the infant's mother) with its cost implications. Fetal blood (HbF), acidosis and temperature dysregulation can all affect the oxygen dissociation curve in the

Table 4.2 Normal values for blood gases during the first week for healthy term infants

Age (hours)	1–4	12–24	24	48–168
PaO$_2$ (mmHg)	50–75	60–80	65–85	70–85
PaCO$_2$ (mmHg)	30–45	30–40	30–40	30–38
Arterial pH	7.30–7.34	7.30–7.35	7.35–7.30	7.35–7.40

Table 4.3 Metabolic and respiratory conditions with the characteristic features evident on blood gas analysis

Metabolic failure				
	Metabolic acidosis (UC)	Metabolic acidosis (C)	Metabolic alkalosis (UC)	Metabolic alkalosis (C)
pH	↓	N	↑	N
pCO$_2$	N	↓	N	↑
HCO$_3$	↓	↓	↑	↑
BE	↓	↓	↑	↑
Respiratory failure				
	Respiratory acidosis (UC)	Respiratory acidosis (C)	Respiratory alkalosis (UC)	Respiratory alkalosis (C)
pH	↓	N	↑	N
pCO$_2$	↑	↑	↓	↓
HCO$_3$	N	↑	N	↓
BE	N	↑	N	↓

UC = uncompensated; C = compensated

infant. It is necessary to know the range of normality before one can diagnose the abnormal state. The normal range of values for blood gases in healthy infants as reported by Fleming et al.[2] are listed in Table 4.2.

By 6 months of age, much of the HbF has been replaced by adult haemoglobins and the parameters remain constant, although the interpretation of blood gases can still be challenging. Listed in Table 4.3 is a series of metabolic and respiratory conditions with the characteristic features evident on blood gas analysis.

ARTERIAL BLOOD GAS SAMPLING

There are a limited number of sites for arterial blood sampling. The primary sites are the radial, posterior tibial and dorsalis pedis arteries. The brachial, femoral and temporal arteries should be avoided where possible because of the risk of reflex spasm and embolization. Indeed, brachial artery puncture is associated with a 2% incidence of complications.[3]. Immediate limb pain or paraesthesia occurs in 1.1% of the patients while the onset of symptoms, mainly from haematoma formation, can be delayed by 24 h in up to 0.9% of patients. Generally speaking, the radial artery is the safest and most accessible site for arterial puncture in children.[4]

Vessel spasm, intraluminal clotting and bleeding with the formation of peri-arterial clot are all potential side effects of arterial blood sampling.[5-7] It is important to choose the arterial puncture site that has collateral blood flow should the artery get obstructed or go into spasm. As 1.6% of children have their hand perfused primarily by the radial artery, a simple test to assess collateral circulation in the radial artery (Allen's test) should routinely be performed.[8]

It can be difficult to palpate and stabilise the artery in young children who may have an abundance of subcutaneous fat. The role of an assistant is vital in this regard. A comforting but firm hold of the child will not only expedite the test but also reduce the chances of unsuccessful attempts. Where time permits, topical anaesthetic creams should always be applied 45 min prior to the procedure. Alternatively, as the initial part of the procedure, the skin should be infiltrated with a local anaesthetic. In neonates, caution should be exercised when using local anaesthetic in excessive volumes or frequently as recurrent and prolonged seizures have been reported.[9] Generally, a 25 French gauge needle is advanced at a 45° angle to the longitudinal path of the vessel until there is a 'flash back' of blood which passively fills the heparinised syringe. Conversely, some people prefer to transfix the artery with the needle after the flashback and then withdraw slowly, allowing the syringe to fill. Given adequate blood pressure and the correct placement of the needle tip in the artery, it is usually unnecessary to draw back on the plunger of the syringe in order to obtain the sample.

A recent development has seen the advent of continuous intra-arterial blood gas monitoring. It has recently been evaluated and shown to be useful and reliable.[10] With the important advantage of continuous monitoring, it is may soon become standard clinical practice in the intensive care setting.

ARTERIALISED CAPILLARY SAMPLES

If the child is stable in terms of the cardiopulmonary status, the correlation between arterial PO_2, PcO_2 and pH and arterialised capillary blood is good.[11] This has obvious advantages in being simpler to perform, less invasive and less uncomfortable than the arterial blood analysis. As it requires one-tenth as much blood as a formal arterial blood sample (100 µl), it has distinct advantages in neonates as well as in the sleep and exercise laboratories.

A highly vascularised capillary bed such as the earlobe, heel, great toe or finger can be used. Pre-warming of the site using warm towels may aid the blood collection. Arterialised capillary samples are only accurate in the setting of cardiopulmonary stability and when the peripheral perfusion is good.[12] If these criteria are not satisfied, an arterial blood sample is required.

VENOUS SAMPLES

Acid/base status can be monitored by the use of peripheral venous blood.[13] However, venous levels of oxygen and carbon dioxide cannot be relied upon to reflect, consistently, arterial and alveolar levels. This is due to variations in vasomotor tone and arteriolar resistance in local organ systems. Given these limitations, the two settings where venous carbon dioxide measures may be useful are: (i) in the management of metabolic disorders such as diabetic keto-acidosis (low CO_2), where acid/base status is most important; and (ii) in the assessment of sleep hypoventilation (raised CO_2 upon waking), when arterial sampling may be difficult to obtain.

The recent development of the Paratrend 7 monitor has enabled continuous monitoring of the pH and PCO_2 using a peripheral venous catheter. This monitor provides a clinically acceptable correlation with arterial values.[14]

POTENTIAL ERRORS IN BLOOD GAS MEASUREMENTS

Pre-laboratory errors

The commonest errors in this category are time delay; air bubbles in the sample; small sample size and blood clots in the sample.

The blood samples need to be stored in an iced container should there be a delay greater than 15 min before testing.[15] If the sample is iced, the testing can be delayed for up to 60 min. A delay in analysing the blood would decrease the PO_2. Air bubbles need to be removed prior to storing the sample in ice.[16] If there is insufficient anticoagulant in the syringe, the sample will clot. If the sample size is small, the relative excess of heparin anticoagulant will result in a falsely alkaline reading.

Calibration errors

Calibration is important to ensure accuracy and consistency. Two point calibration checks should be performed every 8 h or every 50 gas measurements.[17] The pH, PO_2, and PCO_2 parameters should each be calibrated against two reference points. A detailed discussion on calibration techniques is beyond the scope of this article but the readers are directed to the report by Holmes et al.[18]

Summary

1. Arterial blood samples remain the gold standard when assessing blood gases.
2. Pre-analytic errors can lead to inaccuracies and results which are inconsistent with the clinical state of the child should be repeated.
3. Venous gases are useful in the management of metabolic diseases (e.g. diabetic ketoacidosis) when monitoring acidosis is necessary.
4. Arterialised capillary samples can be used to analyse blood gases if the child is well perfused and haemodynamically stable.

TRANSCUTANEOUS GAS MONITORING

How does it work?

The human skin comprises of the stratum corneum, the epidermis and the dermis. The dermis contains numerous dermal capillaries located within the dermal papillae which loop up into the epidermal layer. The oxygen concentration is lower at the tip of the dermal papillae due to the diffusion out of oxygen at this level. When the skin is heated to greater than 41°C, the lipids in the stratum corneum melt and the speed of gas diffusion through the skin is greatly enhanced.[19] If the perfusion of the skin is diminished, as with oximetry, the transcutaneous oxygen value will underestimate the circulating PaO_2.

In neonates, while the correlation coefficient is approximately 0.95 between $PtcO_2$ and PaO_2,[20] the $PtcO_2$ may over estimate the PaO_2 by 10%.[21] By the age of 1 year, $PtcO2$ consistently underestimates the PaO_2.[22] As expected, the correlation is dependent on the adequacy of skin perfusion.[23]

Clinical applications

Transcutaneous gas monitoring has obvious advantages as a non-invasive, continuous measure of PaO_2 and $PaCO_2$. Continuous monitoring is of particular use in the neonatal and paediatric intensive care settings where repeated arterial blood gas sampling may give rise to a sampling anaemia. Episodes of hypoxia and hypercapnea can be detected (e.g. episodes of pulmonary hypertension occurring during endotracheal suctioning) which were previously missed due to the temporal nature of arterial blood gas sampling. Similarly, transcutaneous gas monitoring can be more reliable than apnoea monitors in detecting apnoea.[24] Whereas end tidal CO_2 monitoring can also provide a continuous assessment of $PaCO_2$, $TcCO_2$ has the distinct advantage of providing the same information in the unintubated child. This is of particular benefit in monitoring the sick unventilated child.[22] Furthermore, when compared directly, $TcCO_2$ was a more accurate measure of $PaCO_2$ than end tidal CO_2.[25]

Non-invasive ventilation, most often with positive end expiratory pressure (PEEP) or bilateral positive airway pressure (BiPap) therapy is being increasingly in children. It is used acutely with severe upper airway obstruction and in life-threatening asthma and chronically in children with neuromuscular diseases, obstructive sleep apnoea and chronic respiratory failure (e.g. cystic fibrosis). $PtcCO_2$ is very useful in the titration of pressure settings for PEEP therapy.[26,27]

Transcutaneous gas monitoring is of particular use in the intra-operative anaesthetic management of children. Hypoxia and airway obstruction – such as a kinked endotracheal tube, right main stem bronchus intubation and accidental extubation – can be readily detected by transcutaneous gas monitoring.[28,29] Nonetheless, oximetry remains the mainstay of intra-operative oxygen monitoring and has been deemed mandatory in many countries since the mid-1980s.

Transcutaneous gas monitoring can monitor intravascular volume depletion and the fluid resuscitation. Skin perfusion can be assessed using the $PtcO_2$ index. The formula $PtcO_2/PaO_2$ derives this.[23] In early shock, the $PtcO_2$ index is reduced and provides a sensitive early sign of decreasing tissue perfusion. Studies have shown that if this index remains low after fluid resuscitation, the risk of cardiac arrest in the subsequent 45 min is greatly increased.[9]

A less common use of transcutaneous oxygen monitoring is to assess the adequacy of surgical skin flaps and autografts.[30,31] Patients with vascular disease (e.g. arteritis, occlusive disease) may be detected using PtcO$_2$ using the PtcO$_2$ index.[32,33]

Clinical disadvantages

The most significant disadvantage of PtcO$_2$ use is potential blistering of the skin. If severe, this can even lead to second-degree burns. Changing the site of attachment every 4 h and avoiding its use in hypothermic patients can prevent this side effect. Its use in the haemodynamically unstable child is very limited.

Summary

1   Transcutaneous gas monitoring is a continuous, non-invasive and sensitive measure of PaO$_2$ and PaCO$_2$.

2   It can also be used in assessing the effect of fluid resuscitation and skin perfusion in skin graft surgery.

3   The main problem with PtcO$_2$ measurements is the potential for blistering of the skin which can be prevented by frequent changing of the attachment site.

PULSE OXIMETRY

Pulse oximetry has provided a major advancement in the estimation of blood oxygen status. Since its introduction into clinical practice in the 1980s, its role has expanded dramatically. Initially intended as an inexpensive, rapid, non-invasive screen for hypoxia in the operating theatre and emergency room, its role has expanded to incorporate continuous monitoring in intensive care units, respiratory and sleep laboratories and in the home setting for oxygen-dependent patients. The essential features of oximetry are summarised in Table 4.4.

Table 4.4 Essentials of oximetry

Purpose	Rapid, non-invasive detection of hypoxia
Clinical uses	Operating theatres, emergency rooms, intensive care units, hospital wards, sleep laboratories, respiratory laboratories
Advantages	Non-invasive, reliable, reproducible, robust, appropriate for all ages, minimal knowledge required to operate an oximeter, reading is easily interpreted, inexpensive
Accuracy	Optimal (± 2%) when SpO$_2$ > 90%, but considerably less accurate when SpO$_2$ < 80%
Limitations	Extraneous energy sources, poor peripheral perfusion, penumbra effect, raised carboxyhaemoglobin, electromagnetic interference

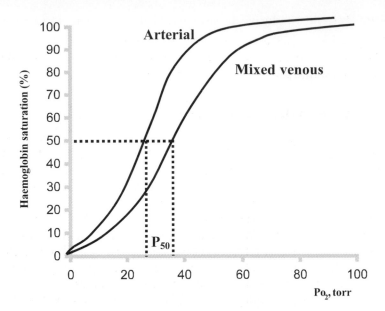

Fig. 4.1 Oxyhaemoglobin dissociation curves for arterial and mixed venous blood. Adapted from the Ohmeda 3000 pulse oximeter users' manual (Madison, WI, USA: Ohmeda, 1989: 22).

What does a pulse oximeter measure?

The oximeter measures the percentage haemoglobin oxygen saturation in arterial blood. It is not a partial pressure of dissolved oxygen (units are kPa, mmHg or torr). However, the partial pressure of oxygen is related to the SaO_2 in the oxygen dissociation curve (Fig. 4.1). The oxygen dissociation curve differs for each type of haemoglobin (e.g. HbF shifts the curve to the left and HbSS shifts the curve to the right when compared to the predominant type, HbA). The curve is altered by a number of variables including blood acid/base status (pH), $PaCO_2$ and body temperature. A clinically relevant difference between the haemoglobins is the partial pressure of oxygen at which the haemoglobin is 50% saturated (P_{50}). However, it is also known that the mixed venous P_{50} is higher than the arterial P_{50} because the pH is lower and the $PaCO_2$ is higher resulting in a rightward shift of the curve (Fig. 4.1). The P_{50} for HbA is 26.5 kPa.

How does a pulse oximeter work?

Pulse oximeters determine oxygen saturation by measuring and comparing the amount of light transmitted at two different wavelengths, typically 650 nm and 940 nm. Light is scattered through a tissue bed to a photodetector from two light emitting diodes. An algorithm is included which distinguishes the pulsatile component of the measurement cycle ('arterial') from the background reading (light absorption due to arterial blood, venous blood and tissue). The beat to beat inflow of arterial blood affects the intensity of transmitted light (Fig. 4.2). The ratio of the absorption of the pulsatile component of the signal at the two light wavelengths corresponds to the ratio of HbO_2 to Hb.

Nomenclature

To differentiate the value of arterial oxygen saturation by blood gas analysis using the co-oximeter (SaO_2), the value for the oximeter derived estimation of arterial oxygen saturation is correctly designated SpO_2.

How accurate is an oximetry reading?

Most manufacturers quote an error of ± 2% for SpO_2 readings above 90% and progressively larger errors at SpO_2 < 90%.[34,35] Comparisons have been performed between brands of oximeters, suggesting that results may differ slightly (approximately 2%) because of the algorithms used to calculate the value.[34] A major limitation of some oximeters is the absence of a displayed pulsatile waveform which may preclude the differentiation of a low reading attributable to a poor trace from a true hypoxic event. Moreover, there exist concerns about the averaging time used in some oximeters which is of clinical relevance in the estimation of oxygen desaturation complicating obstructive sleep hyponoeas and apnoeas (OSA) during polysomnography. Farre et al.[36] demonstrated that by prolonging the oximeter averaging time from 3 to 12–21 s, one could underestimate the degree of oxygen desaturation by up to 60% in adults with severe obstructive sleep apnoea. In contrast, Levy et al.[37] used an averaging time of 12 s in a similar group of adults with OSA successfully, although they concentrated on apnoeas with SpO_2 < 90%. However, standard practice in our sleep laboratory is to use a shorter oximetry averaging time (3 s)

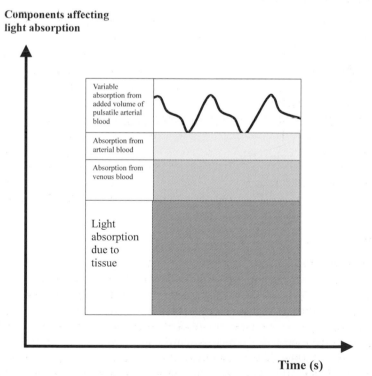

Fig. 4.2 Components affecting light absorption in pulse oximetry.

as infants and young children may rouse from REM sleep in order to protect themselves from greater falls in oxygenation.[38]

Clinical applications

The most useful contribution of oximetry has been to facilitate the detection of mild hypoxemia (SaO_2 90–94%), such as may occur in acute exacerbations of asthma, laryngotracheobronchitis and pneumonia. The documentation of hypoxia may have a profound influence upon treatment strategies, at times prompting hospital admission. Indeed, it can be extremely difficult to determine mild degrees of oxygen desaturation. Factors such as skin pigmentation, circulatory state, anaemia, ambient light intensity and colour may confound accurate estimations.[39]

Situations where oximetry is most useful

1. This is an essential tool for continuous monitoring of patients in the operating theatre whilst under general anaesthesia or heavy sedation.
2. The emergency department where it is used both as a screening tool for patients at risk of hypoxia (e.g. laryngotracheobronchitis, asthma, decreased level of consciousness with hypoventilation following trauma, seizure or drug ingestion).
3. The intensive care unit for continuous monitoring of patients.
4. The polysomnography laboratory: continuous SpO_2 monitoring is an essential component for the detection of hypoxia related to sleep disordered breathing.[40] It is most useful when combined with $PtcCO_2$ where it can be used for the detection of hypoventilation complicating obstructive sleep apnoea or congenital central alveolar hypoventilation syndrome (Ondine's curse). In addition, it can be used for the back titration of oxygen therapy in infants with chronic neonatal lung disease[38] and the adjustment of non-invasive ventilation.

Limitations of oximetry

As with any investigation, it is important to determine whether the oximetry reading appears consistent with the clinical scenario. A **poor trace** may reflect inadequate application of the sensor rather than poor peripheral perfusion. To help the clinician, many oximeters have visual and audible alarms to highlight the problem of a suboptimal reading.[41] A common example of this arises with movement artefact. Another problem has been electromagnetic interference (EMI) from radio frequency diathermy in operating theatres and cellular telephones positioned close to oximeter microprocessors. Another example of EMI is the intense magnetic field near magnetic resonance imaging or nuclear magnetic spectroscopy equipment. To overcome the problem, special pulse oximeters have been developed in which the photodetectors (in the sensor) and the light emitting display on the screen are placed inside the shell of the apparatus and the energy is transmitted between the patient and the photodetector by optical fibres.[41]

The calibration of the oximeter is based upon data derived from fit healthy adults who were sequentially desaturated to a minimum SaO_2 of 80%. Values of SpO_2 < 80% represent extrapolations from the accurately measured SpO_2 > 80% and so are less accurate.[42]

The importance of the delay between a physiological event occurring and the reading appearing on the oximeter is noteworthy. The time delay, often up to 10–20 s may reflect in-built averaging algorithms which produce more accurate but slower results. In the clinical setting, this may reflect an important delay in the detection of hypoxia. This is well demonstrated in standard polysomnography tracings, especially for obstructive apnoea related falls in oxygenation.[36,37]

There are unexpected limitations from extraneous energy sources. Firstly, bright visible or infrared lights may overload the semiconductor detector in the probe resulting in an erroneous value of 85%. This occurs because a ratio of red/infrared of one light is equivalent to an SpO_2 of 85%. Similarly, the penumbra effect has been described in young children.[43] This occurs when the sensor may over or under read due to there being a different path length of tissue for each of the wavelengths because of the precarious placement of an inappropriate (adult or older child) probe on the tip of a digit. This has largely been overcome with the introduction of specific probes for infants. Alternatively, if the infant probe is not readily available, as an interim measure, one can cover the probe area with a towel or an empty alcohol wipe wrapper. Additionally, dependent positioning of the monitoring site may cause venous pooling and cause a lower reading from enhanced venous pulsations. Another consideration is the use of nail polish (especially blue nail polish) which may cause lower SpO_2 measurements by absorbing light of the wavelength used by the pulse oximeter. Consequently, nail polish should be removed before applying the oximeter probe as a normal pulsatile waveform will be still be detected.

The issue of dyshaemoglobins is an important one. Specifically, carboxy-haemoglobin may give an erroneous result because the pulse oximeter does not differentiate carboxyhaemoglobin from HbO_2. Consequently, the oximeter over-estimates the true HbO_2 fraction. In this situation, the patient needs blood gas analyses using an octameter.

CASE STUDIES

Case 1

A 12-year-old boy is ventilated after a motor vehicle accident in which he sustained a severe head injury.

An initial arterial blood gas (ABG) on FiO_2 of 0.45:

pH	7.42	HCO_3	23 mM
PCO_2	33 mmHg	BE	–2
PO_2	139 mmHg		

Consequently, the FiO_2 is reduced to 0.35 and the gases are repeated 30 min later. There is no obvious change in the clinical state of the patient. The repeat ABG demonstrates:

pH	7.47	HCO_3	16 mM
PCO_2	15 mmHg	BE	–13
PO_2	140 mmHg		

What is the cause?
Pre analytic error is most likely. An excess of sodium heparin or a delay in running analysis could explain these results.

Case 2

A 7-year-old known asthmatic girl presents with a 4 day history of wheezing precipitated by a viral upper respiratory tract infection. She has been using frequent bronchodilators with minimal benefit. There is widespread expiratory wheeze on auscultation of the chest. The ABG in room air demonstrates:

pH	7.39	HCO_3	17 mM
PCO_2	28 mmHg	BE	−7
PO_2	54 mmHg		

This is compensated respiratory alkalosis due to chronic alveolar hyper-ventilation with hypoxia.

Case 3

A 2-year-old girl presents dehydrated with tachypnoea and accessory muscle use. A blood gas in room air reveals:

pH	7.01	HCO_3	5 mM
PCO_2	23 mmHg	BE	−30 mM
PO_2	102 mmHg		

This is a severe metabolic acidosis. The glucose was 5 2 mM and the child was diagnosed with diabetic ketoacidosis.

Case 4

A 15-year-old boy with cystic fibrosis and long-term home oxygen use presents with increasing cough and sputum production. A blood gas in an FiO_2 of 0.35 showed:

pH	7.34	HCO_3	33.5
PCO_2	78 mmHg	BE	12
PO_2	54 mmHg		

This is compensated respiratory acidosis with hypoxia. The boy is in chronic respiratory failure and non-invasive ventilation was commenced.

Case 5

A 2-month-old male infant presents with a history of vomiting after feeds and dehydration.

pH	7.50	HCO_3	30 mM
PCO_2	36 mmHg	BE	16
PO_2	77 mmHg		

This infant has an uncompensated metabolic alkalosis. The serum chloride was 71 mmol/l and a pyloric tumour was palpable after a test feed. This diagnosis is pyloric stenosis.

Key points for clinical practice

- Arterial blood gases are the gold standard for the assessment of hypoxaemia and acid-base status.

- Arterial blood gases must always be interpreted in the light of the clinical setting as sampling errors and delayed processing may provide erroneous results. If a result is out of keeping with the clinical expectations, it should be repeated.

- Transcutaneous oxygen monitoring provides a useful continuous estimate of arterial oxygenation with acceptable accuracy.

- Transcutaneous monitoring is most widely used in the neonatal intensive care unit.

- Continuous oximetry is the mainstay of assessment of oxygenation in the operating theatre, intensive care unit, emergency department and on general hospital wards.

- Oximetry is susceptible to misinterpretation if one is not confident about the position of the probe, adequacy of the arterial tracing and the perfusion of the area.

- Oximetry is most reliable ($\pm$ 2%) for values of SpO_2 > 85%.

References

1 Carruthers DM, Harrison BD. Arterial blood gas analysis or oxygen saturation in the assessment of acute asthma? Thorax 1995; 50: 186--188

2 Fleming PJ, Spieled BD, Marrow N, Dunne PM. A neonatal Vader – Mecca, 2nd edn. London: Edward Arnold, 1991

3 Okeson GC, Wulbrecht PH. The safety of brachial artery puncture for arterial blood sampling. Chest 1998; 114: 748–751

4 Sackner MA, Avery WG. Sokolowski J. Arterial puncture by nurses. Chest 1971; 59: 97–98

5 Eriksen HC, Sorenson HR. Arterial injuries: iatrogenic and non iatrogenic. Acta Chir Scand 1969; 135: 133–136

6 Mortensen JD. Clinical sequelae from arterial needle puncture cannulation and incision. Circulation 1967; 35: 1118–1123

7 Mathieu A, Dalton B, Fischer JE, Kumar A. Expanding aneurysm of the radial artery after frequent puncture. Anaesthesiology 1973; 38: 401–403

8 Allen EV. Thromboangitis obliterans: methods of diagnosis of chronic occlusive arterial lesions distal to the wrist with illustrative cases. Am J Med Sci 1929; 178: 237–244

9 Resar LM, Helfar MA. Recurrent seizures in a neonate after lidocaine administration. J Perinatol 1998; 18: 193–195

10 Pappert D, Rossaint R, Lewandowski K et al. Preliminary evaluation of a new continuous intra arterial blood gas monitoring device. Acta Anaesthesiol Scand 1995; 107 S: 60-67

11 Bannister A. Comparison of arterial and arterialised capillary blood in infants with respiratory disease. Arch Dis Child 1969; 44: 726–728

12 Siggard-Andersen O. Acid base and blood gas parameters: arterial or capillary blood ? Scan J Clin Lab Invest 1968; 21: 289–294

13 Gambino SR, Thiede WH. Comparisons of pH in human arterial, venous and capillary blood. Am J Clin Pathol 1959; 32: 298–305

14 Tobias JD, Meyer DJ, Helikson MA. Monitoring of pH and PCO_2 in children using the paratrend in a peripheral vein. Can J Anaesth. 1998; 45: 81–83

15 Shapiro BA, Harrison RA, Cane RD, Templin R. Clinical Applications of Blood Gases, 4th edn. London:Year Book Medical Publishers, 1996

16 Mueller RG, Lang GE, Beam JM. Bubbles in samples for blood gas determinations. Am J Clin Pathol 1976; 65: 242–249

17 Moran RG. External factors influencing blood gas analysis: quality control revisited. Am J Med Tech 1979; 45: 1009–1011

18 Holmes PL, Green HC, Lopez-Majano V. Evaluation of methods for calibration of O_2 and CO_2 electrodes. Am J Clin Pathol 1970; 54: 566–569

19 Van Duzee BF. Thermal analysis of human stratum corneum. J Invest Dermatol 1975; 65: 404

20 Lucey JF. Clinical uses of transcutaneous oxygen monitoring. Adv Pediatr 1981; 28: 27–56

21 Huch R, Lubbers DW, Hutch A. Reliability of transcutaneous monitoring of arterial PO_2 in newborn infants. Arch Dis Child 1974; 49: 213–218

22 Monaco F, Nickerson BG, McQuilty JC. Continuos transcutaneous oxygen and carbon dioxide monitoring in the paediatric ICU. Crit Care Med 1982; 10: 765–766

23 Tremper KK, Shoemaker WC. Transcutaneous oxygen monitoring of critically ill adults with and without low flow shock. Crit Care Med 1981; 9: 706

24 Peabody JL, Gregory GA, Willis MM. Failure of conventional monitoring to detect apnoea resulting in hypoxemia. Birth Defects 1979; XV: 274–282

25 Tobias JD, Meyer DJ. Non invasive monitoring of carbon dioxide during respiratory failure in toddlers and infants: end tidal versus transcutaneous carbon dioxide. Anesth Analg 1997; 85: 55–58

26 Halden L; Monitoring of optimal oxygen transport by the transcutaneous oxygen tension method. Acta Anaesthesiol Scand 1982; 26: 209–212

27 Murray IP, Modell JH, Gallagher JJ et al. Titration of PEEP by the arterial minus end tidal carbon dioxide gradient. Chest 1984; 85: 100–104

28 Marshall TA, Kattwinkel J, Bevry FA et al. Transcutaneous oxygen monitoring of neonates during surgery. J Pediatr Surg 1980; 15: 797–804

29 Tremper KK Waxman KS, Bowman R. Continuous transcutaneous oxygen monitoring during respiratory failure, cardiac decompensation, cardiac arrest and CPR. Crit Care Med 1980; 8: 377–381

30 Keller HP, Klaye P, Hockerts T; Transcutaneous PO_2 measurement on skin transplants. Birth Defects 1979; XV: 511–516

31 Achauer BM, Blacks KS, Beran AV. Transcutaneous PO_2 monitoring of flap circulation following surgery. Birth Defects 1979; XV: 517–522

32 Burgess EM, Matsen FA, Wyss CR et al. Segmental transcutaneous measurements of PO_2 in patients requiring below knee amputation for peripheral vascular insufficiency. J Bone Joint Surg 1982; 64A: 373–382

33 White RA, Nolan L, Harley D et al. Noninvasive evaluation of peripheral vascular disease using transcutaneous oxygen tension. Am J Surg 1982; 144: 68–75

34 Thilo EH, Andersen D, Wasserstein ML, Schmidt J, Luckey D. Saturation by pulse oximetry: comparison of the results obtained by instruments of different brands. J Pediatr 1993; 122: 620–626

35 Ralston AC, Webb RK, Runciman WB. Potential errors in pulse oximetry. Anaesthesia 1991; 46: 202–206

36 Farre R, Montserrat JM, Ballester E, Hernandez L, Rotger M, Navajas D. Importance of the pulse oximeter averaging time when measuring oxygen desaturation in sleep apnea. Sleep 1998; 21; 386–390

37 Levy P, Pepin JL, Deshcaux-Blanc C, Paramelle B, Brambilla C. Accuracy of oximetry for detection of respiratory disturbances in sleep apnea syndrome. Chest 1996; 109: 395–399

38 Fitzgerald D, Van Asperen P, Leslie G, Arnold J, Sullivan C. Higher SaO$_2$ in chronic neonatal lung disease: does it improve sleep? Pediatr Pulmonol 1998; 26: 235–240

39 Moyle JTB. Uses and abuses of pulse oximetry. Arch Dis Child 1996; 74: 77–80

40 Yamashiro Y, Kryger MH. Nocturnal oximetry: is it a screening tool for sleep disorders? Sleep 1995; 18: 167–171

41 Wukitsch MW, Petterson MT, Tobler DR, Pologe JA. Pulse oximetry: analysis of theory, technology and practice. J Clin Monit 1988; 4: 290–301

42 Clark JS, Votteri B, Ariagno RL et al. State of the art: non-invasive assessment of blood gases. Am Rev Respir Dis 1992; 145: 220–232

43 Kelleher JF, Ruff RH. The penumbra effect: vasomotion-dependent pulse oximeter artifact due to probe malposition. Anaesthesiology 1989; 71: 787–791

Monitoring oxygen in the blood

Michelle Shouldice Dirk Huyer

Non-accidental rib fractures

Rib fractures in infancy are uncommon and, when present, are strongly suggestive of non-accidental injury. Reports have described a frequency of 15–21% when abused children under the age of 2 years are imaged.[1,2] This may represent an underestimate of the true incidence, since fractures in this area are often missed with chest X-ray alone. Additional techniques during death investigation have demonstrated rib fractures in as many as 35% of abused infants.[3] In this group of infants who died with inflicted injury, rib fractures were second in frequency only to metaphyseal fractures. In this chapter, we will discuss the clinical presentation and radiological appearance of non-accidental rib fractures in childhood, the force and mechanism of injury required to produce these fractures and potential alternate diagnoses.

CLINICAL PRESENTATION

Rib fractures are not common during infancy and childhood. When accidental, they result from significant, high velocity trauma which is easily identified on history, such as motor vehicle accident or fall from a significant height. Non-accidental rib fractures are generally occult, typically without external signs of injury. The majority are found incidentally when chest X-rays are done for other clinical indications. Alternatively, fractures may be found on skeletal surveys performed during an abuse evaluation.

The majority of non-accidental rib fractures occur in preverbal infants and children. History of preceding events is, therefore, unattainable from the child

Michelle Shouldice BScH MSc MD FRCPC, Suspected Child Abuse and neglect (SCAN) Program, The Hospital for Sick Children, Toronto, Ontario M5G 1X8, Canada

Dirk Huyer MD, Suspected Child Abuse and neglect (SCAN) Program, The Hospital for Sick Children, 555 University Avenue, Toronto, Ontario M5G 1X8, Canada (for correspondence)

and symptoms such as chest pain cannot be elicited. In fact, infants with rib fractures may display few signs related directly to the fracture. Clinical signs, if present, are non-specific, such as irritability or mild respiratory distress. There are likely several factors which contribute to the paucity of clinical indicators of rib fractures, including: splinting of fractures by intercostal muscles, increased use of abdominal muscles for breathing leading to decreased chest wall excursion and the frequent undisplaced, greenstick nature of the fractures. In addition, abusive rib fractures are usually caused by indirect forces, with no resultant overlying bruising or soft tissue swelling. Occasionally, crepitus over the fractured area may be felt by a caregiver or medical provider. Pneumothorax, haemothorax and pulmonary contusions may rarely complicate inflicted rib fractures. Traumatic chylothorax secondary to lymphatic disruption from rib fractures has been reported as the presenting feature of child abuse.[4-6] Rib fractures can be lethal, as in the case of an infant who developed a secondary pneumonia, dehydration and sepsis as a complication from rib fracture-related pulmonary contusions. When rib fractures are present, symptoms displayed generally reflect other accompanying injuries, including limb fractures or brain injury.

In studies comparing accidental and non-accidental rib fractures in children, several differences between the two groups are evident. Accidental rib fractures occur with a clear history of preceding significant, high velocity trauma. Motor vehicle accidents with child pedestrians represent the most frequent cause of rib fractures, followed by falls from a significant height.[7,8] Accidental injuries occur most commonly in ambulatory children greater than 2 years old. Children sustaining accidental trauma with sufficient force to fracture ribs are more likely to have associated intrathoracic injuries such as pulmonary contusions, pneumothorax or haemothorax.[8]

In contrast, the majority of non-accidental rib fractures occur in infants under 1 year of age.[9] There is generally no history of preceding injury and the fractures are found incidentally. Associated intrathoracic injury is less common, but there may be accompanying unexplained extrathoracic injury. Abusive rib fractures in infants are commonly multiple, bilateral and occur in groups of adjacent ribs.[9] Different stages of healing may be evident, reflecting several episodes of injury.

When rib fractures are found, particularly during infancy, strong consideration must be given to the possibility of abuse. The history obtained from care-givers should be carefully documented. A thorough physical examination is necessary, and should include growth parameters, head circumference, neurological assessment, ophthalmological examination for retinal haemorrhages, and a careful skin examination for evidence of recent or past injury. Further imaging may be necessary to evaluate for evidence of other fractures. At a minimum, a skeletal survey must be obtained. This imaging should **not** be a 'babygram' which provides a view of the full body of the infant on one or two films, but a skeletal survey, a series of X-rays which carefully documents each area of the body separately.[10] In our hospital, views include: AP and lateral of skull, AP and lateral spine, AP of both humeri, and of radius and ulna, PA of both hands and wrists, AP of pelvis, AP of both femora, of both tibia/fibula and both feet and AP and lateral chest views for ribs. If there is evidence of other organ involvement, further investigations may be indicated, such as head imaging to look for intracranial bleeding or ophthalmological assessment for retinal haemorrhages. Finally, if non-accidental injury is suspected, local child protective services must be notified.

SHAKEN BABY SYNDROME

As will be discussed further, rib fractures typically result from thoracic compression. This mechanism of injury may occur during violent shaking of children, producing the clinical features observed in shaken baby/shaken impact syndrome. This injury occurs when an assailant holds an infant, commonly using the chest as a handle, and violently shakes the infant forwards and backwards. The relatively large head, which is poorly supported by the developing neck muscles and the limbs flail back and forth during this

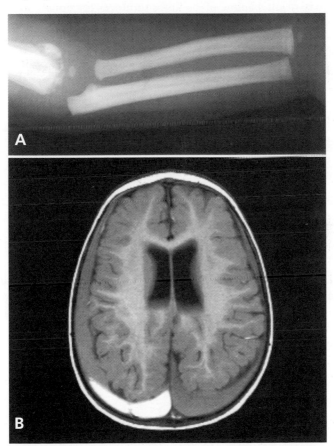

Fig. 5.1 This 9-month-old infant presented with a history of a fall from a couch. Multiple fractures and intracranial bleeding were found on imaging. Eye examination revealed retinal hemorrhages. **(A)** Lateral radiograph of the forearm demonstrating a healing fracture of the distal humerus with peri-osteal reaction and a bucket handle fracture of the distal radial metaphysis. **(B)** MR imaging of the head demonstrated subdural haemorrhage of different age, reflecting more than one abusive episode.

application of force. Impact of the head may occur during shaking as the head collides with a solid surface or when the infant is thrown down or against a wall. Angular acceleration/deceleration forces are generated during shaking. These forces are applied to the brain as it rotates on its axis within the skull. This results in diffuse brain injury and tearing of bridging veins with resultant intracranial bleeding. Clinical presentation is often with non-specific symptoms of irritability, lethargy, poor feeding or vomiting relating to brain injury. More severe injury may result in seizures, apnoea or impaired consciousness. The fontanelle may be full, reflecting intracranial bleeding or cerebral oedema.

In addition to the brain injury, other associated clinical features are observed in the syndrome.[11] Ophthalmological examination reveals retinal haemorrhages in the majority of infants with shaken baby syndrome. These may be unilateral or bilateral. There may be associated retinoschisis or detachment. Significant visual loss may result. Flailing of the limbs produces tractional force application to the limbs, which may cause metaphyseal corner or bucket handle fractures of the long bones (Fig. 5.1). Intracranial bleeding may be subdural or subarachnoid with a frequent predilection for the interhemispheric (parafalcine) region. Fractures at different stages of healing or intracranial bleeding of different ages may indicate more than one traumatic event.

RIB FRACTURES

Treatment of rib fractures

No treatment is indicated for rib fractures themselves. Treatment of associated intrathoracic and extrathoracic injuries may be frequently indicated.

Mechanism of injury

The production of rib fractures in infancy and childhood requires the application of significant force. The infant rib cage is elastic and pliable and, therefore, able to withstand significant compressive force before fractures occur. As indicated

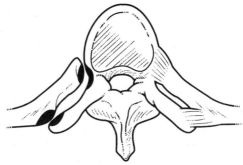

Fig. 5.2 The costovertebral relationship involving the rib head articulation with the vertebral body and rib tubercle articulation with the vertebral transverse process. Ligamentous attachments at both articulations hold the medial rib in place. With posterior levering of the rib on the transverse process, fractures occur in the posteromedial location.

previously, accidental rib fractures result from violent trauma. The magnitude of the force required to produce rib fractures is reflected in the mortality rate of 42% described in one study of children with blunt thoracic trauma causing fractures, compared with 18% in those without rib fractures.[7] In abused children with thoracic injury, the mortality rate may be as high as 50%.[12] It is well recognized that injuries occurring during typical childhood play and falls from low heights do not cause rib fractures.

There is ample evidence that posterior rib fractures result from indirect forces produced by a lever mechanism involving the rib and its adjacent vertebrae. The rib head is relatively fixed by its ligamentous attachments at the articulation with the costal facet of the vertebral body. As the rib curves posteriorly, its tubercle meets and articulates with the vertebral transverse process (Fig. 5.2). This anatomical arrangement results in localization of the largest force to the rib head and neck as the ribs are levered posteriorly during thoracic compression, producing fractures of the posteromedial ribs.[13,14]

Evidence supporting this mechanism is provided by experimental, clinical and pathological data. Sternotomy in adult cadavers results in fractures located at or medial to the costotransverse articulation due to posterior levering of the ribs.[14] Pathological evaluation of posterior rib fractures demonstrates greater separation of fracture margins anteriorly, consistent with levering on the fulcrum of the transverse process.[13,14] Anterior-posterior compression of post-mortem rabbit rib cages held by hands encircling the rabbit's chest, produced posterior rib fractures near the costovertebral articulation.[14] During the squeezing of the rabbit's chest, CT scanning demonstrated the ribs levered posteriorly over the vertebral transverse process. Imaging of the excised fractures demonstrated posterior impaction and anterior separation of the fracture fragments. When the rabbit was placed on a flat surface and the chest compressed at the sternum, simulating CPR, posterior migration of the ribs did not occur and no fractures were identified.

The indirect forces causing the levering mechanism responsible for posterior rib fractures are produced by forceful squeezing of the thorax. This may accompany vigorous shaking of the infant held with the chest used as a handle. In fact, multiple posteromedial rib fractures have been described in infants where a clear history of shaking was obtained during confession of the assailant.[15] Acute posterior rib fractures found during autopsy of abused infants demonstrate features consistent with this mechanism. These fractures have been shown histologically and on specimen radiography to occur in the anterior portion of the rib opposite the costotransverse articulation, with the posterior periosteum remaining intact.[16]

The described morphological, experimental and clinical information demonstrates that indirect forces causing posterior levering of the rib over the vertebral transverse process produce rib fractures at the posteromedial location in infants. Any other accidental mechanism suggested to explain fractures in this location must involve such posterior levering. For example, posterior rib fractures have been demonstrated from motor vehicle accidental injuries, when children were struck anteriorly or hurled forwards against a dashboard, leading to compression of the chest and resultant posterior angulation of the ribs.[14]

Lateral rib fractures in infants are similarly thought to result from indirect trauma applied during compression of the chest, causing bending of the ribs

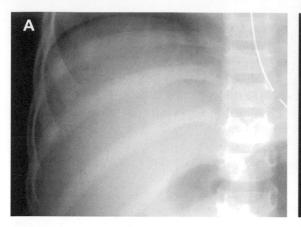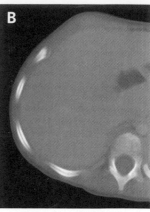

Fig. 5.3 A 2-year-old child with abusive abdominal trauma. (**A**) Chest X-ray showing anterior rib fractures. (**B**) CT scan improves visualization of the fractures.

and eventual fracture. Imaging and pathological studies show buckling of the inner surface of the fractured rib with separation of the fracture fragments at the external surface.[17] These fractures tend to occur in groups of adjacent ribs.

Fractures of the anterior ribs occur at the costochondral junction at the location of the growth plate in the anterior rib end.[15] The anatomy in this location during infancy is similar to the long bone metaphysis. Thus, little new bone growth occurs with healing in this region, making these fractures difficult to detect, both by imaging (Fig. 5.3) and pathological assessment.[3] They are, therefore, likely to be more common than described in the literature. When excised anterior rib fractures from abused infants were studied using specimen radiography and histological assessment, the posterior surface of the periosteum was seen to be disrupted, with the fracture fragment displaced inwards.[3,15] This is consistent with an external compressive force depressing the costochondral joints inwards. Therefore, anterior rib fractures likely also result from external compression.

Imaging

Rib fractures, particularly those in the posterior arc near the costovertebral articulation, are difficult to identify on chest X-ray. In fact, these fractures are commonly not seen until healing callus appears (Fig. 5.4). In a series of infants who died with inflicted injuries, only 26% of the rib fractures were found on pre-autopsy skeletal survey. The remainder were seen on autopsy with visual examination, or histopathology; (Fig. 5.5) or by imaging of excised ribs.[3] When radiological and pathological features were compared, factors affecting visibility of the fractures were identified.[16] The location of posterior arc fractures is such that the image of the transverse process often overlies the fracture site. The fracture line is frequently oblique to the plane of the X-ray, making acute identification difficult. As discussed above, the levering mechanism produces an anterior fracture, maintaining the posterior periosteum, with little displacement or angulation of the fracture fragments. Furthermore, imaging of rib fractures involves the shadows of lung, blood

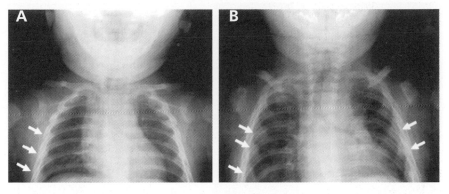

Fig. 5.4 A 3-month-old infant who presented with a spiral fracture of the femur. Skeletal survey demonstrated multiple fractures. (**A**) Angulation of several right lateral ribs (arrows) reflecting acute fractures. A metaphyseal fracture of the right proximal humerus was also seen on the chest X-ray. (**B**) Follow up skeletal survey 2 weeks after the injury. The right lateral rib fractures are more easily identified by the healing callus (arrows). Previously unidentified fractures of the left lateral ribs can now be identified.

vessels, heart, soft tissues and bone being superimposed upon one another. Oblique views of the ribs may increase detection of rib fractures by re-orienting the fracture line with respect to the X-ray beam and permitting greater exposure of the fractured area. A follow-up skeletal survey completed 2 weeks after injury has been shown to increase the radiological detection of rib fractures (Fig. 5.4). Kleinman et al. showed that repeat skeletal surveys revealed fractures not seen acutely or confirmed questionable acute fractures.[18]

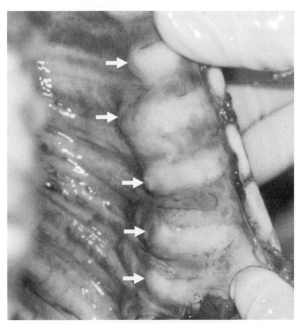

Fig. 5.5 A 13-month-old child who died from direct traumatic head injury. Pathological examination revealed several healing rib fractures (arrows).

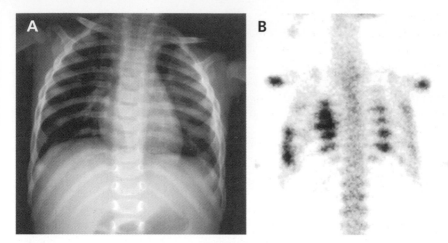

Fig. 5.6 A 7-month-old infant who presented with respiratory symptoms. Rib fractures were found incidentally on chest X-ray. (**A**) Chest X-ray reveals multiple rib fractures of various ages. (**B**) Radionuclide bone scan reveals posterior and lateral rib fractures not easily identified on plain film imaging.

Of the additional 19 fractures found in the 23 infants assessed, 42% were rib fractures. In addition, the repeat assessment provided valuable information regarding the age of injuries seen.

A number of studies have demonstrated the increased sensitivity of bone scan compared with plain film imaging in identifying rib fractures in infants.[19–21] Rib fractures detectable by bone scan may be missed, or the number underestimated using X-ray alone (Fig. 5.6). However, radionuclide bone scanning has several disadvantages. Sedation of the infant is often necessary. Success of fracture detection depends on the technical quality of the study and the expertise of the interpreting radiologist. Abnormalities seen on bone scan are non-specific and may be secondary to injury, infection or neoplasm. In contrast, X-rays provide information regarding the type of fracture, stage of healing and changes of metabolic bone diseases that is unavailable through bone scanning alone.

The use of bone windows during CT scanning may increase the sensitivity of radiological detection of rib fractures in infancy (Fig. 5.3). CT scanning may also provide clearer documentation of the configuration of the fracture and the degree of healing. Occasional reports of the use of CT scan for the detection of rib fractures appear in the literature,[14,15] but no formal assessment of this mode of imaging for bony injury in abused infants or children has been reported to date. The value of MRI in assessing rib fractures in children is unknown.

When investigating the possibility of physical abuse in infants and young children, a skeletal survey must be completed to evaluate for occult acute and/or healing fractures. As discussed above, acute posterior rib fractures which are highly suggestive of abusive injury may be poorly visualized on chest X-ray. If abuse is strongly suspected, bone scan should be considered, in addition to a follow up skeletal survey.

Dating rib fractures

As previously discussed, rib fractures are usually occult and not accompanied by clinical signs or symptoms. Determining the age of the injury, therefore, is difficult clinically. Radiological dating is commonly relied upon to provide information regarding the timing of fractures. However, there are no reports in the literature documenting dating of fractures in axial skeleton resulting from inflicted injury in children.

For reasons previously discussed, acute rib fractures may not be seen on initial chest X-ray. They may be visible on bone scan within a few hours of injury, although false negative scans may occur within the first 48 h of injury.[22] Radiological features used in dating rib fractures are extrapolated from patterns seen in long bones. These features include: clear visibility of the fracture line (acute to 14 days after injury), time to periosteal reaction (4 days to 2 weeks after injury) and callus formation (10 days to 3 months after injury).[23] Kleinman indicates that callus is visible in the region of the rib neck 7–10 days after injury.[15] It appears that the dating of rib fractures radiologically can be an approximation only. Infants who have compressive injury to the bony thorax may experience more than one abusive episode, leading to acute injury superimposed on chronic fractures. This could lead to persistence of the visibility of a fracture line, a feature commonly used to date acute fractures, within an extensive callus and contribute to difficulties in dating. Follow-up skeletal surveys not only help to identify fractures which may have gone undiagnosed acutely, but may also contribute to a greater understanding rib fracture healing in infancy.

Alternative explanations for rib fractures

Cardiopulmonary resuscitation

Rib fractures are described in adults as a complication of closed chest cardiopulmonary resuscitation (CPR), leading some authors to suggest this aetiology for rib fractures in infants and children. However, the chest wall, particularly in infancy, is elastic and flexible, permitting greater compression without bony injury. This physiological flexibility of the infant rib cage is protective during the birth process and results in a much lower incidence of rib fractures in this age group.

A number of studies have been evaluated for a possible link between injury and CPR in children. In a series of 50 CPR survivors, Feldman found no infants or children with radiographic evidence of acute rib fractures.[9] Healing fractures were also absent in the 18 patients who had follow-up X-rays done at least 2 weeks after CPR. Similarly, Spevak found no X-ray or autopsy evidence of rib fractures.[24] Thomas reviewed 10,000 infant chest X-rays and identified 25 infants with rib fractures in 91 infants without suspicion of abuse who underwent CPR before death.[25] The author postulated that some of these fractures could have been caused by resuscitation or physiotherapy. However, information regarding which of these infants required CPR and why, was not provided. Similarly, those infants receiving physiotherapy were not identified. In addition, all of the infants with rib fractures not identified as abusive in cause were premature, low birth weight or had evidence of metabolic bone disease. Bush described bilateral rib fractures at the sternochondral junction, found at autopsy in a 3-month-old infant whose cause of death was identified as SIDS.[26] CPR was provided for 75 min in this case by several different people. The circumstances of this infant's death and the extent of investigation for non-accidental injury were not described. In particular, the authors do not indicate whether skeletal survey and autopsy were done. Betz and Liebhardt reviewed 94 cases of non-traumatic death in infancy and childhood where CPR was performed prior to death. They describe a 2-month-old infant and a 5-year-old child with anterolateral rib fractures after CPR.[27] The cause of death was ascribed to SIDS in the infant and drowning in the 5-year-old child. Again, the circumstances of these deaths and the extent of investigation for non-accidental injury are not detailed.

In the typical positioning for CPR utilized in North America, with the child supine on a hard, flat surface, the chest is compressed between the sternum and the table. The solid surface on which the child lies prevents posterior levering of the ribs. CPR, therefore, does not produce the mechanism necessary to cause posterior rib fractures. Anecdotal information provided to the authors suggests that, in some countries, the method of CPR differs, in that the provider's hands encircle the chest with the fingers stabilizing the infant's chest posteriorly and the thumbs overlapping anteriorly to provide sternal compression. Complications of this method of CPR are unknown.

In summary, there is no biomechanical or clinical evidence to suggest that CPR causes posterior rib fractures in infants without bone disease. Caution should be used in attributing rib fractures in any location to CPR in infants. Rib fractures in older children are uncommonly attributable to CPR. In cases where rib fractures are observed following CPR, further investigations, such as skeletal survey and pathological assessment in the case of death, must be considered in order to assess for possible non-accidental aetiology.

Birth trauma

Birth trauma has been proposed as a possible mechanism for rib fractures in infants. There are a few case reports in the literature to support birth as a mechanism for rib fractures, although large studies assessing birth injuries have failed to show fractures in this location.[28–31] It is, therefore, likely that birth-related rib fractures are uncommon in neonates. However, difficulties with the acute detection and the lack of specific clinical signs and symptoms related to rib fractures may have resulted in an underestimate of their frequency.

Case reports describing rib fractures in neonates ascribed to the birth process suggest that traumatic delivery and large birth weight are contributing factors. Rizzolo describes a 3300 g neonate with posterolateral rib fractures diagnosed by imaging at 9 h of age. When examined for respiratory distress, crepitus was palpated over the infant's back.[32] The labour and delivery were complicated by fetal distress, vacuum extraction and shoulder dystocia. A skeletal survey was negative for bony abnormalities and further fractures. A number of risk factors for child maltreatment were present, but the injury was not felt to have been inflicted by the mother. In his review of 10,000 chest X-rays in infants, Thomas reported healing fractures in one 3-week-old baby, thought to be produced by birth trauma.[25] The baby was macrosomic with a birth weight of 5686 g and was delivered by mid-forceps. Hartmann described posterior rib fractures in two large for gestational age neonates, discovered when crepitus was felt over the infrascapular region.[33] Both neonates were clinically well, with no respiratory distress. A 9-hour-old infant, weighing 5020 g was found by Barry and Hocking to have posterior fractures of 5 ribs after presenting with crepitus over the back.[34]

In our hospital, an infant who remained admitted from the time of birth for investigation of persistent neonatal hypoglycaemia, was found on chest X-ray to have fractures of the 7th and 8th ribs posteriorly at 13 days of age. The history was of full-term gestation with a birth weight of 3575 g. Labour and delivery were uncomplicated. Interestingly, the mother participated in the child's birth by helping to deliver the infant's body with her hands. The obstetrician described mother holding the infant under the axillae while he supported the body. He described never having seen complications previously with this method of delivery which he commonly uses. The baby remained in the special care nursery and was alone with her mother only for breast feeding when she was surrounded by a curtain. No history of trauma related to hospitalization was evident upon investigation. A skeletal survey showed no additional fractures and no changes consistent with bone disease. Although non-accidental injury during hospitalization could not be entirely ruled out, it was determined to be unlikely.

The infant rib cage is flexible and able to withstand significant compressive force before fracture occurs. Compression of the infant's rib cage does occur during delivery and the birth-related rib fractures described above are thought to occur during thoracic compression and flexion against the symphysis pubis. The paucity of case reports of rib fractures secondary to birth injury suggests this is a rare occurrence and, when present, rib fractures are likely related to large size and traumatic delivery.

Coughing

There are no convincing reports in the literature of cough-related rib fractures in infants and children. In the authors' clinical experience, rib fractures caused by coughing have not been seen, including in young infants hospitalized at length for pertussis with apnoea related to severe paroxysms of coughing. Cough should not be determined to be the cause of rib fractures in infancy.

Bone diseases

Rib fractures have been reported in the clinical setting of rickets. However, confusion with non-accidental injury does not usually occur because the radiological features of rickets are easily identified if sufficient bone loss to predispose for fractures has occurred.

Prematurity and low birth weight are risk factors for both the development of metabolic bone disease and for child abuse. Amir et al. describe a series of 973 premature infants who required neonatal intensive care and survived for greater than 6 months.[35] In this series, 12 patients were found to have fractures during their hospitalization. None of these were felt to have resulted from birth injury. Rib fractures were found in 7 of these infants and were described as primarily anterolateral in location. All infants with rib fractures were born at less than 32 weeks gestation or were of low birth weight (< 1500 g). One patient was determined biochemically to have rickets. Risk factors reported for the development of metabolic bone disease were: cholestatic jaundice, parenteral nutrition for greater than 3 weeks, chronic lung disease or diuretic therapy for longer than 2 weeks. All infants with rib fractures had at least 2 of these risk factors. With sufficient bone loss to predispose to pathological fractures, osteopenia is evident radiologically.[15] There is no evidence in the literature to suggest that prematurity or low birth weight result in fractures with normal handling after discharge from hospital. A study of children under the age of 6 years presenting to emergency with fractures did not reveal an increased risk of fracture related to prematurity.[36] This suggests that an increased risk of fractures related to prematurity does not persist into childhood.

Osteogenesis imperfecta (OI) is a rare disorder of collagen synthesis which leads to bone fragility and easy fracture. Of the subtypes of OI, types II and III are very severe and unlikely to be confused with child abuse. Types I and IV exhibit autosomal dominant inheritance, with spontaneous mutations not uncommon. A family history of frequent fractures, hearing loss and dental problems may be elicited. Physical examination may reveal blue sclerae, however, this finding may be observed in normal infants. Fractures in OI occur mainly in the long bones and are typically accompanied by generalized osteoporosis and bowing in weight-bearing bones. Wormian bones may be found on skull X-ray. Rib fractures are rare in OI. Kleinman reports that rib

---

Key points for clinical practice

- Non-accidental rib fractures in infancy are usually found incidentally on X-ray and are unlikely to be associated with external signs of injury, such as bruising or soft tissue swelling.

- Clinical, experimental, anatomical and pathological information demonstrate that rib fractures in infancy result from indirect forces produced during anterior-posterior compression of the thoracic cage.

- Production of rib fractures during infancy requires significant force since the infant rib cage is pliable and withstands significant compressive pressure before fracture occurs.

- Any accidental injury resulting in rib fractures, therefore, must have a preceding history of significant violent trauma, such as a motor vehicle accident or fall from a significant height.

- Non-accidental rib fractures result from forceful squeezing of the infant's rib cage between the assailant's hands or during vigorous shaking of the infant held by the chest.

- Investigation of an infant found to have rib fractures without a history of preceding violent trauma must include a skeletal survey to look for associated occult fractures.

- Acute rib fractures are difficult to visualize on chest X-ray. Radionuclide bone scanning and follow-up skeletal survey increase the sensitivity of imaging for the diagnosis of rib fractures.

- Rib fractures in infants and young children without a history of preceding violent trauma are highly suggestive of child abuse. When prematurity and bone diseases are ruled out, the majority of these fractures are due to non-accidental injury.

fractures from minor trauma in OI are seen in cases where the ribs are obviously thin or osteopenic.[15] Therefore, OI alone should not be accepted as an explanation for rib fractures in infants.

References

1 Kogutt M, Swischuk L, Fagan C. Patterns of injury and significance of uncommon fractures in the battered child syndrome. AJR 1974; 121: 143–149

2 Merten D, Radkowski M, Leonidas J. The abused child: a radiological reappraisal. Radiology 1983; 146: 377–381

3 Kleinman P, Marks S, Richmond J, Blackbourne B. Inflicted skeletal injury: a postmortem radiologic-histopathologic study in 31 infants. AJR 1995; 165: 647–650

4 Geismar S, Tilelli J, Campbell J, Chiaro J. Chylothorax as a manifestation of child abuse. Pediatr Emerg Care 1997; 13: 386–389

5 Green H. Child abuse presenting as chylothorax. Pediatrics 1980; 66: 620–621

6 Guleserian K, Gilchrist B, Luks F, Wesselhoeft C, DeLuca F. Child abuse as a cause of traumatic chylothorax. J Pediatr Surg 1996; 31: 1696–1697

7 Garcia V, Gotschall C, Eichelberger M, Bowman L. Rib fractures in children: a marker of severe trauma. J Trauma 1990; 30: 695–700

8 Schweich P, Fleisher G. Rib fractures in children. Pediatr Emerg Care 1985; 1: 187–189

9 Feldman K, Brewer D. Child abuse, cardiopulmonary resuscitation, and rib fractures. Pediatrics 1984; 73: 339–342

10 Kleinman P, Blackbourne B, Marks S, Karellas A, Belanger P. Radiologic contributions to the investigation and prosecution of cases of fatal child abuse. N Engl J Med 1989; 320: 507–511

11 Duhaime A, Christian C, Rorke L, Zimmerman R. Nonaccidental head injury in infants – the 'shaken-baby syndrome'. N Engl J Med 1998; 338: 1822–1829

12 Peelet MH, Newman KD, Eichelberger MR, Gotschall CS, Garcia VF, Bowman LM. Thoracic trauma in children: an indicator of increased mortality. J Pediatr Surg 1990; 25: 961–966

13 Kleinman P, Marks S, Spevak M, Richmond J. Fractures of the rib head in abused infants. Radiology 1992; 185: 119–123

14 Kleinman P, Schlesinger A. Mechanical factors associated with posterior rib fractures: laboratory and case studies. Pediatr Radiol 1997; 27: 87–91

15 Kleinman P. Bony thoracic trauma. In: Kleinman P, ed. Diagnostic Imaging of Child Abuse, 2nd edn. Missouri: Mosby, 1998; 113

16. Kleinman P, Marks S, Adams V, Blackbourne B. Factors affecting visualization of posterior rib fractures in abused infants. AJR 1988; 150: 635–638

17 Kleinman P, Marks S, Nimkin K, Rayder S, Kessler S. Rib fractures in 31 abused infants: postmortem radiologic-histopathologic study. Radiology 1996; 200: 807–810

18 Kleinman P, Nimkin K, Spevak M et al. Follow-up skeletal surveys in suspected child abuse. AJR 1996; 167: 893–896

19 Jaudes P. Comparison of radiography and radionuclide bone scanning in the detection of child abuse. Pediatrics 1984; 73: 166–168

20 Smith F, Gilday D, Ash J, Green M. Unsuspected costo-vertebral fractures demonstrated by bone scanning in the child abuse syndrome. Pediatr Radiol 1980; 10: 103–106

21 Sty J, Starshak R. The role of bone scintigraphy in the evaluation of the suspected abused child. Radiology 1983; 146: 369–375

22 Rosenthall L, Hill R, Chuang S. Observation on the use of 99mTc-phosphate imaging in peripheral bone trauma. Radiology 1976; 119: 637–641

23 O'Connor J, Cohen J. Dating fractures. In: Kleinman P, ed. Diagnostic Imaging of Child Abuse, 2nd edn. St Louis: Mosby, 1998; 168–177

24 Spevak M, Kleinman P, Belanger P, Primack C, Richmond J. Cardiopulmonary resuscitation and rib fractures in infants. JAMA 1994; 272: 617–618

25 Thomas P. Rib fractures in infancy. Ann Radiol 1977; 20: 115–122

26 Bush C, Jones J, Cohle S, Johnson H. Pediatric injuries from cardiopulmonary resuscitation. Ann Emerg Med 1996; 28: 40–44

CHAPTER

5

Recent Advances in Paediatrics 18

27 Betz P, Liebhardt E. Rib fractures in children - resuscitation or child abuse? Int J Legal Med 1994; 106: 215–218

28 Bhat B, Kumar A, Oumachigui A. Bone injuries during delivery. Indian J Pediatr 1994; 61: 401–405

29 Nadas S, Gudinchet F, Capasso P, Reinberg O. Predisposing factors in obstetrical fractures. Skeletal Radiol 1993; 22: 195–198

30 Cumming W. Neonatal skeletal fractures: birth trauma or child abuse? J Can Assoc Radiol 1979; 30: 30-33

31 Rubin A. Birth injuries: incidence, mechanisms, and end results. J Obstet Gynecol 1964; 23: 218-221

32 Rizzolo P, Coleman P. Neonatal rib fracture: birth trauma or child abuse? J Fam Pract 1989; 29: 561–563

33 Hartmann R. Radiological case of the month. Rib fractures produced by birth trauma. Arch Pediatr Adolesc Med 1997; 151: 947–948

34 Barry P, Hocking MD. Infant rib fracture: birth trauma or non-accidental injury. Arch Dis Child 1993; 68: 250

35 Amir J, Katz K, Grunebaum M, Yosipovich Z, Wielunsky E, Reisner S. Fractures in premature infants. J Pediatr Orthop 1988; 8: 41–44

36 Dahlenburg S, Bishop N, Lucas A. Are preterm infants at risk for subsequent fractures? Arch Dis Child 1989; 64: 1384–1385

Paul L.P. Brand

Practical interpretation of lung function tests in asthma

WHY MEASURE LUNG FUNCTION IN ASTHMA?

A child with asthma and significant airways obstruction may express no symptoms at all, or be very short of breath. Taking a history of respiratory symptoms,[1] or doing a physical examination of the chest[2] may fail to identify airways obstruction.

What the clinician needs is an objective measure of the severity of disease in the airways of asthmatic subjects, i.e. a test of lung function. Every paediatrician caring for children with asthma should be able to interpret simple lung function test results within the clinical context. The aim of this review is to provide the paediatrician with both the basic and the practical knowledge required to do this.

In this chapter, the different possible ways of studying lung function in asthma will be reviewed concisely, followed by an in-depth discussion of spirometry, flow-volume curves, peak expiratory flow, and airways hyper-responsiveness as the most easily and commonly applied tests of lung function in asthma. A number of case histories of patients are presented, along with lung function test results, showing some of the answers provided (and questions raised!) by doing lung function tests in a paediatric asthma clinic.

LUNG FUNCTION TESTS IN ASTHMA – AN OVERVIEW

There are countless ways to assess lung function. For practical purposes, the following groups of lung function tests can be distinguished.

Paul L.P. Brand MD PhD, Consultant Paediatric Pulmonologist, Isala Clinics, De Weezenlanden Hospital, PO Box 10500, 8000 GM Zwolle, The Netherlands

Tests aiming at assessing airways inflammation

Because asthma is an inflammatory disorder,[3] one would like lung function tests to reflect the severity of asthmatic airways inflammation. The only direct way to assess asthmatic airways inflammation is through bronchoscopy, taking bronchial mucosal biopsies or performing bronchoalveolar lavage. Because this is not feasible in children, a number of methods have been developed recently that attempt to measure airways inflammation indirectly.

Measuring compounds in exhaled air

The advantages of analysing exhaled air are that is easily collected and that it comes straight from the site of the disease, i.e. the lungs and airways. Over the past few years, tests have been described that measure several compounds in exhaled air, such as nitric oxide,[4] hydrogen peroxide,[5] and carbon monoxide.[6] Although promising, a number of methodological issues need to be worked out before these tests can be implemented in clinical practice.[7] For example, because the exhaled nitric oxide level is highly dependent on air flow,[7] during the measurement procedure subjects must exhale at a constant flow, which is impossible for many children, especially young ones.

Induced sputum

Another 'exhaust' product of the airways, which can be examined for the nature and severity of inflammation, is sputum. Sputum expectoration may be enhanced after inhaling hypertonic (4.5%) saline (for 0.5–10 min, with a normal jet nebulizer), and this method of sputum induction has been introduced in children.[8] At present, only cell counts can be measured reliably in sputum, and the degree of overlap between asthmatics and non-asthmatics is considerable.[9] Measurements of inflammatory cytokines and mediators in sputum are disturbed quite strongly by compounds used to process the sputum before analysis, such as agents that dissolve sputum plugs.

Eosinophilic proteins and leukotrienes

The eosinophil, one of the key inflammatory cells in asthma, produces toxic proteins such as eosinophilic cationic protein and eosinophil protein X which can be quantified in blood and in urine.[10,11] Although significant differences between asthmatic and healthy children have been found, the degree of overlap precludes any usefulness in individual patients in clinical practice. The same applies to the measurement of leukotrienes, other mediators of the asthmatic inflammation, in urine or nasal lavage fluid.[12]

Assessing airways inflammation in children — state of the art

At present it is impossible to assess airway inflammation in children reliably. New developments in this exciting field are to be expected, but implementation in daily clinical practice still has a long way to go.

Lung flows, volumes, and capacities

Definitions

During normal inspiration and expiration under resting conditions, tidal volume (Vt) is breathed in and out. With maximal effort, inspiratory reserve volume

Table 6.1 Lung volumes and capacities – abbreviations

Vt	*Tidal volume*: volume of air inspired and expired during normal quiet breathing
IRV	*Inspiratory reserve volume*: volume of air that can be inspired during maximal inhalation over and above tidal volume
ERV	*Expiratory reserve volume*: volume of air that can be expired during maximal exhalation over and above tidal volume
RV	*Residual volume*: amount of air left in the lung after maximal expiration
VC	*Vital capacity*: amount of air that can be maximally inhaled after full expiration: or exhaled after full inspiration
TLC	*Total lung capacity*: total amount of air in the lungs after maximal inhalation
FEV_1	*Forced expiratory volume in one second*: amount of air that can be maximally expired in one second, after complete inhalation
PEF	*Peak expiratory flow*

Practical interpretation of lung function tests in asthma

(IRV) and expiratory reserve volume (ERV) can be added to tidal volume. After complete exhalation, there will be some air left in the lungs, the residual volume (RV) (*see* Fig. 6.1 and Table 6.1).

Combinations of two or more lung volumes are called lung capacities. Tidal volume plus the inspiratory and expiratory reserve volumes comprises vital capacity (VC) – the maximal volume that can be exhaled after full inspiration. VC plus RV constitutes total lung capacity (TLC).

These static lung volumes yield information on the amount of air in the lungs under certain conditions. Thus, they reflect lung function in the true sense of the word. However, they provide no insight on function of the airways through which air is transported into and out of the lungs. The speed with

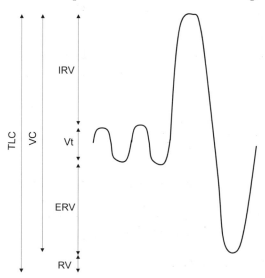

Fig. 6.1 Schematic representation of lung volumes and capacities (see text). Vt = tidal volume; IRV = inspiratory reserve volume; ERV = expiratory reserve volume; VC = vital capacity; RV = residual volume; TLC = total lung capacity.

which air can be moved out of the lung is relevant in a variety of airway disorders, particularly in asthma. This air flow can be quantified by measuring the volume of air that can be maximally expired in a given amount of time, usually the forced expiratory volume in one second (FEV_1). The FEV_1 can be expressed as a percentage of the VC (FEV_1 /VC ratio or Tiffenau index), in order to correct the FEV_1 to a certain degree for the patient's lung volume. The maximal air flow generated during forced exhalation is called peak expiratory flow (PEF).

Spirometers and pneumotachographs

Spirometry is the technique used to measure VC and FEV_1. Traditionally, this was done with a water-sealed spirometer. This instrument consists of an air-filled bell hanging upside down in a container of water. Tubing connects the air inside the bell with the patient's mouth, a nose clip occluding nasal air flow. With exhalation, the bell moves upward; with inhalation, it moves downward. Movements of the bell are recorded with a pen on paper and quantified with a ruler. Carbon dioxide is removed from the expiratory gas by an absorber, and oxygen is supplied to the inspiratory gas to compensate for oxygen consumption during the procedure.

Great care should be given to calibration of the instrument and to standardization of the measurement conditions, including to ATPS-BTPS corrections (ATPS: ambient, and BTPS: body temperature-pressure-saturation with water vapour).[13]

Water-sealed spirometers are quite bulky, and measurements can be made by hand only. No 'trend registration' of lung function changes over time, which is important in patient follow-up, is available. These drawbacks have been circumvented in newer instruments, called pneumotachographs, which primarily measure flow (in various ways), which is then integrated to volume. Modern pneumotachographs are fully computerized, facilitating calibration, ATPS-BTPS corrections, comparison to reference values, and creating print-outs of results, including trend registration over time.

Both the water-sealed spirometer and the pneumotachograph will yield information on VC and FEV_1 in a single manoeuvre of forced expiration from full inspiration (TLC level) to complete expiration (RV level, Fig. 6.1).

Reduced VC suggests reduction of lung volume (restrictive lung disease). Strictly speaking, restrictive lung disease may only be diagnosed if TLC is reduced.[14] RV and TLC, however, can not be measured with a single forced expiration, but require more complicated techniques such as gas dilution or body plethysmography. From a practical point of view, therefore, reduction of VC is commonly interpreted as reflecting restrictive lung disease. In this paper, the term 'restrictive lung disease' is used to describe a situation in which VC is diminished.

Reduced FEV_1 suggests narrowing of airways (obstructive lung or airways disease) which is commonly present in patients with symptomatic asthma, but also in cystic fibrosis and other disorders. Both for diagnostic and therapeutic purposes, it may be useful to assess the change in FEV_1 after inhalation of a bronchodilator. Interpretation of such a bronchodilator response or reversibility test should always take prebronchodilator FEV_1 and the clinical situation into account.[15]

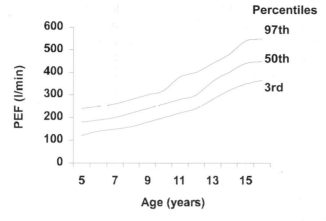

Fig. 6.2 PEF in a population healthy boys, aged 5–16 years. Lines represent 3rd, 50th, and 97th percentiles of the distribution of PEF in this population, respectively. Note considerable variation in PEF levels between these healthy children. Adapted from Taylor (1994)[16], with permission.

Comparison to reference values

Lung function is considered to be abnormal in a patient when it is below the reference value. Such reference (or predicted) values of lung function are collected in populations of healthy non-smoking subjects. Lung function in such populations is highly variable. Even after correction for obvious confounders such as age, height, and gender, considerable variation remains between healthy subjects with respect to, for example, PEF, VC and FEV_1 (Fig. 6.2).[16] The 'reference values' recorded in tables, formulae, and lung function software, are the mean values of, say, FEV_1, for a healthy population of a certain age, height, and gender (comparable to the 50th percentile of a growth chart). An FEV_1 equalling this population mean can certainly be normal, but might also be low for a certain patient whose FEV_1 usually is way above the reference value. This is why the term 'normal values' should be avoided. It also emphasizes that the true power of measurement of lung function lies in its repetition, looking at patterns of change over time in individual patients.

By agreement, lung function levels are considered to be reduced when being below the 90% confidence limit of the mean population value (i.e. 1.64 standard deviation scores (SDS) below the reference value; 1.96 SDS below the reference value corresponds to the 95% confidence limit).[14] In clinical practice, the expression 'percentage of the reference (or predicted) value' (%pred) is commonly favoured, because clinicians feel comfortable with its use and because it is felt to be more easily calculated.[17] Thus 80%pred is commonly used as guideline to consider level of lung function to be normal (> 80%pred) or abnormal (< 80%pred). Unfortunately, the lower 90% confidence limit equals a different percentage of the predicted value in patients of different ages, heights, and genders. Therefore, expressing lung function levels in SDS (as is done in growth curves) is preferable.[17] Because most lung function software will print out %pred but not SDS, the %pred will be used throughout this text. It should be emphasized that a single measurement only tells you something about that particular patient's level of lung function at that particular time point.

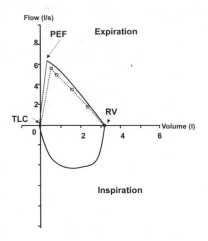

Fig. 6.3 Example of a normal flow-volume loop in a healthy individual. The X-axis represents volume (L) (the difference between TLC and RV being VC); the Y-axis represents flow (l/s). The expiratory part of the curve is above the X-axis, the inspiratory part is below it. The dashed line represents a connection between reference values for PEF (first open square), midexpiratory flows at 25%, 50%, and 75% of VC (second, third, and fourth open squares), and VC (open square on X-axis). The solid line is the patient's flow-volume loop. The FEV₁ can not be read from the curve.

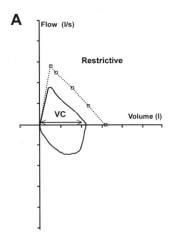

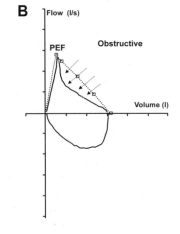

Fig. 6.4 (A) Example of a flow-volume curve of a patient with **restrictive lung disease**. VC is reduced considerably. The shape of the flow-volume curve in restrictive lung disease is almost identical to that of a normal subject, the only difference being its smaller size in restrictive lung disease (further details, see text). **(B)** Example of a flow-volume curve of a patient with **obstructive lung disease**. These patients usually have normal VCs. Hence, the final part of the expiratory loop of the curve will cut through the X-axis at or around the predicted value. Air flow is reduced, as is apparent from the concave shape of the flow-volume curve (arrows). Reduced flows at high lung volumes (close to TLC, shortly after the beginning of expiration) reflect large airways obstruction, whereas flows at lower lung volumes (closer to RV, later in expiration) indicate obstruction of smaller airways. Note that PEF is (almost) normal in this patient. PEF is mainly determined by the calibre of large airways. It is, therefore, entirely possible that a patient has severe airways obstruction with normal PEF. Further details, see text.

Flow-volume loops: principle of use in children with asthma

PEF and FEV1 only tell you what happens in early expiration. Much valuable information can be obtained from events in mid- and end-expiration, and to do this we look at flow-volume loops (Fig. 6.3). These are clinically highly relevant because mid- and end-expiratory flows are largely independent of driving pressure (i.e. effort) once a threshold value of driving pressure is exceeded (i.e. the patient does his best to blow a good manoeuvre). The shape of the maximal expiratory flow-volume curve is highly indicative of the nature and severity of lung disease, for example in asthma. This is illustrated in Figure 6.4.

Firstly, the VC can easily be read from the curve as the distance on the volume (or X) axis between the two ends of the expiratory (upper) part of the flow-volume loop (Fig. 6.4A). It is quite easy to see, even without looking at the numerical value of VC in relation to its reference value, that the VC is reduced considerably in the flow-volume-loop depicted in the upper panel of Figure 6.4. This curve represents restrictive lung disease. A patient with such restricted lung volume will have difficulty in generating enough expiratory force to blow normal peak expiratory flow, which explains why PEF is usually below the reference value in restrictive lung disease. From PEF, there is a steady, almost straight-lined decline of expiratory flow towards zero during the entire expiration. As a result, the shape of the flow-volume curve in restrictive lung disease (Fig. 6.4A) is almost identical to that of a normal subject (Fig. 6.3), the only difference being its smaller size in restrictive lung disease (Fig. 6.4A).

By contrast, the shape of the flow-volume curve in obstructive lung disease (Fig. 6.4B) is completely different from that observed in healthy subjects (Fig. 6.3). Patients with airways obstruction usually have normal VCs. Hence, the final part of the expiratory loop of the curve will cut through the X-axis at or around the predicted value. The main problem in obstructive airways disease is getting the air out of the lungs. During normal expiration, air flows out of the lung because pressure at the mouth is lower than pressure in the alveoli. Because the airways are closer to the mouth than the surrounding lung parenchyma (mainly consisting of the alveoli), during normal expiration pressure in the airways is a bit lower than that in the lung parenchyma surrounding it. As a result, intrathoracic airways tend to collapse slightly during normal expiration. Any intrathoracic airways obstruction will, therefore, manifest itself firstly in the expiratory phase of the breathing cycle. Due to the obstruction of the airways, it takes longer to move the same amount of air (for example, the VC) out of the lungs, and expiratory time is prolonged. The flow-volume-loop does not contain a time axis, and the prolongation of expiration can not be appreciated from it. However, air flow (which is volume divided by time) is highly dependent on expiratory time: if expiration is prolonged, flow will be reduced, and this can be read from the flow-volume loop.

In addition, the flow rate at different levels of expiration can be read directly from the curve. These are clinically highly relevant because reduced flows at high lung volumes (close to TLC, shortly after the beginning of expiration) reflect large airways obstruction, whereas flows at lower lung volumes (closer to RV, later in expiration) indicate obstruction of smaller airways. The added value of the flow-volume loop over and above a numerical value for, say, FEV_1, therefore, is that the flow-volume curve not only provides information on the severity of airways obstruction, but also on its site.

Take for example the flow-volume curve in Figure 6.4B. This patient has severely reduced mid-expiratory flows, indicated by the arrows. This means that his (or her) small and medium-sized airways are obstructed considerably. Because the flow-volume-curve passes through the X-axis at normal VC level (there is no evidence of restrictive lung disease), expiratory flow approaches predicted levels again as it gets closer to the end of expiration. It is noteworthy that PEF is (almost) normal in this patient. PEF is mainly determined by the calibre of large airways. It is, therefore, entirely possible that a patient has severe airways obstruction with normal PEF (as is the case with the patient in Fig. 6.4B). The (relatively) well maintained PEF, together with severely reduced mid-expiratory flows and more or less normal end-expiratory flows results in a concave shape of the expiratory part of the flow-volume curve that is so characteristic of obstructive airways disease (Fig. 6.4B).

The beauty of flow-volume curves from a clinician's point of view, therefore, is that eyeballing such a curve will yield lots of information on current severity of obstruction and restriction in a patient with lung disease. The computer software gives the clinician the numerical values of important variables from the curve, such as PEF, VC, FEV_1, and midexpiratory flow (summarized as MEF_{25-75}, which is the mean expiratory flow between 25% and 75% of expired VC), both in absolute terms and in %pred. The latter expression allows for tracking lung function over time. There are now many commercial systems available which will store a patient's previous levels of lung function in memory, and provide a print-out of changes of these levels over time in individual patients.

After the age of 6 years, almost every child can reliably blow a maximal expiratory flow-volume curve after a little bit of training which should take no longer than 15–30 min. The principal drawback of flow-volume loops is that most children younger than 5 years will not be able to do the manoeuvre in any clinically meaningful way. At present, there is no routinely available method of measuring lung function in asthmatic patients below that age, although new developments are evolving rapidly.[18] It is worth noting that when obstructive airways disease (asthma) is suspected, the expiratory part of the flow-volume loop is the most important part. It is, therefore, not necessary to obtain a full and reliably blown inspiratory loop of the curve in children with asthma.

Home peak expiratory flow monitoring

Any test of lung function in a laboratory is a reflection of lung function at that time point only. Informative as this may be (see practical examples), this is a

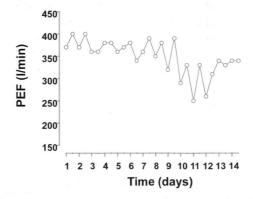

Fig. 6.5 Chart showing PEF values recorded at home in a 12-year-old boy with asthma. PEF is blown twice daily (in the morning and late in the afternoon), before inhaling medication. There is a clinically important reduction in PEF on days 10–12, following a day of cleaning up a dusty attic. This event helped in establishing that this boy had house dust mite allergy (a skin prick test performed 5 years earlier had not shown any response to house dust mite allergy; a repeated test after this event did). Adapted from Brand et al (1997)[19], with permission.

drawback in a disease with large day-to-day variability, such as asthma. The portable peak expiratory flow (PEF) meter is a simple device allowing the patient to monitor the variation of his or her own lung function daily at home, which may prove very useful in identifying impending exacerbations or their triggers (Fig. 6.5).[19] Portable PEF meters are fitted with a spring (attached to a scale) which expands when the patient exhales forcefully into the meter. Such PEF measurements are highly effort-dependent. In addition, PEF is a measure of large airways calibre – thus, significant asthmatic obstruction of medium-sized and small airways may exist in the presence of normal PEF (Fig. 6.4).[20] PEF levels may vary considerably between healthy subjects (Fig. 6.2). Measurement of a single PEF level, therefore, is of limited value – PEF monitoring is more useful as trend registration. That is why asthma self-management plans commonly incorporate some sort of home PEF monitoring.[21,22] Typically, the patient establishes his 'personal best' PEF during a good phase of his/her disease, and a written action plan is agreed upon between patient and physician to increase/alter treatment when PEF levels drop below a predefined percentage of the patient's personal best PEF level (by giving bronchodilators, increasing the dose of inhaled corticosteroids, or some other intervention such as admission to hospital or starting oral corticosteroids). Although evidence is accumulating that such modern self-management plans reduce asthma morbidity,[21,22] it is unknown whether the patient education or the home PEF monitoring is responsible for the beneficial effects.[23]

Airways hyper-responsiveness

Airways hyper-responsiveness, the exaggerated response of the airways to various sorts of environmental stimuli, is considered to be one of the hallmarks of asthma. In asthmatic children, airways obstruction and symptoms may be induced by numerous triggers, such as exercise, cold, tobacco smoke, fog, food, chemicals, exposure to airborne allergens, and viral respiratory infections. Although this increased expression of asthmatic signs and symptoms is probably caused by upregulated asthmatic airways inflammation, the underlying mechanisms of this upregulation is likely to differ between stimuli, and between patients. The lack of a single underlying mechanism of 'airways hyper-responsiveness' in asthma makes it impossible to do a single test for overall hyper-responsiveness.[24] The most common approach to quantify airways hyper-responsiveness is to determine the degree of airway narrowing after application of an airway constrictor. Constrictor stimuli can induce airway narrowing directly or indirectly.

Direct stimuli to assess airways hyper-responsiveness
Nebulized agents that act directly on airway smooth muscle, such as histamine and methacholine, are inhaled in doubling concentrations, until a predefined deterioration in lung function occurs (usually a 20% drop in FEV_1). The concentration or the cumulative dose of histamine or methacholine that causes such a 20% drop in FEV_1 is called the PC_{20} or PD_{20}, respectively. In addition to this sensitivity to the stimulus, the degree of maximal airway narrowing that can be induced by the stimulus is thought to be a critical feature distinguishing mild or episodic asthma from severe or life-threatening asthma (Fig. 6.6).[25]

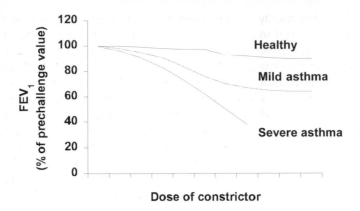

Fig. 6.6 Graph showing changes in FEV_1 during provocation with increasing doses of a constrictor stimulus (e.g. histamine), in healthy children (top line) and in children with mild and severe asthma, respectively (middle and bottom lines). Even in healthy children, constrictor stimuli have some effect. Children with asthma respond to lower doses of constrictor stimuli with a decrease in FEV_1 than do healthy children. This sensitivity is expressed as the concentration (or dose) of constrictor that leads to a 20% decrease in FEV_1 (PC_{20} or PD_{20}). In children with mild asthma, a plateau of FEV_1 is reached at high doses of constrictor, (the maximum degree of airway narrowing is limited). In contrast, in children with severe asthma such a plateau is not reached and these children can respond with very severe (even life-threatening) decreases in FEV_1 with increasing doses of constrictor.

Although methods to assess 'direct hyper-responsiveness' are both well standardized and reproducible,[26] it is impossible to correct for age-related differences in lung size and aerosol distribution, which makes comparison of results between children of different ages and sizes very difficult.[27]

Most symptomatic asthmatic children have low values for PD_{20} or PC_{20} (i.e. moderate or severe airways hyper-responsiveness),[28] but these may vary considerably over time within subjects, not necessarily parallel with changes in symptoms or lung function.[29] In population studies, a large degree of overlap in PD_{20} values has been found between healthy and asthmatic children.[30] Thus, the power of a direct challenge test for airways hyper-responsiveness to discriminate between healthy children and those with asthma is limited. In children with respiratory symptoms but without a clinical diagnosis of asthma, a negative test of hyper-responsiveness is sometimes helpful in excluding asthma. In most children with asthma, tests of airways hyper-responsiveness are not needed to monitor the severity of the disease or to guide changes in therapy. In clinical trials, tests of hyper-responsiveness are very useful because they improve to a greater extent and continue to do so for a longer period of time than do symptoms, PEF, or FEV_1.[31]

Indirect stimuli to assess airways hyper-responsiveness

These stimuli are thought to induce airways obstruction through interaction with activated inflammatory cells or via neuronal pathways. Because of this, these tests were initially assumed to distinguish better between asthmatics and non-asthmatics,[32] although later studies have shown that the degree of overlap between asthmatic and healthy children for these indirect tests is comparable to that of direct tests for airways hyper-responsiveness.[33]

Perhaps the most commonly applied indirect challenge is the exercise test.[34] This test can be very useful in clinical practice when a patient presents with 'dyspnoea' during exercise, and the further history does not support or exclude the diagnosis of exercise-induced asthma. Measuring FEV_1 before and after exercise will then help to differentiate exercise-induced asthma (where FEV_1 drops by > 10%) from other causes of 'breathlessness' or 'dyspnoea' during exercise (where no or little deterioration of FEV_1 will be observed), including poor effort, poor training, or hyperventilation. Comparable to direct challenge tests, however, the test is not very useful as a screening test for asthma in general. Thus, an exercise test can not be recommended in the routine work-up for a child with asthma. Similar to methacholine or histamine provocation tests, exercise tests can be useful in clinical trials because they tend to improve considerably during treatment with anti-inflammatory agents.[35]

Increasingly, challenges with hypertonic saline are used in clinical and epidemiological studies of childhood asthma[9,36] This approach offers the advantage of combining an indirect challenge test for airways hyper-responsiveness with a method of obtaining sputum for cell counts. At present, however, neither of these applications of hypertonic saline challenge are sufficiently evaluated to allow for implementation in clinical practice.

THE ROLE OF LUNG FUNCTION TESTING IN THE MANAGEMENT OF CHILDHOOD ASTHMA

The first prerequisite for using tests of lung function in clinical management of asthma is that the test results are reliable and reproducible. Getting patients to blow optimal lung function test results is a skilled task, even more so in children. Results obtained by untrained personnel are useless. It takes at least 6 weeks of training before interested personnel (such as physiotherapists, asthma clinic nurses, or physicians) are able to supervise simple lung function tests (spirometry and flow-volume loops) and get more or less reliable results. However, lung function test results obtained by fully qualified lung function technicians are invariably more reliable. The American Thoracic Society recommends 6 months of supervised training time before technicians are allowed to perform spirometry independently.[13] In The Netherlands, 3 years of full-time theoretical and practical training are required before registration as a board-certified lung function technician.

Standardization of equipment and procedures

The lung function equipment must perform according to published standards.[13,37] These include the following components:

1. *Technical requirements*: requirements for the accuracy, linearity, and response time of lung function equipment have been outlined in detail. Daily calibration with a high-precision calibration syringe is recommended to assure that reliable results are obtained.

2. *Written procedure protocols*: each lung function laboratory should have written protocols on each and every aspect of lung function testing.

These protocols should be very detailed indeed. For example, the following factors have all been shown to exert a significant influence on test results and must, therefore, be standardized: position of the patient (standing or sitting), position of the neck (flexed or extended), wearing a nose clip, withdrawal of bronchodilator medication, use of caffeinated beverages prior to measurement, resting prior to the measurement, room temperature, etc. (Table 6.2)

Table 6.2 Example of a protocol on withdrawal of asthma medication prior to a histamine challenge test or exercise test

Bronchodilators	
Ipratropium bromide	8 h
Fenoterol, salbutamol, terbutaline	8 h
Formoterol, salmeterol	24 h
Theophyllines	48 h
Inhaled corticosteroids	
Beclomethasone, budesonide, fluticasone	8 h
Antihistaminic agents	48 h
Except: astemizole	2 months
Ketotifen	1 week

This list (with the associated brand names) is given to children when an appointment is made for a histamine challenge or exercise test. Patients and their parents are asked to withhold medication for the time period mentioned above prior to the test. If this is not possible due to increased symptoms, patients are asked to contact the laboratory to reschedule the appointment, or to do the test 'under required medication'. All patients are tested after at least 15 min of quiet seated resting.

3. *Instructions to patients*: these must be standardized as well, because it has been shown that, for example, the volume history (i.e. the number and nature of respiratory manoeuvres performed by patients) and the breath hold time prior to any lung function measurement can affect the results significantly.

4. *Personnel qualifications*: as stated above, highly trained personnel are very important in obtaining reliable lung function test results.

5. *Reproducibility*: every spirometric or flow-volume manoeuvre must be repeated at least three times, until results are within 5% or 200 ml of each other, whichever is smaller.[13] Only if this condition is met **and** the technician is satisfied with the patient's performance can results be printed. In young and/or inexperienced children, a remark on the performance of the child, jotted down on the lung function print-out by the technician, is essential in interpreting the test result.

The best way for clinicians to get a feeling for the measurements, their drawbacks and limitations, the standardization procedures, and for their usefulness, is to visit the lung function laboratory frequently, to talk to the technicians, to show an interest, and to do the manoeuvres themselves.

PRACTICAL EXAMPLES OF LUNG FUNCTION TESTS AND THEIR INTERPRETATION

The case histories in this section are based on real patients. Each case starts with a brief introduction to the history and physical findings, followed by the lung function test results, either as numbers or as a graph with numbers. After each lung function test result, please interpret the information given on your own and try either to answer the questions posed, or to work out a diagnosis and a therapeutic strategy on your own before moving on to the case discussion. The names are fictitious. In all flow-volume loops, the thick solid lines are the results before bronchodilator, and the thin solid lines are the results after inhaling bronchodilators.

Case A

Cynthia, 6 years of age, is referred for evaluation of bronchitis. Over the past year she has had 5 courses of antibiotics for episodes of cough, 'full chest', and wheeze following upper respiratory tract infections. She says she has no symptoms now. The physical examination is normal apart from a prolonged expiratory phase. She goes to the lung function laboratory for her first lung function test ever. Data from our lung function laboratory are shown below and in Figure 6.7:

	Value	*% of predicted*
FEV$_1$	1.08 l	89
FVC	1.45 l	93
FEV$_1$/FVC	0.75	87
PEF	137 l/min	74

Discussion. At first glance, the results do not look so bad: FEV$_1$, VC, and FEV$_1$/FVC ratio are all in the range that one would consider to be 'normal'. Only PEF is low,

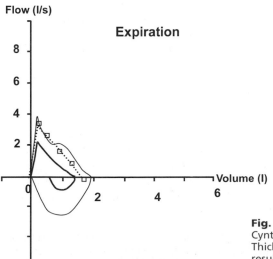

Fig. 6.7 Flow-volume loop of Cynthia, a 6-year-old girl (case A). Thick line: prebronchodilator results; thin line: postbronchodilator results; dotted line with open squares: reference values.

but it does not seem to fit with the other values obtained. There are three important lessons to be learnt from this case.

Firstly, a first spirometry test result is hardly ever a good one. The child has not had time to familiarize with the apparatus and the technicians. The manoeuvres are not that easy to master at the first attempt, and prolonged repetition of the manoeuvres at a single occasion leads to boredom and poor performance. With repeated efforts at subsequent occasions, the reliability of lung function test results in children improves (learning effect).[38]

Secondly, the flow-volume curve (Fig. 6.7) reveals more information than the numbers and percentages of predicted. Taken at face value, the curve (thick solid line) looks 'restrictive' (compare to Fig. 6.4A). The lack of any concavity confidently rules out any relevant obstruction. Could it be that this girl blew a poor manoeuvre? Yes it could. Now examine the curve after bronchodilator (the thin solid line in Fig. 6.7). The β_2 agonist really worked magic here: now this girl blows a supranormal curve with an FEV_1 of 138 %pred and a VC of 134 %pred. The improvement in FEV_1 is 55% of the baseline value! Yet, it doesn't mean that there was airways obstruction that reversed after a bronchodilator – the curve tells you that there was poor performance that improved upon repetition. The curious shape of the postbronchodilator curve indicates suboptimal effort still. All in all, these curves and results can not be interpreted reliably. This could have been predicted by the lung function technician who was probably aware of Cynthia's difficulties blowing a good test, and should have reported that to you.

Thirdly, even with this suboptimal procedure, Cynthia outblows the reference values easily. This shows that there are many, many children out there with 'supranormal' lung function test results.

Case B

Kevin, 12 years old, has episodic lower respiratory symptoms (cough and wheeze) for about 2 weeks each time, whenever he has a cold. In between these

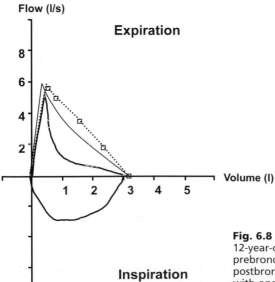

Fig. 6.8 Flow-volume loop of Kevin, a 12-year-old boy (case B). Thick line: prebronchodilator results; thin line: postbronchodilator results; dotted line with open squares: reference values.

episodes, Kevin occasionally wheezes on exertion. He has been treated with cough syrup and antihistaminic agents, without much of an effect. On physical examination, Kevin's chest sounds normal. He comes back the next day for his first lung function test ever. Data from our lung function laboratory are shown below and in Figure 6.8:

	Prebronchodilator		Postbronchodilator	
	Value	% of predicted	Value	% of predicted
FEV$_1$	2.10 l	74.2	2.70 l	95
FVC	3.05 l	97	3.10 l	100
FEV$_1$/FVC	0.69	82	0.87	105
PEF	320 l/min	91	345 l/min	99

'Good effort by Kevin: optimal technique', the experienced technician has written on the report.

Discussion: Here, the numbers are rather straightforward: there is airways obstruction (low FEV$_1$, normal VC) which is completely reversible after inhaling a bronchodilator. The remark by the technician tells you that this can not be the result of poor effort or insufficient training. The curve, however, shows the obstruction much more dramatically than do the numbers. As a result, the curve can be used in patient education. This can be particularly helpful to convince teenagers (who rather wish to believe that they have no disease at all) that they do have a serious health problem. The curve also shows that PEF may be normal in the presence of significant obstruction. The case teaches us how variable asthma may be: completely normal (symptom-free, normal auscultation) on one day, significant airways obstruction on the next. This patient needs to start prophylactic inhaled corticosteroids.

Case C

Robert, 11 years of age, has been treated for asthma by his general practitioner for 4 years. He inhales sodium cromoglycate aerosol (5 mg/puff) 3 times daily and salbutamol aerosol (100 µg/puff) prn, both through an Aerochamber®. Robert's mother, a volunteer for the National Asthma Campaign, has asked for a second opinion, for which she comes to you. Robert is doing well. His home peak flow chart shows little variation, the highest and lowest levels being 380 and 350 l/min, respectively. He has never been to a lung function laboratory. Data from our lung function laboratory are shown below and in Figure 6.9:

	Value	% of predicted
FEV$_1$	1.80 l	90
FVC	2.24 l	73
FEV$_1$/FVC	0.80	90
PEF	370 l/min	105

The mother asks you whether this lung function test confirms his asthma, or shows other abnormalities. She is worried that the low VC suggests loss of lung tissue due to his asthma. What do you tell her in reply?

Discussion. The most striking result in Robert's test is the low VC, which is surprising. The numerical results do not suggest airways obstruction. You have learnt to always inspect the flow-volume curve, especially when the patient has never had any lung function test previously. Examination of the curve (Fig. 6.9) confirms that VC is low; in addition, however, the concave shape of the curve indicates some obstruction as well (midexpiratory flow is reduced, FEV_1 is somewhat reduced). It is unusual that expiratory flow drops steeply, from a relatively normal flow at 75% of VC to zero almost immediately thereafter. This suggests that the child finished expiration before reaching RV level (i.e. before exhalation was complete), which is quite common in children who perform spirometry for the first time. Current lung function software contains computer graphics incentives to stimulate the child to exhale forcefully (e.g. blow out candles) and completely (e.g. blow a balloon over a bed of nails). In Robert's case the low VC was probably due to his lack in training to blow out completely, being only accustomed to blowing peak flows where only explosive maximal expiration is taught, but not full and complete expiration to RV level.

It is important to emphasize that all tests based on forced expiration are dependent on the effort and co-operation of the patient. If one wants to, a flow-volume loop of any shape can be blown. Proper training of patients by experienced technicians, aided by the computer incentives outlined above, can help in assuring good effort and reliable flow-volume loops.

So, you can tell Robert's mother that there is no reason to believe that there has been loss of lung tissue due to asthma, but that there is some airways obstruction. When Robert was properly trained in blowing a complete flow-volume loop, his VC was normal.

Case D

You have followed-up Nicola, 12 years of age, from the age of 5 years onwards because of her asthma. Two years ago, her asthma was very stable indeed on

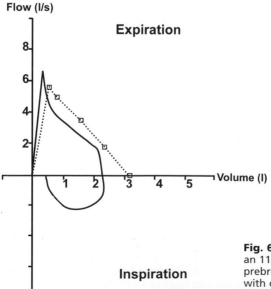

Fig. 6.9 Flow-volume loop of Robert, an 11-year-old boy (case C). Thick line: prebronchodilator results; dotted line with open squares: reference values.

200 μg of inhaled budesonide daily. Since then, she has missed three consecutive follow-up appointments. You invite her to your office because you want to discuss whether or not she should stay in your clinic, or go back to the general practitioner. She has no complaints at all, says she is doing 'terrific'. Proudly, she tells you that she no longer needs any medication whatsoever. Data from our lung function laboratory are shown below and in Figure 6.10:

	Prebronchodilator		Postbronchodilator	
	Value	% of predicted	Value	% of predicted
FEV_1	1.59 l	76.8	1.97 l	95
FVC	2.12 l	87.7	2.26 l	93
FEV_1/FVC	0.75	88.6	0.87	103
PEF	185 l/min	64	266 l/min	91

Discussion. Nicola is a 'poor perceiver': she says she has no symptoms at all, in the presence of considerable airways obstruction. This is not uncommon in childhood asthma.[1] Apparently, children can get used to a certain degree of airways obstruction, without feeling this as shortness of breath. Normal peak flow rates do not rule out this phenomenon.[39] When such children are given a bronchodilator, lung function improves (in Nicola's case almost to 100%pred), and they can sometimes feel the difference as suddenly 'having more air'. This was also the case with Nicola. Upon further asking, she admitted to quitting her sports activities and commonly dropping out of physical education classes because she was short of breath and tired. When she was re-started on inhaled corticosteroids, these complaints disappeared and she was able to perform competitive athletic activities again. When repeated 3 months later, her flow-volume curve was normal.

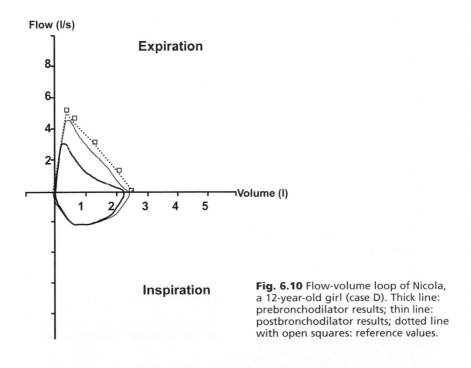

Fig. 6.10 Flow-volume loop of Nicola, a 12-year-old girl (case D). Thick line: prebronchodilator results; thin line: postbronchodilator results; dotted line with open squares: reference values.

Case E

Jeffrey, 14 years of age, is new to your practice: he moved from another part of the country. He comes in for a regular check-up and is disappointed that his case notes have not arrived by mail yet. He has always been under the care of Dr Q, a respected colleague. He tells you confidently that he has bronchial asthma and a house dust mite allergy, that allergen exposure control measures have all been taken, and that he feels that his asthma is perfectly well controlled. He says he uses his budesonide (turbuhaler, 400 µg) twice every day and hardly ever misses a dose. He has needed his terbutaline inhaler only twice during the last 6 months. He is on his school rugby team and never misses a match or a training because of his asthma. He has no nocturnal symptoms. Physical examination is normal. Data from our lung function laboratory are shown below and in Figure 6.11:

	Prebronchodilator		Postbronchodilator	
	Value	% of predicted	Value	% of predicted
FEV$_1$	2.06 l	79.3	2.10 l	80
FVC	3.21 l	103	3.21 l	103
FEV$_1$/FVC	0.64	76.3	0.65	77
PEF	336 l/min	110	335	109

Discussion. Jeffrey's prebronchodilator lung function is quite similar to Nicola's, in that there is considerable airways obstruction. In contrast to Nicola, however, Jeffrey's airways obstruction does not improve after inhaling a bronchodilator. In addition, he is absolutely free from symptoms, even during competitive sports. Either Jeffrey has true irreversible airways obstruction, or there is significant asthmatic inflammation which does not resolve after inhaling a bronchodilator but may respond to aggressive anti-inflammatory therapy. It has been shown in adults that short-term bronchodilator reversibility is a poor predictor of the response to corticosteroids.[40] Already being treated with a relatively high dose of inhaled corticosteroids, this would have to be a course of systemic steroids in Jeffrey's case. This dilemma was discussed with Jeffrey

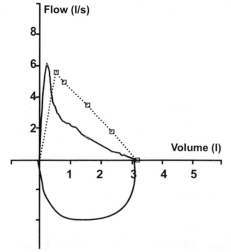

Fig. 6.11 Flow-volume loop of Jeffrey, a 14-year-old boy (case E). Thick line: prebronchodilator results; dotted line with open squares: reference values.

alone and together with his parents, and we decided to give him a course of prednisolone, 30 mg/day, for 14 days. Nothing happened: neither his well-being, nor his lung function improved. From that day, we considered the flow-volume curve in Figure 6.11 to be Jeffrey's best curve. The dose of inhaled corticosteroids was successfully tapered off slowly to 200 μg daily, without a deterioration in symptoms or lung function. Below this dose, symptoms of wheeze increased. From the case notes that arrived later you learnt that Dr Q and his colleagues had stepped up the dose of inhaled steroids repeatedly over the past few years because they were startled by the impressive degree of airways obstruction in Jeffrey's lung function tests. There is very little data in the literature on cases such as Jeffrey's, which could be called 'asymptomatic irreversible airways obstruction'. It is my view that these cases should be managed as if their best lung function level is normal for them, and that inhaled steroids should be stepped down to the lowest effective dose, just as you would do if this 'normal' lung function level was at the predicted normal level.

Case F

Joanna, 9 years of age, is one of your lung function laboratory veterans. She has had asthma from the age of 2 years onwards, and has been difficult to manage. Over the past 2 years or so, however, her asthma has been relatively stable on fluticasone 250 μg and salmeterol 50 μg twice daily by diskhaler. She comes in for a regular check-up. Data from our lung function laboratory are shown below and in Figure 6.12:

	Prebronchodilator		Postbronchodilator	
	Value	% of predicted	Value	% of predicted
FEV_1	1.70 l	89.5	1.75 l	92.6
FVC	2.10 l	94.9	2.08 l	94.7
FEV_1/FVC	0.81	94.9	0.87	102
PEF	190 l/min	70.4	188 l/min	69.4

Discussion. Apart from a relatively low PEF, the lung function test results look normal. The flow-volume curve, however, shows you that something is wrong.

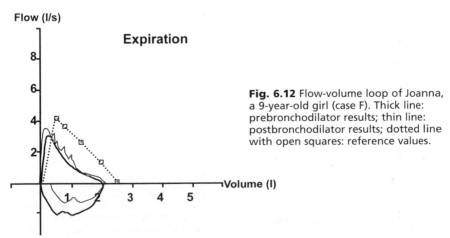

Fig. 6.12 Flow-volume loop of Joanna, a 9-year-old girl (case F). Thick line: prebronchodilator results; thin line: postbronchodilator results; dotted line with open squares: reference values.

The phenomenon of multiple 'ups and downs' in the expiratory part of the curve are due to cough during expiration. The hump in the inspiratory part is caused by swallowing or other muscular movement during inspiration. Joanna had a cold, and increased asthma symptoms caused by it. When the cough resolved she was able to blow a perfectly normal flow-volume curve, as she usually did.

Case G

Muhmad is 10 years of age and has complained of dyspnoea and wheeze on exertion for years. He has a proven house dust mite allergy. Carpets and upholstered furniture have been removed from the house; his mattress and pillow are encased in house dust mite impermeable coverings. Both his parents are asthmatic. His father has had frequent changes of job and the family has moved around the country quite a bit over the years. Two years ago, a colleague started him on fluticasone 100 µg twice daily, which was increased by another colleague to 250 µg twice daily because the low dose did not help. Because the higher dose did not help either and the peak flow remained consistently low at about 140 l/min, a third colleague added salmeterol 50 µg twice daily. Now he comes to you. He brings a thick sheaf of papers including his latest lung function test performed at another hospital:

	Value	% of predicted
FEV$_1$	1.58 l	86
FVC	2.43 l	100
FEV$_1$/FVC	0.65	76
PEF	132 l/min	52

On examination you hear soft breath sounds, with a prolonged expiration and slight wheezing. He says he feels 'as always'.

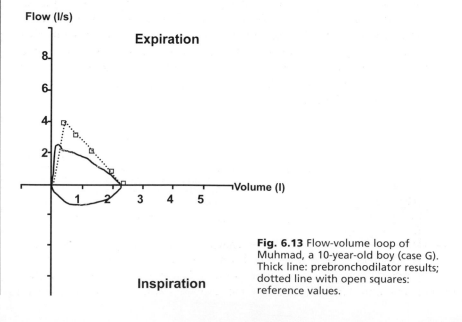

Fig. 6.13 Flow-volume loop of Muhmad, a 10-year-old boy (case G). Thick line: prebronchodilator results; dotted line with open squares: reference values.

Discussion. This lung function test result should raise an eyebrow. Muhmad has been treated for asthma for years, but he says the treatment does not help one bit, and his lung function is indeed quite poor. Either he has significant asthma and very poor compliance to therapy, or he does not have asthma at all. The family insisted that Muhmad's adherence to the treatment schedule prescribed was exemplary. The clue to the diagnosis came when Muhmad blew a flow-volume curve instead of spirometry (Fig. 6.13). This curve showed a very characteristic shape with impressively reduced peak flow and relatively well-maintained mid-expiratory flows. As a result, the shape was not concave at all but rather flat. The inspiratory loop was also flattened. This is the classic curve of obstruction of large intrathoracic airways – an adult chest physician will start looking for an endobronchial tumour if he sees such a curve. Paediatricians tend more to think in terms of congenital abnormalities which Muhmad had: a vascular ring impressing on the trachea. After resection, he said he had more air and his lung function improved. He was able to withdraw all asthma medication altogether.

It is quite curious to note that the shape of such a curve can not be expressed reliably in the numerical parameters that are usually drawn from it. In Muhmad's case, the numerical lung function values had tricked three colleagues into believing Muhmad had asthma. The boy's history – anti-asthma therapy did not work – already suggested that he might not have asthma, and the flow volume loop confirmed this.

Case H

You see Maria, 12 years of age, after an exasperated phone call from a general practitioner who tells you: 'This girl's mother really drives me crazy. She is either on the phone or in my office almost every day because her daughter coughs so badly. I treated her with antibiotics, I treated her for asthma, but nothing works. Now she wants a paediatric consult'. Skin prick tests showed that Maria is allergic to house dust mite, dog, and grass pollen. Her mother tells you that, apart from the troublesome cough, Maria has 3 or 4 'big attacks' each year, during which the cough is even worse and she can not breathe. She uses salbutamol puffs on demand. On physical examination you see a coughing girl with reduced breath sounds and soft wheezing. She does not appear to be in much distress. Data from our lung function laboratory are shown below and in Figure 6.14:

	Prebronchodilator		Postbronchodilator	
	Value	*% of predicted*	*Value*	*% of predicted*
FEV$_1$	0.92 l	44.9	1.61 l	78.6
FVC	1.38 l	57.6	2.03 l	84.9
FEV$_1$/FVC	0.67	78.9	0.79	93.3
PEF	125 l/min	43.4	170 l/min	58.1

Discussion. Underdiagnosis of asthma still occurs although the increased public awareness and professional training have reduced the rate of underdiagnosis and undertreatment considerably over the last two decades. Every now and again, however, one comes across a classical case of underdiagnosis or undertreatment of asthma such as Maria's. The prebronchodilator lung function is impressively abnormal, even though she does not appear to be in much distress. Adaptive as children are, Maria was on her way to becoming a poor perceiver. The postbronchodilator lung function, impressively improved as it is, is still far from optimal. From the shape of the curve (which is restrictive more than it is obstructive, see Fig. 6.4) it appears that this is more due to improper technique (which should improve after training) or poor general condition (which should improve after proper treatment) than to 'irreversible airways obstruction'. This underscores the limitations of the one-occasion-only test of reversibility of airways obstruction. Indeed, Maria's lung function abnormalities were completely reversible after proper treatment with budesonide at a relatively low dose of 400 μg daily by dry powder inhaler.

Case J

Angela, 12 years of age, had asthma diagnosed when she was 3-years-old. She has always been treated by a colleague who has recently retired. She is on inhaled beclomethasone by metered dose inhaler, 200 μg daily, and requires bronchodilators only occasionally. When you ask her whether she has had any other medical problems, her mother answers gladly, 'Oh no, doctor, she's been quite well this winter, she only had two courses of antibiotics'. These are very familiar events for Angela, who reportedly has had repeated bouts of pneumonia every winter ever since she was a toddler. It always starts with a cold, but 'when the sputum gets green and the cough gets wet, we call the GP for a prescription'. Angela is very reliable in keeping peak flow records, and she brought along one of the peak flow charts obtained during such an episode (Fig. 6.15).

Discussion. Angela's type of asthma is rather common among school-age children and teenagers: relatively mild asthma that is well controlled on low-dose inhaled

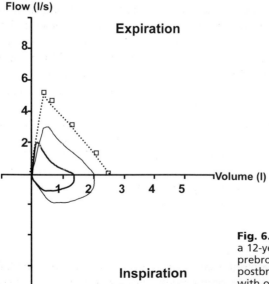

Fig. 6.14 Flow-volume loop of Maria, a 12-year-old girl (case H). Thick line: prebronchodilator results; thin line: postbronchodilator results; dotted line with open squares: reference values.

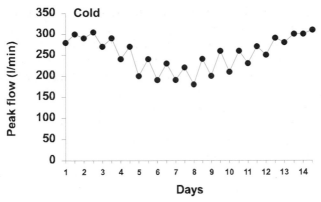

Fig. 6.15 Chart showing home recorded PEF values of Angela, a 12-year-old girl (case J). There is a marked and prolonged reduction of PEF values following a viral upper respiratory tract infection.

corticosteroids, with troublesome prolonged episodes of increased pulmonary symptoms induced by common colds. Such episodes are exacerbations of asthma, as is obvious from the peak flow diary card (Fig. 6.15): there is a drop in peak flow to less than 70% of the patient's best value in this diary. Such drops in peak flow are commonly preceded by viral upper respiratory tract infections in children,[41] but may also be caused by exposure to aero-allergens (this was the case with the patient in Fig. 6.5) or tobacco smoke. Peak flow diaries can be very useful in identifying such drops in lung function and their triggers.

Exacerbations of asthma have nothing to do with bacterial infections. Treating such episodes with antibiotics is wrong because it is not necessary and it does not work. Angela's last exacerbation had been 'treated' with three courses of antibiotics: first amoxicillin for one week, when that did not work she was given cefradine for one week, and when that did not work she was prescribed azithromycin because the 'pneumonia', in the reasoning of the GP, was atypical. This behaviour of treating asthma exacerbations with antibiotics comes from an era when bronchiectasis and bacterial infections were frequently encountered as complications of asthma. Fortunately, these days are over. It has been shown that asthmatics are not at increased risk of developing bacterial lower respiratory tract infections,[42] and that treating asthma exacerbations with antibiotics does not improve recovery.[43] A green colour of sputum does not necessarily indicate a bacterial cause and does not, by itself, justify the use of antibiotics. When a respiratory infection does not respond to antibiotics it is more likely to be caused by a virus than by a resistant strain of bacteria. If in doubt, a bacterial culture of sputum can be helpful. Usually, however, the history (little, if any, fever, no general sickness) and physical examination (no localized breath sound abnormalities) will be sufficient to rule out bacterial lower respiratory tract infection. The use of antibiotics for viral respiratory tract infections is dangerous because it will lead to increased resistance of bacteria.[44]

Case K

Jimmy, 12 years of age, presented to his GP with dyspnoea on exertion. The GP, thinking of asthma, asked Jimmy to keep a peak flow diary (Fig. 6.16). Based

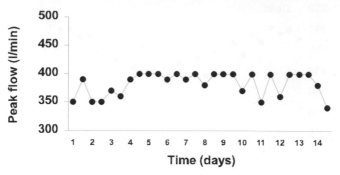

Fig. 6.16 Chart showing home recorded PEF values of Jimmy, a 12-year-old boy (case K).

on these results, Jimmy was considered to have exercise-induced asthma and started on inhaled corticosteroids. Because his symptoms did not resolve, he was referred to you.

Discussion. Jimmy's peak flow diary shows some variation but the pattern is haphazard. Jimmy had no idea why he blew better on one day than on another, he was not able to identify any triggers that caused his peak flow to drop. This is unusual in adolescents with asthma who are usually remarkably capable of identifying the things that make them wheeze. The calculated variability of peak flow was 12.5%, which made the GP think of asthma. Although various cut-off levels for 'increased variability' of peak flow circulate, the scientific basis for these is very weak indeed. In fact, the few studies published to date that examined peak flow variability in healthy children showed variations up to 30%.[45]

The only trigger that induced Jimmy's dyspnoea was exercise. This had started three months previously. Before that, he had never had wheeze nor troublesome cough, nor any evidence of atopic disease. None of his siblings or parents had asthma. Physical examination was unremarkable. Based on this, I doubted the diagnosis of asthma, and sent Jimmy for an exercise test. During the test, his FEV_1 did not change, but he said he felt dyspnoea, dizziness, and headache. The lung function technician found he was hyperventilating and his pCO_2 level was indeed low at 3.4 kPa. After he visited the physiotherapist for breathing exercises his 'dyspnoea' resolved and he never had to use anti-asthma medication again.

Case L

Priscilla was 7-years-old when she made her first visit ever to the GP. She was quite sick, with high fever and a full cough. She was given amoxicillin; the fever improved after 3 days but the cough did not. She was then provided with a peak flow meter and produced the following diary record (Fig. 6.17). The reference value on the peak flow package insert was 290 l/min. Because of this low lung function, Priscilla was diagnosed as having asthma and prescribed inhaled corticosteroids, which did not work either. Then, she was referred to you.

Discussion. Making a diagnosis of asthma on the basis of reduced peak flow levels only is a mistake. Firstly, there is a very wide range of 'normal' peak flow levels

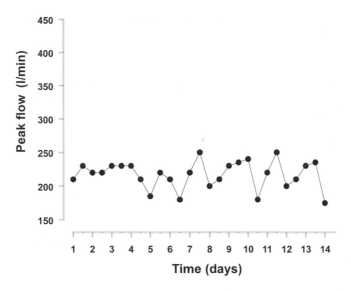

Fig. 6.17 Chart showing home recorded PEF values of Priscilla, a 7-year-old girl (case L).

in healthy children (Fig. 6.2). Secondly, in many diseases other than asthma, peak flow may be reduced (see previous cases). Thirdly, even in asthma with significant airways obstruction, peak flow may be normal (see previous cases). Thus, a peak flow diary is not a very reliable instrument to make or rule out a diagnosis of asthma. Common sense tells you that this girl does not have asthma: she has never had any respiratory problems up to now, and she presents with classical signs of a respiratory infection (malaise, fever, cough). Serology tests showed that this girl had had influenza. After she fully recovered (which took 3 weeks) she was perfectly able to blow normal peak flows.

Case M

John, 6 years of age, was referred to you for analysis of his asthma. He complains of wheeze and cough on exposure to animals, dust, fog, and during colds. He has no symptoms now. He uses inhaled bronchodilators on demand, about twice weekly. Allergy to cat, dog, and house dust mite has been established, and allergen exposure reduction measures have been taken. There is no smoking in the household.

Data from our lung function laboratory are shown below and in Figure 6.18:

	Value	*% of predicted*
FEV$_1$	1.13 l	97
FVC	1.42 l	104
FEV$_1$/FVC	0.80	93
PEF	175 l/min	105

Discussion. These numbers apparently reflect perfectly 'normal' lung function, which is quite normal in childhood asthma during symptom-free episodes. The catch here is that there was some airways obstruction after all, which was apparent from the shape of the flow-volume curve, and that John's lung function improved considerably to 'supra-normal' levels after inhaling a bronchodilator (Fig. 6.18). This shows that numerical values of FEV_1, FEV_1/VC, and PEF do not adequately describe the whole flow-volume curve. In John's case, the low midexpiratory flows (70% of predicted) would have suggested airways obstruction. Now these numerical values can be printed of course, but with the same effort, machinery, and software, you can print the whole flow-volume curve, which, as is hopefully obvious now, contains more information than the numerical data. Additionally, this case nicely underscores the limitations of predicted values in individual cases. Although John's prebronchodilator level of lung function was at or near the predicted level, this was clearly below normal for him. The almost convex postbronchodilator flow-volume curve in Figure 6.18 is quite common in young school-age children, and flattens off with increasing age. Such a convex normal shape of the flow-volume curve does not occur in adults – an example that children do not behave like little adults, and that lung function results in children should be evaluated by paediatricians, not by chest physicians.

Case N

Nicole is 9 years old and has moved from another town. Her parents tell you that Nicole is a very atopic girl, who has had severe eczema and cow's milk allergy during the first years of life, and frequent asthmatic attacks until the age of 6 years. After that, she has been symptom-free for years. Two months before the family moved Nicole had had an annoying episode of wheeze and cough. Since then, her symptoms of wheeze and dyspnoea have recurred, on exertion and during fog and cold weather. In the office, she is symptom-free; physical examination is normal, as is her flow-volume curve, both before and after a bronchodilator. The results of the methacholine provocation test are given in Figure 6.19.

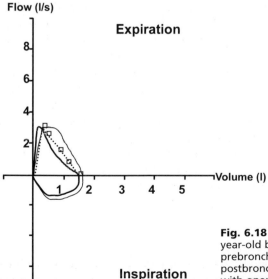

Fig. 6.18 Flow-volume loop of John, a 6-year-old boy (case M). Thick line: prebronchodilator results; thin line: postbronchodilator results; dotted line with open squares: reference values.

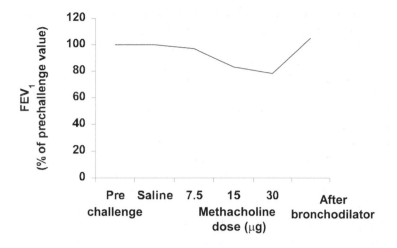

Fig. 6.19 Graph showing results of a methacholine challenge test in Nicole, a 9-year-old girl (case N). There is a decrease in FEV$_1$ of > 20% at low doses of methacholine. PD$_{20}$ is 27.1 μg, indicating severe airways hyper-responsiveness. After this 20% decrease in FEV$_1$, the challenge was terminated and a bronchodilator was given, and FEV$_1$ returned to the prechallenge value.

Discussion. Nicole has severe airways hyper-responsiveness to methacholine: PD$_{20}$ is low at 27.1 μg. In our laboratory and with our methacholine challenge protocol,[31] a PD$_{20}$ of < 150 μg is considered to be abnormal, indicating airways hyper-responsiveness. A PD$_{20}$ of 100–150 μg is arbitrarily defined as 'mild' hyper-responsiveness; a PD$_{20}$ < 100 μg as 'moderate', and a PD$_{20}$ < 50 μg as 'severe' hyper-responsiveness.

Even without symptoms and in the presence of normal prechallenge lung function, Nicole's airways are easily constricted. In our experience, a methacholine challenge is quite a useful teaching instrument: children often recognize the chest tightness induced by methacholine as the same feeling they encounter in daily life (children who do not feel wheezy or chest tight when their FEV$_1$ drops by 20% may be viewed as poor perceivers). It is assumed that the airways of children with low PD$_{20}$ levels are also easily constricted in daily life.[46] This is not always the case: there are children with low PD$_{20}$ levels who are absolutely symptom-free on the one hand, and children with severe asthmatic symptoms and hardly any evidence of airways hyper-responsiveness during methacholine challenge.[29,30] During therapy with inhaled corticosteroids, PD$_{20}$ improves more dramatically and continues to do so for a longer period of time than do symptoms, FEV$_1$, and peak flow.[31] Thus, PD$_{20}$ methacholine may be used as a guide to titrate the dose of inhaled corticosteroids. Nicole's airways hyper-responsiveness improved considerably after institution of inhaled corticosteroid therapy: her PD$_{20}$ increased to 120 μg after 6 months, and she remained symptom-free.

Case O

Gareth was 15-years-old when he was referred to you because his asthma symptoms had come back. Having had asthma as a young child, he had been

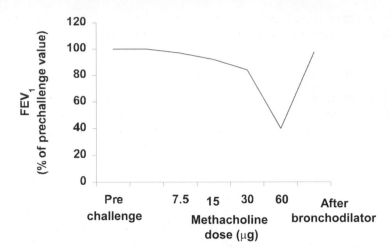

Fig. 6.20 Graph showing results of a methacholine challenge test in Gareth , a 15-year-old boy (case O). There is a decrease in FEV_1 of > 50% at low doses of methacholine. PD_{20} is 27.1 µg, indicating severe airways hyperresponsiveness and, possibly, severe maximal airway narrowing. After this severe and steep decrease in FEV_1, the challenge was terminated and a bronchdilator was given, and FEV_1 returned to the prechallenge value.

symptom-free for 6 years, without any medication. Now he complained of wheeze and cough on exertion, in the fog, and when stroking a cat. Allergy to house dust mite, dog and cat had been demonstrated. He inhaled β_2 agonists on demand. In your office Gareth was very shy, answering only in short sentences such as 'OK', 'I guess', and 'Don't know'. His mother told you that Gareth's learning abilities were limited. He had always wanted to become a house painter.

On examination, he had no signs or symptoms of airways obstruction. His flow-volume curve, both before and after bronchodilator were normal. The results of his methacholine challenge are presented in Figure 6.20.

Discussion. Similar to Nicole, Gareth had few symptoms but was severely hyper-responsive. Gareth's fall of lung function with increasing doses of methacholine was steeper and deeper than Nicole's, suggesting the possibility of sudden severe airways obstruction. Of course, Gareth was started on inhaled steroids maintenance therapy, in addition to his bronchodilators on demand. The main dilemma here, however, was whether or not to advise Gareth to give up his wish to become a painter. Painters have an increased risk of developing occupational asthma, due to exposure to vapours of solvents and thinners in paint. For a boy with such severe hyper-responsiveness, I thought it might be wise to consider a career that carried a lower risk of occupational asthma. Should he become a painter and develop serious painter's asthma, it would be very difficult for a boy with his limited learning capabilities to re-train for a different profession, and find a new job. On the other hand, Gareth insisted that during paint jobs he had no wheeze or dyspnoea at all, and this was confirmed by his school teachers. And painting really was the only thing he wanted to do. I really struggled with this dilemma, and decided to let Gareth make his own choice. He's studying to become a painter now, and only time will tell if I made the right decision.

Case P

Edward was 14 years old when he was referred to our asthma clinic for what might be considered to be a fourth opinion. Edward had had very troublesome asthma from infancy, with repeated hospitalizations for severe exacerbations. Remarkably, an allergy had never been established (total IgE 20 kU/l, RAST results to inhalant and food allergens negative). He was on high-dose inhaled steroids, long-acting β_2 agonists, and short-acting β_2 agonists on demand. Next to having asthma, he also had a deficiency of IgA, IgG2, and IgG4, and had been found to be incapable of producing antibodies against encapsulated bacteria (e.g. *Pneumococcus*). Therapy with repeated immunoglobulin infusions had not been successful. He had been evaluated at a university paediatric pulmonology clinic; admission to an asthma centre had been terminated prematurely because of homesickness. He was referred now because he had been feeling dyspnoeic and incapable of any activities for weeks on end. On admission, he was breathless at rest; on auscultation, breath sounds were reduced. Data from our lung function laboratory are shown below and in Figure 6.21:

	Prebronchodilator		Postbronchodilator	
	Value	% of predicted	Value	% of predicted
FEV$_1$	1.13 l	37.0	1.25 l	40.9
FVC	2.11 l	57.6	.22 l	60.9
FEV$_1$/FVC	0.53	63.1	0.56	66.7
PEF	156 l/min	41.1	188 l/min	48.9

Discussion. The numerical data indicate severe airways obstruction **and** a low VC, with little reversibility after inhaling a bronchodilator. The flow-volume

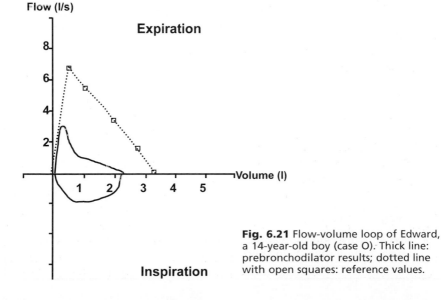

Fig. 6.21 Flow-volume loop of Edward, a 14-year-old boy (case O). Thick line: prebronchodilator results; dotted line with open squares: reference values.

curve Edward blew on admission to our hospital shows why these low values were obtained. The curve was extremely concave, with the so-called 'check valve' phenomenon: after peak flow, a sudden steep drop of flow, with severely reduced midexpiratory flows and relatively well-maintained end-expiratory flows. This pattern is characteristic of severe small airways obstruction as can be encountered in emphysema. A high-resolution CT scan made previously, however, had ruled out emphysema, and α_1-antitrypsin levels were normal. Thus, we reasoned, the airways obstruction and reduced VC, together with the reduced breath sounds, could only be caused by severe airways obstruction with air trapping. Indeed, this was found to be true as total lung capacity (measured with a helium dilution method) was normal (105%pred) but residual volume was extremely increased at 57% of total lung capacity (normal < 10%). Airways resistance, as measured in a body plethysmograph, was strongly elevated (372%pred).

At bronchoscopy, we observed inflamed oedemateus mucosa throughout the lungs, with plugs and casts of tenacious mucus obstructing segmental and

Key points for clinical practice

- Because respiratory symptoms and physical examination of the chest are unreliable predictors of the severity of airways obstruction, lung function testing should be part of routine clinical management in every child with asthma old enough to perform the test reliably (usually aged 6 years or older).

- A single lung function test only tells the clinician something about the condition of the patient's respiratory system at that particular point in time. Repeated testing of lung function over time helps in elucidating triggers of exacerbations, the course of disease over time, and response to therapy.

- By examining the shape of the full expiratory flow-volume curve, the present site and severity of airways obstruction and of restrictive lung disease can be assessed quickly and reliably. The shape of the curve is more informative than the numerical expression of FEV_1, VC, and PEF alone, either in absolute terms or as a percentage of predicted.

- Well-trained and highly motivated lung function technicians are essential to get children to perform reliable and optimal lung function tests. Tests of lung function must be performed according to rigorously standardized written protocols.

- In the majority of cases, simple lung function tests (such as flow-volume curves, peak flow diaries, and tests of airways hyper-responsiveness) are sufficient to differentiate asthma from other causes of cough, dyspnoea, and wheeze, and to follow up asthma and guide changes in therapy.

- Home monitoring of peak flow alone is not sufficient to reliably assess asthma severity in children.

smaller airways. Bronchoalveolar lavage showed an increased amount of eosinophils and T helper lymphocytes, with normal neutrophil counts. These findings are suggestive of asthma – because of the lack of demonstrable allergy this would have to be called intrinsic asthma in Edward's case. Edward was treated with high-dose prednisolone, and received intensive physiotherapy aimed at mucus clearance from the lungs. The latter was continued; the former was changed back to high-dose inhaled corticosteroids after 4 weeks. His lung function returned to predicted normal.

CONCLUDING REMARKS

Edward's case shows the value of comprehensive lung function testing. This is particularly useful in complicated cases, or in the unusual event of difficult differential diagnoses. In the vast majority of cases, however, simple lung function tests (such as flow-volume curves, peak flow registration, and tests of airways hyper-responsiveness), are sufficient to: (i) reliably distinguish asthma from other causes of cough, dyspnoea, and wheeze; and (ii) reliably follow-up asthma and guide changes in therapy.

References

1 Canny GJ, Levison H. Pulmonary function abnormalities during apparent clinical remission in childhood asthma. [Editorial]. J Allergy Clin Immunol 1988; 82: 1–4
2 Spiter MA, Cook DG, Clarke SW. Reliability of eliciting physical signs in examination of the chest. Lancet 1988; 1: 873–875
3 The British Thoracic Society, The National Asthma Campaign, The Royal College of Physicians of London in association with the General Practitioner in Asthma Group, The British Association of Accident and Emergency Medicine, The British Paediatric Respiratory Society, The Royal College of Paediatrics and Child Health. The British guidelines on asthma management: 1995 review and position statement. Thorax 1997; 52 (Suppl 1): S2–S21
4 Nelson BV, Sears S, Woods J et al. Expired nitric oxide as a marker for childhood asthma. J Pediatr 1997; 130: 423–427
5 Jöbsis Q, Raatgeep HC, Hermans PWM, de Jongste JC. Hydrogen peroxide in exhaled air is increased in stable asthmatic children. Eur Respir J 1997; 10: 519–521
6 Zayasu K, Sekizawa K, Okinaga S, Yamaya M, Ohrui T, Sasaki H. Increased carbon monoxide in exhaled air of asthmatic patients. Am J Respir Crit Care Med 1997; 156: 1140–1143
7 Kharitonov S, Alving K, Barnes PJ. ERS task force report. Exhaled and nasal nitric oxide measurements: recommendations. Eur Respir J 1997; 10: 1683–1693
8 Twaddell SH, Gibson PG, Carty K, Woolley KL, Henry RL. Assessment of airway inflammation in children with acute asthma using induced sputum. Eur Respir J 1996; 9: 2104–2108
9 Gibson PG, Wlodarczyk JM, Hensley MJ et al. Epidemiological association of airway inflammation with asthma symptoms and airway hyperresponsiveness in childhood. Am J Respir Crit Care Med 1998; 158: 3641
10 Hoekstra MO, Hovenga H, Gerritsen J, Kauffman HF. Eosinophils and eosinophil-derived proteins in children with moderate asthma. Eur Respir J 1996; 9: 2231–2235
11 Kristjánsson S, Strannegård I-L, Strannegård Ö, Peterson C, Enander I, Wennergren G. Urinary eosinophil protein X in children with atopic asthma: a useful marker of antiinflammatory treatment. J Allergy Clin Immunol 1996; 97: 1179–1187
12 Balfour-Lynn IM, Valman HB, Wellings R, Webster AD, Taylor GW, Silverman M. Tumour necrosis factor-α and leukotriene E_4 production in wheezy infants. Clin Exp Allergy 1994; 24: 121–126

13 American Thoracic Society. Standardization of spirometry – 1994 update. Am J Respir Crit Care Med 1995; 152: 1107–1136

14 Quanjer PH. Standardized lung function testing (report of working party on Standardization of Lung Function Tests of the European Community for Coal and Steel). Bull Eur Physiopathol Respir 1983; 19 (Suppl. 5): 1–95

15 Waalkens HJ, Merkus PJFM, van Essen-Zandvliet EEM et al. Assessment of bronchodilator response in children with asthma. Eur Respir J 1993; 6: 645–651

16 Taylor MRH. Asthma: audit of peak flow rate guidelines for admission and discharge. Arch Dis Child 1994; 70: 432–434

17 Miller MR, Pincock AC. Predicted values: how should we use them? [Editorial]. Thorax 1988; 43: 265–267

18 Kraemer R. Assessment of lung function in infants and young children with lung disease. Eur J Pediatr 1995; 154 (Suppl 3): S13–S17

19 Brand PLP, Duiverman EJ, Postma DS, Waalkens HJ, van Essen-Zandvliet EEM, Dutch CNSLD Study Group. Peak flow variation in childhood asthma: relationship to symptoms, atopy, airways obstruction and hyperresponsiveness. Eur Respir J 1997; 10: 1242–1247

20 Klein RB, Fritz GK, Yeung A, McQuaid EL, Mansell A. Spirometric patterns in childhood asthma: peak flow compared with other indices. Pediatr Pulmonol 1995; 20: 372–379

21 Charlton I, Antoniou AG, Atkinson J et al. Asthma at the interface: bridging the gap between general practice and a district general hospital. Arch Dis Child 1994; 70: 313–318

22 Madge P, McColl J, Paton J. Impact of a nurse-led home management training programme in children admitted to hospital with acute asthma: a randomised controlled study. Thorax 1997; 52: 223–228

23 Fishwick D, Beasley R. Use of peak flow-based self-management plans by adult asthmatic patients. Eur Respir J 1996; 9: 861–865

24 Wilson N, Silverman M. Bronchial responsiveness and its measurement. In: Silverman M (ed) Childhood Asthma and other Wheezing Disorders. London: Chapman & Hall, 1995; 141–174

25 de Pee S, Timmers MC, Hermans J, Duiverman EJ, Sterk PJ. Comparison of maximal airway narrowing to methacholine between children and adults. Eur Respir J 1991; 4: 421–428

26 Sterk PJ, Fabbri LM, Quanjer PH et al. Airway responsiveness. Standardized challenge testing with pharmacological, physical and sensitizing stimuli in adults. Eur Respir J 1993; 6 (Suppl 16): 53–83

27 LeSouëf PN. Validity of methods used to test airway responsivenesss in children. Lancet 1992; 339: 1282–1284

28 Murray AB, Ferguson AC, Morrison B. Airway responsiveness to histamine as a test for overall severity of asthma in children. J Allergy Clin Immunol 1984; 68: 119–124

29 Clough JB, Williams JD, Holgate ST. Effect of atopy on the natural history of symptoms, peak expiratory flow, and bronchial responsiveness in 7- and 8-year-old children with cough and wheeze. Am Rev Respir Dis 1991; 143: 755–760

30 Pattemore PK, Asher MI, Harrison A, Mitchell EA, Rea HH, Stewart AW. The interrelationship among bronchial hyperresponsiveness, the diagnosis of asthma, and asthma symptoms. Am Rev Respir Dis 1990; 142: 549–554

31 van Essen-Zandvliet EEM, Hughes MD, Waalkens HJ et al. Effects of 22 months of treatment with inhaled corticosteroids and/or β_2-agonists on lung function, airway responsiveness, and symptoms in children with asthma. Am Rev Respir Dis 1992; 146: 547–554

32 Godfrey S, Springer C, Noviski N, Maayan C, Avital A. Exercise but not methacholine differentiates asthma from chronic lung disease in children. Thorax 1991; 46: 488–492

33 Riedler J. Nonpharmacological challenges in the assessment of bronchial responsiveness. Eur Respir Mon 1997; 5: 115–135

34 West JV, Robertson CF, Roberts R, Olinsky A. Evaluation of bronchial responsiveness to exercise in children as an objective measure of asthma in epidemiological surveys. Thorax 1996; 51: 590–595

35 Waalkens HJ, van Essen-Zandvliet EEM, Gerritsen J et al. The effect of an inhaled corticosteroid (budesonide) on exercise- induced asthma in children. Eur Respir J 1993; 6: 652–656

36 Riedler J, Gamper A, Eder W, Oberfeld G. Prevalence of bronchial hyperresponsiveness to 4.5% saline and its relation to asthma and allergy symptoms in Austrian children. Eur Respir J 1998; 11: 355–360

37 Quanjer PH, Helms P, Bjure J, Gaultier C. Standardization of lung function tests in paediatrics. Report of the working party 'Standardization of Lung Function Tests in Paediatrics' of the working group 'Paediatrics'. Eur Respir J 1989; 2: 121s–264s

38 Studnicka M, Frischer T, Neumann M. Determinants of reproducibility of lung function tests in children aged 7 to 10 years. Pediatr Pulmonol 1998; 25: 238–243

39 Ferguson AC. Persisting airway obstruction in asymptomatic children with asthma with normal peak expiratory flow rates. J Allergy Clin Immunol 1988; 82: 19–22

40 Kerstjens HAM, Overbeek SE, Schouten JP, Brand PLP, Postma DS, Dutch CNSLD Study Group. Airways hyperresponsiveness, bronchodilator response, serum IgE, and smoking habit predict improvement in FEV1 during long-term inhaled corticosteroid treatment. Eur Respir J 1993; 6: 868–876

41 Johnston SL, Pattemore PK, Sanderson G et al. Community study of role of viral infections in exacerbations of asthma in 9–11 year old children. BMJ 1995; 310: 1225–1229

42 McIntosh K, Ellis EF, Hoffman LS, Lybass TG, Eller JJ, Fulginiti VA. The association of viral and bacterial respiratory infections with exacerbations of wheezing in young asthmatic children. J Pediatr 1973; 82: 578–590

43 Graham VAL, Milton AF, Knowles GK, Davies RJ. Routine antibiotics in hospital management of acute asthma. Lancet 1982; i: 418–420

44 Dowell SF, Marcy SM, Phillips WR, Gerber MA, Schwartz B. Principles of judicious use of antimicrobial agents for pediatric upper respiratory tract infections. Pediatrics 1998; 101: 163–165

45 Quackenboss JJ, Lebowitz MD, Krzyzanowski M. The normal range of diurnal changes in peak expiratory flow rates: Relationship to symptoms and respiratory disease. Am Rev Respir Dis 1991; 143: 323–330

46 Carey VJ, Weiss ST, Tager IB, Leeder SR, Speizer FE. Airways responsiveness, wheeze onset, and recurrent asthma episodes in young adolescents: the East Boston childhood respiratory disease cohort. Am J Respir Crit Care Med 1996; 153: 356–361

Practical interpretation of lung function tests in asthma

Stephen M. Schexnayder

Family support when a child is critically ill

Few life events generate more emotion than the serious illness or injury of a child. While the effects may be most pronounced on the parents, the emotional effects extend to not only the immediate family, but also to extended family, friends, and the health care providers. Paediatric health care professionals have a fundamental responsibility to not only care for the medical needs of the child, but must make support of the family an integral part of the paediatric health care environment.

Parents are subject to many stressors in the paediatric intensive care unit. Recognition of the causes of stress may seem trivial, but is a prerequisite for successfully minimizing the stress. The vast array of technology in modern intensive care units, complete with many different alarms and warnings, is a source of major stress to both patients and their families. Emotional responses from the child, in response to pain, procedures, or simply being in an unfamiliar environment leads to heightened anxiety on the part of both families and care-takers. Parents may also be concerned about the appearance of the child and the need for isolation practices. Financial concerns, because of both direct medical costs and the loss of wages from a job are other sources of concern, as are transportation difficulties. One of the most serious issues for families is sleep deprivation, as excessive fatigue impairs the coping abilities. Recent work has shown the most significant sources of stress for families were the painful procedures conducted on their children, the sights and sounds of the PICU, and the child's behaviour and emotional response to the intensive care.[1] Parents may also have great difficulty accepting that their duties as a parent are temporarily revised, as health care providers assume most of basic care functions. The ongoing needs of other siblings may also be a source of great stress to families while their children are PICU patients.

Stephen M. Schexnayder MD
Associate Professor of Pediatrics and Internal Medicine, University of Arkansas for Medical Sciences and
Arkansas Childen's Hospital, 800 Marshall St, Slot 900, Little Rock, AR 72202, USA

FAMILY COPING

While the coping mechanisms for no two families are exactly the same, a number of predictable behaviours are seen. Some choose reliving the events up to the crisis, seeking information, staying near the patient, or blaming themselves or others. Other families may cope by turning to others for support, minimizing the seriousness of the illness or injury, or comparing their own circumstances to that of families in more serious situations. It is particularly important for staff members to recognize these behaviours as coping mechanisms, as they can generate emotional reactions from the care-givers as well, which can sometimes interfere with their relationships with the families. Anger toward the care-givers is a frequently seen reaction, and is often very difficult for the health care team. Care must be taken not to heighten the stress by responding with anger. Attempting to understand that reason behind the anger can be very helpful, as it is frequently some ungrounded fear that must be addressed. It is frequently best to deal with such situations in an open, non-threatening way with another key support person such as the child's nurse or social worker becoming a part of the discussions. Some institutions have a specifically designated liaison whose job is to represent the families and communicate their concerns with the health care team when the family members are reluctant to express these concerns.

It is also important for staff to realize that, while the most vocal families may demand considerable attention, other families who react differently may require just as much care. The most common example would be the family member who withdraws from the situation, and may choose to spend a very limited amount of time at the child's bedside. An assigned social worker for the intensive care area can greatly facilitate identifying such families, and can direct other staff members toward meeting the needs of the family in this situation.

Intensive care providers can enhance family coping mechanisms by providing information on many levels: about the child's condition, the PICU environment, the care plan, and services that are available to them in the institution.

VISITING

Perhaps one of the greatest 'advances' in providing family centred care has been the liberalization of visiting policies in intensive care units. Intensive care units have historically had much more restrictive visiting than other areas of the hospital, but most paediatric critical care providers have realized the benefits of increasing parental presence. Many paediatric intensive care units have adopted an open visitation policy, where parents may come and go at their leisure. Sibling visitation, and even pet visitation, has been recognized as having potential benefits to some patients, although most experience is anecdotal. Studies have not shown adverse outcomes, however, such as an increase in infection.[2] Resistance by staff to a change in visiting policies is common, but most reasons against liberalizing visiting are attitudes, rather than supported by data.[3]

Preparation of parents and other family members for their first visit may help to reduce stress by helping them understand what they will see and hear. This is particularly important when they saw the child prior to the placement of monitoring and therapeutic devices. When siblings visit, they also should have age-appropriate information beforehand about what they will see.

For families whose children have a scheduled admission to the PICU after major surgery, a pre-operative visit can reduce stress by establishing some familiarity with the environment. For families whose children are admitted on an emergency basis, a brief orientation video can serve as a less formal tour to orient them to the PICU in a time of major stress. Providing written information about unit operating procedures and the availability of support services helps ensure that consistent information is given to all families, even during busy times.

COMMUNICATION

Establishing open lines of communication with the staff at all levels is perhaps the single most important intervention that can be offered to support families. Parents desire to have honest answers to their questions, but also wish to retain hope, even in the most dismal situations. Communication should be clear and be given in language that is appropriate for the family.[4] They should be notified of any change in their child's condition and should get a daily update. They also should be informed of major diagnostic studies and therapeutic interventions before they occur, unless they must be undertaken in an emergency. In a teaching institution with multiple trainees and consultants, it is important that they understand the roles of various team members. Our PICU has recently adopted a simple bedside board where the names of the patients' medical team are listed and is a source of ready reference. This is particularly important in PICUs where staff changes frequently, as frequent staff changes has been identified as a stress factor for families.[1]

Communication by all members of the health care team can help families to cope with their child's hospitalization. Frequently, a concern will be expressed to one staff member that is not readily apparent to other members of the child's health care team, and this information can be used to improve the lines of communication at all levels. Active listening is as important as giving out information, and can easily be forgotten in the fast-paced intensive care unit.[5] Care should also be taken to include older children and adolescent patients, as their level of anxiety may heightened if they believe they are excluded from conversations about their condition.

INVOLVING PARENTS

Because loss of the parental role has been shown to be an important source of stress for most parents,[6] involving them in the care of their children can be an important mechanism in helping them cope with the illness. All parents can assist in such tasks as bathing and diapering small children, and providing breast milk from nursing mothers can be a source of pride and comfort to nursing mothers.[7] Other roles that parents can assume are holding, soothing, providing stimulation, and performing physiotherapy. Involving parents in the care of the child can help reduce their perceived need to watch the patient's physiological monitors, which should be discouraged.

Some parents wish to be present while staff perform procedures, and staff attitudes toward such an approach are quite variable. In a teaching institution, it can be a source of stress for both the family and staff during a very difficult procedure. Many clinicians are very comfortable with this approach, however, and regularly offer it to families. Some institutions permit family presence at all times, even during cardiopulmonary resuscitation. Surveys of families who have recently experienced the death of a child have shown most families would like the option of being present during resuscitation,[8] although staff opinions on this issue vary widely.[9]

Open visitation policies will frequently expose family members to the death of a child other than their own in a busy PICU, most often by encountering parents during bereavement. While unit designs and staff attempts to maintain privacy can help minimize this, there is no practical way to eliminate such stress. Support for 'the other child's' family during this time is an important part of the ongoing care for families, and can help reduce some of their fears and anxiety.[10]

FAMILY SUPPORT

Supporting parents is best accomplished through a multidisciplinary approach. Our local model includes a social worker, chaplain, a psychologist, nurses, respiratory care practitioners, and physicians. While all of these professionals work independently, they occasionally make rounds as a team and share information about patients and families that better enables each individual to address issues and provide ongoing support. One individual will frequently identify an issue than impacts all of the team, and can make others more effective in supporting the family. Having a psychologist trained in issues regarding critically ill children can be a major source of support to families after they leave the PICU, as such an individual can follow the patient throughout the hospitalization and even provide outpatient follow-up for ongoing support and therapy.

Family support groups are another avenue to help express emotions, and can decrease anxiety and tension.[11,12] Even if no formal group exists with a facilitator, families are frequently seen supporting each other in the waiting areas.

For parents who cannot stay at the hospital, they should be provided with some type of phone access, preferably toll-free, so they may check on their child at all times.[7] In rural areas were transportation can be difficult for some families and ongoing needs of other children require they must be away from the hospital, such a resource can be invaluable in helping families stay connected with the critical care team.

Attention to detail in the supporting environment can also be helpful to families during critical illness. Because families vary considerably in their desires, having small zones in a waiting room can be helpful to minimize tension between families about issues such as noise, television, and telephones.[13] A variety of comfortable seating is desirable.[14] A hospital volunteer or family service associate can help orient families to the available services and comfort them after their initial arrival at the hospital. A family sleeping area near the PICU is highly desirable, and should offer personal care facilities such as showers and the ability to do laundry. Lockers and kitchenettes can be an asset to such an area.

Because having some time away from the PICU is needed for nearly all families, effective communication systems make families feel more secure about leaving their child. Having pagers or cellular phones available can provide an effective communication link for families at all times.

DIFFICULT PARENTS

Difficult parents are felt to be one of the major sources of stress for providers in the PICU setting, and frequently lead to conflict between staff if not recognized. Many every day occurrences in the PICU can lead to hostile families. These include inconvenience, worsening of the patient's condition, and the lack of communication by staff members, particularly physicians. When such hostility occurs, it is particularly important that the staff members do not react with anger, but rather in a caring manner. It is important that staff members realize the importance of non-verbal communication, as a defensive attitude can be projected by posture, lack of eye contact, facial expression, and gestures, and can worsen already strained relationships. Listening to the family concerns is one of the most effective interventions in such situations.

The behaviour from a persistently difficult family member often represents an underlying personality disorder.[15] A number of personality traits have been described such as 'obsessive', 'hysterical', 'denying', 'dependent', 'demanding', and 'help-rejecting'. Grooves and Beresin have recently published suggestions for intervention in these situations.[15]

THE DYING CHILD

Few, if any, situations are more stressful for a family than the loss of a child and are extremely intense for the critical care team. Withdrawal of support is the most frequent manner of death in PICUs. This may take the form of active discontinuation of support such as mechanical ventilation or vasopressors, or it may simply be a decision not to escalate care, then allowing the child's condition to deteriorate. While heroic measures are being abandoned, it is crucial for the family and child to sense the ongoing care of the critical care team. Our institution uses the term 'comfort care', rather than 'do not resuscitate' as a reminder of the commitment to provide for the ongoing needs of the child including analgesia and sedation. These patients require significant amounts of staff time and energy. In units with restricted visitation, this policy should be modified for these families to allow the maximal contact with their child.

Palliative care arrangements can be made to begin inside the PICU, and may be continued in another hospital location or at home, should the child survive. Parents need ongoing access to support on a 24 h/day basis. Particular attention should be paid to pain control, with the realization that there is no single dose appropriate for every child, even of the same weight. Many recent recommendations for pain management in this setting are available.[16] Careful titration of analgesia to effect is very important to reduce the child's suffering and stress experienced by the family. In recent years, a number of different scales have been developed and validated to assist practitioners in the assessment of pain in children.[17] If practitioners are uncomfortable with the doses required, they should quickly consult an expert in paediatric pain management. Laxatives are commonly needed to prevent and treat constipation induced by narcotic analgesics. If anxiety is present, the addition of a benzodiazepine is useful. Tolerance to the effects of both narcotics and benzodiazepines may develop rapidly, so care-takers should be informed about the need for increased doses if the therapeutic endpoints are not reached. Patients with underlying neurological conditions may have seizures, which can be extremely frightening to families. Having a supply of rectal diazepam can be quite useful for these patients.

Failure of a family to agree with the recommendations of the critical care team can also be a source of tension with families. The most often occurs when the staff believes the child is terminally ill, and recommends the withdrawal of life support. Such an agreement is rarely, if ever, accomplished in the first meeting with a family. Many families that initially refuse such requests will ultimately grant them when allowed time for the reality of the child's demise becomes apparent as they spend time with the child. It is crucial in such situations that the care-givers do not withdraw from the family, as they may need a substantial amount of explanation to understand the child's ongoing decline. One of the more difficult situations for staff is when the family does not spend time with the child, as care-givers frequently believe they are being forced to provide care for a child that causes pain and discomfort, yet the family is unaware of this. In this situation, firm, repeated insistence that the family meet with the staff can allow these concerns to be expressed; however, when such a meeting does occur, it is important that those concerns are openly expressed. Such a meeting should be multidisciplinary to emphasize the agreement and concern by various staff members.

Religious-based hopes for a miracle are common, and families sometimes view the continuation of such support necessary for a miracle to occur. The involvement of a social worker, chaplain, and the family's own minister can be very helpful in working through such situations. It can be helpful to explain that such a divine miracle would not require the use of human technology such as mechanical ventilators. The explanation works with many families, as it allows them to maintain their belief system, while allowing consent for removal of support.

When death occurs in the hospital setting, families need to be allowed as much control as possible. The staff approach should be one of caring with an unhurried commitment toward fulfilling the family's wishes for privacy and spending time with their child. There is substantial variation in our experience of the wishes of families in this setting. Some prefer to be with the child at every moment, and wish to bathe, clothe, hold, and rock their child, while others may not wish to be with the child after death. Personal items of the child such as favourite toys or animals are important remembrances. Many families appreciate providing a lock of hair and a photograph.

Families should be counselled on what to expect following a death, although many will not recall details given to them near the time of death. For this reason, written bereavement materials should be provided. Many paediatric institutions have developed their own resource materials and bereavement programmes, although the impact of these materials on grief is unknown.[18,19]

AUTOPSY

Requesting a postmortem examination is very stressful to many physicians. While autopsies have traditionally been viewed as a procedure to advance medical science, they may provide families with important information about their child's illness or injury. Autopsies may find unsuspected conditions,[20] even in oncology patients.[21,22] Such information can help families to understand the child's condition, and may provide genetic information that is important for other siblings or subsequent offspring. This is particularly true when an infant death occurs and metabolic disease is suspected.

If consent for a postmortem examination is obtained, it is crucial that families be informed of the results. This is particularly effective in a conference 1–2 months after the child's death, and allows family the opportunity to ask questions that have arisen in the interim. Such a conference also allows clinicians to suggest referral for counselling or therapy when families are struggling with the loss.

BRAIN DEATH

Brain death is a frequent event in most PICUs, and has a set of unique issues that require substantial explanation to families. Many families have difficulty believing their child is dead when there is cardiac activity on a heart monitor, and such families often require multiple discussions about the condition. When brain death appears to be likely at the time of admission, it is our practice to begin discussing the concept with families in initial conferences. Some cultures do not acknowledge brain death, and this issue can be particularly difficult if the child dies in a country with laws recognizing brain death as a legal standard of death.

ORGAN DONATION

If brain death occurs, organ donation offers families the chance to have a positive impact on another's child's life. For some, this is an important positive action during a tragic time. In cases of cardiac arrest, tissue donation is possible, and some countries allow the routine use of organs from non-heartbeating donors.[23]

Recent studies in the US have demonstrated that families are most likely to agree to organ and tissue donation when approached by a team including both the child's medical team and a representative from an organ procurement organization. Federal regulations in the US now require that the person initiating the request either be the organ procurement representative, or an individual who has been trained and approved by the organ procurement agency. This recent change in practice has been met with resistance among physicians who have routinely made such requests, often with substantial success, although there is substantial data that many health care providers do not request donation, or have insufficient knowledge and experience to make such requests.[24]

SEQUELAE

There are a significant number of long-term sequelae after a child's critical illness, particularly if the child dies or has severe disability. Holidays and birthdays are persistently difficult times for families, and a number of emotional problems such as depression, post-traumatic stress disorder, and anxiety are common.[25,26] If a psychologist is part of the critical care team, this person may be able to provide ongoing counselling to families after the illness or death. Siblings may have similar emotional sequelae, and frequently need counselling. Childhood bereavement programmes may help them cope with the loss in a setting of other individuals who have had similar experiences.

When a child survives a critical illness, the event may have long-term consequences for the child including being subject to excessive protection by the family, or even child abuse. Families often experience serious financial consequences including the loss of income and significant expenses, and parents are at high risk for divorce. Resources should be available to these families on a chronic basis, and there should be occasional contact with them to assess their functioning. This can be accomplished by the child's primary paediatrician or their staff.[27]

EFFECT ON HOSPITAL STAFF

Caring for critically ill children is both physically and emotionally difficult. Feelings of staff involved in the care of seriously ill children must be confronted, as they can have serious emotional effects on the staff not only at work, but in their personal lives.[28] Effective support allows staff to continue caring for such children. Meetings involving all members of the critical care team should be encouraged to allow staff members to express their feelings. Acknowledgement of the difficulties in caring for these children by professionals in different disciplines builds staff unity, and promotes trust.

Opportunities to see children that have survived their critical illness allow the staff to see the fruits of their labour. Even after a patient's death, communication with the families provides a source of satisfaction to most practitioners. When an unusually stressful event has occurred, consideration should be given to critical incident stress debriefing session. Such an event

Key points for clinical practice

- Open communication is paramount to providing family-centred care.

- Families cope differently and supporting them requires an individualized approach.

- Visitation policies should be as liberal as possible.

- Parents should be involved in appropriate aspects of their child's care.

- Families of dying children should be allowed enough time to realize the child's terminal condition.

- Palliative care is extremely important, even in intensive care units.

- Postmortem examinations may benefit both families and the health care team, and frequently provide new information.

- Organ donation and tissue donation may be a positive experience for the family and should be offered in appropriate cases.

- Long-term sequelae are common for all family members and may require professional counselling.

- The critical care team also requires support to continue to effective function in a stressful environment.

might be multiple deaths in a short period of time or the death of a staff member. Trained professionals are available in many institutions and can help staff cope with intense feelings that may affect their ability to perform their duties, both at home and work.

References

1 Haines CB, Perger C, Nagy S. A comparison of the stressors experienced by parents of intubated and non-intubated children. J Adv Nurs 1995; 21: 350–355

2 Maloney MJ, Ballard JL, Hollister L. A prospective, controlled study of scheduled sibling visits to a newborn intensive care unit. J Am Acad Child Psychiatry 1983; 22: 565–570

3 Dracup K, Bryan-Brown CW. An open door policy in the ICU. Am J Crit Care 1992; 1: 16–17

4 Todres ID, Earle J, Jellinek MS. Enhancing communication: the physician and family in the intensive care unit. Pediatr Clin North Am 1994; 16: 1395–1404

5 Pearlmutter DR, Locke A, Bourdon S. Models of family-centered care in one acute care institution. Nurs Clin North Am 1984; 19: 173–188

6 Young Seideman R, Watson MA, Corff KE, Odle P, Haase J, Bowerman JL. Parent stress and coping in NICU and PICU. J Pediatr Nurs 1997; 12: 169–177

7 Mahan CK. The family of the critically ill neonate. Crit Care Update 1983; 10: 24–27

8 Meyers TA, Eichhorn DJ, Guzzetta CE. Do families want to be present during CPR? A retrospective survey. J Emerg Nurs 1998; 24: 400–405

9 Jarvis AS. Parental presence during resuscitation: attitudes of staff on a pediatric intensive care unit. Int Crit Care Nurs 1998; 14: 3–7

10 Johnson AH. Death in the PICU: caring for the 'other' families. J Pediatr Nurs 1997; 12: 273–277

11 Fudge C. Helping parents of a baby in a special care baby unit. Med Educ 1983; 2: 596

12 Halm MA. Effects of support groups on anxiety of family members during critical illness. Heart Lung 1990; 19: 62–71

13 Jastremski CA, Harvey M. Making changes to improve the intensive care unit experience for patients and families. New Horiz 1998; 6: 99–109

14 Harvey MA. Critical Care Unit Design and Furnishing. Anaheim, CA: Society of Critical Care Medicine; 1993

15 Groves JE, Beresin EV. Difficult patients, difficult families. New Horiz 1998; 6: 331–343

16 Goldman A. ABC of palliative care. Special problems of children. BMJ 1998; 316: 49–52

17 Morton NS. Pain assessment in children. Paediatr Anaesth 1997; 7: 267–272

18 Steen KF. A comprehensive approach to bereavement. Nurse Pract 1998; 23: 54,9–64,6–8

19 Nesbit MJ, Hill M, Peterson N. A comprehensive pediatric bereavement program: the patterns of your life. Crit Care Nurs Q 1997; 20: 48–62

20 Goldstein B, Metlay L, Cox C, Rubenstein JS. Association of pre mortem diagnosis and autopsy findings in pediatric intensive care unit versus emergency department versus ward patients. Crit Care Med 1996; 24: 683–686

21 Burton EC, Troxclair DA, Newman 3rd WP, Autopsy diagnoses of malignant neoplasms: how often are clinical diagnoses incorrect? [see comments]. JAMA 1998; 280: 1245–1248

22 Kumar P, Taxy J, Angst DB, Mangurten HH. Autopsies in children: are they still useful? Arch Pediatr Adolesc Med 1998; 152: 558–563

23 Koogler T, Costarino Jr AT, The potential benefits of the pediatric nonheartbeating organ donor. Pediatrics 1998; 101: 1049–1052

24 Siminoff LA, Arnold RM, Caplan AL. Health care professional attitudes toward donation: effect on practice and procurement. J Trauma 1995; 39: 553–559

25 Friedman SB. Psychological aspects of sudden unexpected death in infants and children. Pediatr Clin North Am 1974; 21: 103–111

26 Lauer ME, Mulhern RK, Schell MJ, Camitta BM. Long-term follow-up of parental adjustment following a child's death at home or hospital. Cancer 1989; 63: 988–994

27 Wessel MA. The role of the primary pediatrician when a child dies [editorial; comment]. Arch Pediatr Adolesc Med 1998; 152: 837–838

28 Sawatzky JA. Stress in critical care nurses: actual and perceived. Heart Lung 1996; 25: 409–417

Isabelle Rapin

Diagnosis and management of autism

Up to a dozen years ago, autism was viewed as a rare and esoteric disorder. Accelerating research has shown that, if one takes into account the entire range of disorders on the autistic spectrum and their very variable severity, they are, in fact, frequent as they occur in 1–4/1000 individuals, with boys up to 4 times more likely to be affected than girls.[1,2] The autistic spectrum is referred to as pervasive developmental disorder (PDD) in the 10th edition of the *International Classification of Diseases* (ICD 10)[3] and 4th edition of the *Diagnostic and Statistical Manual of Mental Disorders* of the American Psychiatric Association (DSM IV).[4] Autism is not a disease with a specific aetiology, it is a behaviourally-defined syndrome that affects the following aspects of behaviour: (i) sociability; (ii) language and communication; and (iii) range of interests and activities. Research has thoroughly discredited the theory that autism is an emotional disorder attributable to inadequate parenting; it has shown that it is a developmental disorder of brain function that shares characteristics with others such as developmental language disorders, dyslexia, attention deficit disorder, Tourette syndrome, and others.

THE AUTISTIC SPECTRUM: SUBTYPES

DSM IV and ICD 10 distinguish roughly equivalent subtypes of PDD (Table 8.1), which are based on age at onset, and number and distribution of reported or observed behavioural abnormalities among those listed in Table 8.2. Especially for research purposes, there are several other questionnaires and observation schedules to differentiate 'autistic disorder' (classic autism) from other disorders on the autistic spectrum.[5-7] Paediatricians may want to use the

Professor Isabelle Rapin MD, Kennedy Building 807, Albert Einstein College of Medicine, 1300 Morris Park Avenue, Bronx, NY 10461, USA

Table 8.1 The pervasive developmental disorder (PDD) subtypes

DSM-IV[4]	ICD-10[3]
Autistic disorder	Childhood autism
Asperger's disorder	Asperger's syndrome
Childhood disintegrative disorder	Other childhood disintegrative disorder
Rett's disorder	Rett's syndrome
PDD-NOS*	Atypical PDD; other PDD; PDD, unspecified
(No corresponding DSM-IV diagnosis)	Overactive disorder with mental retardation, with stereotyped movements

*PDD-NOS = Pervasive developmental disorder – not otherwise specified.

brief *Checklist for Autism in Toddlers* (CHAT)[8] to identify children as young as age 18 months at risk for an autistic spectrum disorder. Note that, in this report, the term autism refers to the entire autistic spectrum, not just to autistic disorder.

Autistic disorder

The diagnosis of DSM IV autistic disorder requires the endorsement of no less than 6 of the 12 descriptors in Table 8.2, with at least two in sociability, and one each in language and communication and in range of interests and activities. It also requires onset before age 3 years of at least one of the following: (i) social interaction; (ii) language as used in social communication; or (iii) symbolic or imaginative play.

Full-blown autism is an easy diagnosis in non-verbal children who seem oblivious to what is going on around them, have no interest in play, walk around clutching a toy or a stick, do not look up when called, flap their arms when excited, flip light switches, chew their shirts, and resist any activity introduced by another person. It is less obvious in school-age children able to speak who look at you – at least briefly – have learned some play routines, and may pass as overly shy or eccentric. In such children, the history provides crucial clues, notably reports of such abnormalities in infancy as being undemanding and arching of the back when cuddling was attempted, delayed speech followed by unusually rapid progress to full sentences, excess rigidity in food choices, poorly consolidated sleep, toe-walking, tantrums, unprovoked aggression, rejection by peers and a preference for solitary activities, perhaps with an unusual interest in and knowledge of dinosaurs or makes of cars.

The sensorimotor abnormalities of autism have not been well studied. The most striking are persistent toe-walking without evidence of spasticity, and motor stereotypies such as finger flicking or twisting, arm flapping, and whirling. Clumsiness, and increased joint mobility or muscular hypotonia in the absence of classic signs of cerebellar dysfunction are common. Sensory abnormalities may consist of a combination of hyper- and hyposensitivity to a variety of stimuli: decreased response to pain and intolerance for innocuous tactile sensations, failure to respond to some loud sounds, yet covering the ears or distress to sounds others barely notice, fascination with rotating wheels and

Table 8.2 DSM-IV behavioural descriptors for the PDDs[4]

---

1. **Qualitative impairment in social interaction**
   i   marked impairment in the use of multiple non-verbal behaviours such as eye-to-eye gaze, facial expression, body postures, and gestures to regulate social interaction
   ii Failure to develop peer relationships appropriate to developmental level
   iii A lack of spontaneous seeking to share enjoyments, interests, or achievements with other people (e.g. by a lack of showing, bringing, or pointing out objects of interest)
   iv Lack of social or emotional reciprocity

2. **Qualitative impairments in communication**
   i   Delay in, or total lack of, the development of spoken language (not accompanied by an attempt to compensate through alternative modes of communication such as gestures or mime)
   ii In individuals with adequate speech, marked impairment in the ability to initiate or sustain a conversation with others
   iii Stereotyped and repetitive use of language or idiosyncratic language
   iv Lack of varied, spontaneous make-believe play or social imitative play appropriate to developmental level

3. **Restricted repetitive and stereotyped patterns of behaviour, interests, and activities**
   i   Ecompassing pre-occupations with one or more stereotyped and restricted patterns of interest that is abnormal either in intensity or focus
   ii Apparently inflexible adherence to specific, non-functional routines or rituals
   iii Stereotyped and repetitive motor mannerisms (e.g. hand or finger flapping or twisting, or complex whole-body movements)
   iv Persistent pre-occupation with parts of objects

---

shadows on the wall and gazing out of the corner of the eyes, smelling food and people, and rejecting all but a few foods because of their texture or taste.

Pre-school children with autism have several types of language disorders[9] and are unaware of the power of language to alter others' behaviour on their behalf. Early on they lack the drive to communicate by pointing – replaced by dragging by the hand when a desired object is out of reach – and later by jargoning or chatting to no one in particular, rather than engaging in conversation or making verbal demands. The children have difficulty interpreting and producing the communicative gestures, tone of voice, facial expressions, and body postures that clarify communicative intent.

Almost all pre-schoolers with autism speak late and have comprehension deficits. Some have inordinate difficulty decoding acoustic language and, when they start to speak, utter sparse, short, distorted, agrammatical utterances. Children in whom this type of deficit is severe remain non-verbal, with extremely limited comprehension and, often, severe mental retardation. Others also speak late but then may either progress extremely rapidly to full well-formed sentences, often with unusual word choices, or go through a period when they produce a fluent, well-modulated, unintelligible jargon. Such children's comprehension deficit is not at the level of the auditory code of language but at the level of the sentence, and is often marked by immediate echolalia (repeating what has just been said before responding). Some articulate overlearned phrases or scripts (delayed echolalia) which they may use to good effect to compensate for their difficulty with word retrieval or formulation of discourse. Typically, such children do not understand open-ended questions or discourse and may respond to a word in the sentence rather than to the gist of what was said, resulting in loosely chained communication. Verbal perseveration and rhetorical questioning are other tell-tale signs of lack of comprehension or impaired verbal formulation. Monotonous, uninflected, robotic speech, or a high pitched, sing-song or rising tone of voice is sometimes salient.

Cognitive incompetence is not a diagnostic criterion for autism, although cognitive deficits are often prominent and handicapping.[10] Over half of the children fall into the mild-to-moderate level of mental retardation on formal IQ tests, even when tested by competent psychologists familiar with the disorder. The cognitive profile is usually quite uneven, with profound deficits in verbal abilities and sparing of some skills like rote memory or visual-spatial ability, such as reproducing block patterns in the face of overall incompetence. A low comprehension subscore despite adequate vocabulary indexes the language deficit. Specialized tests of cognitive planning and mental flexibility are characteristically deficient,[11] as are tests that require the subject to imagine what another person would infer in a complex situation – so-called theory of mind tests.[12] Autistic persons have characteristically poor insight into the feelings of other people, may lack empathy and be blind to the effects of their behaviour on others.

Autism is often associated with distressing behaviour problems, such as temper tantrums, hyperactivity, unprovoked aggressive outbursts, wanton destructiveness, poor judgement, lack of appreciation of danger, and self-injury . A high level of anxiety and unusual fears, for example of elevators or flushing toilets, may be troublesome. Affect may be blunted or overly labile, although it is rare for children with autism to lack affection completely; rather they are affectionate on their terms and, in fact, some are overly clingy. Perseverance, increased tolerance for monotony, distractibility, and remarkable trouble focusing on an activity introduced by another person make children with autism difficult to live with and educate.

Other disorders on the autistic spectrum

A major advance in the past decade has been the identification of individuals with disorders other than classic autism which still put them on the autistic spectrum.

Rett syndrome

One disorder, Rett syndrome,[13] is a neurologically defined disorder of girls whose brain ceases normal growth after birth and who become symptomatic in infancy or as toddlers. The growth curve of the head circumference flattens and prominent hand stereotypies such as wringing, clapping or licking appear, with impaired or lack of hand use for holding, eating, pointing, and playing. These girls are generally severely retarded, non-verbal and autistic, and many are non-ambulatory. Those who are wheelchair-bound typically have small, cold, blue feet. Many later develop scolioses, epilepsy, and episodes of hyperventilation or aerophagia. Rett syndrome is not a degenerative disease of the brain as a few women survive to old age and some girls become less autistic as they mature. It is thought to be an X-linked disorder lethal in males.

Disintegrative disorder

Disintegrative disorder refers to children whose development, including speaking in sentences, gives no cause for concern until, between ages 2 and 10 years, they undergo an unexplained, catastrophic regression of language, sociability, cognition, and often of such skills as dressing and toilet training.[14] Some parents report psychotic-like behaviours that suggest hallucinations. Some children, like those with classic acquired epileptic aphasia or Landau-Kleffner syndrome,[15] may have almost continuous spike/wave complexes in the EEG during the slow-wave phase of sleep, with or without clinical epilepsy. Long-term prognosis is generally poor. The biological relationship of disintegrative disorder to the much more common autistic regression, discussed later, remains undefined.

Asperger syndrome

Another disorder on the autistic spectrum, rarely diagnosed before mid-childhood, is Asperger syndrome.[16] It applies to boys, mostly, without language delay or mental retardation whose sociability is impaired and who have a particularly narrow range of interests. They often speak like little professors who use long words when short ones would do and are socially exacting and rigid in their demands. They are gauche and remarkably socially obtuse. Whereas they may pass as normal in well defined social environments, their deficits become glaring in circumstances that call for adaptability and 'horse sense'.

Pervasive disorder not otherwise specified

Pervasive disorder not otherwise specified (PDD-NOS) is used for individuals who have fewer than the required number of behavioural descriptors for autistic disorder or do not have them in the required distribution, and who do not fulfil criteria for any of the other disorders on the spectrum. These children are generally less severely affected than children with autistic disorder. By school-age, the differential diagnosis between Asperger syndrome and PDD-NOS often hinges primarily on cognitive level and whether or not language development was delayed.

AUTISTIC REGRESSION, EPILEPSY

About one-third of the parents of children with autism report that their child, who was developing normally – or at least much better than currently – underwent a regression in language and behaviour at a mean age of about 21 months.[17,18] In most cases, the regression was insidious and without an apparent trigger. In a few cases, it was sudden and followed some non-specific illness, or perhaps an immunization or potentially traumatic life event, like the absence of a parent or a hospitalization.[19] The regression may be severe and the child may become non-verbal with markedly defective comprehension of speech and loss of interest in toys. Regression of gross motor skills is unusual in the face of severely compromised cognitive competence and ability to function in every-day life. The usual course after the regression is a plateau, in some cases with fluctuating language and other abilities, which lasts from a few weeks to many months, followed by gradual improvement but rarely full recovery. Occasionally, the regression is associated with the emergence of epilepsy or of subclinical epileptiform activity during the slow phases of sleep.

There are two reasons to consider the potential role of epilepsy in children who undergo an autistic regression. Firstly, a third of individuals with autism, especially among those with significant mental deficiency or motor deficits,[17] will develop epilepsy (i.e. at least two unprovoked seizures) by adolescence. Secondly, unexplained loss of language, usually associated with impaired comprehension of speech (language presented to the auditory channel), is the key feature of the Landau-Kleffner syndrome or acquired epileptic aphasia.[15,17,18] This diagnosis requires that the child's earlier language has been adequate, and that there be either clinical epileptic seizures or a frankly epileptiform EEG, usually with spike/waves in a centro-temporal distribution, that is over the language areas of the neocortex. Unless there are associated seizures, few children come to medical attention close to the time of the autistic regression because, typically, it occurs in toddlers when language is just emerging and verbal skills vary a great deal. Consequently, the frequency and potential importance of subclinical epilepsy as a cause or concomitant of autistic regression is unknown. Family physicians and paediatricians need to be aware that any report of language or behavioural regression in a toddler mandates immediate referral for EEG monitoring, even though the efficacy of steroids or anticonvulsants in the classic Landau-Kleffner syndrome is unpredictable: clinical seizures generally respond and, in a few children, language improves rapidly, whereas in others, the drugs' efficacy for language recovery is questionable or altogether lacking.[15] As in autistic regression and disintegrative disorder, the neurological basis of acquired epileptic aphasia is not understood.

Another unanswered question is whether disintegrative disorder (some times referred to as Heller's syndrome) is but a later and more severe variant of autistic regression, or whether it is a distinct disorder.[14,20] Prognosis in disintegrative disorder is even more dismal than in earlier autistic regression, as cognition and adaptive skills are invariably severely affected and the children often develop distressingly aberrant behaviours. In a few cases, regression is associated with almost continuous spike/wave discharges in slow wave sleep.[21] Longitudinal follow-up is needed to make certain that none of these children is suffering from an insidious degenerative disease of the brain.

CAUSES OF AUTISM

Autism is a behavioural, not a medical diagnosis. It has many causes. In some 10–30% of cases there is an identifiable aetiology.[22,23] Some of the frequently quoted causes are herpes simplex encephalitis which involves one or both temporal lobes, intra-uterine cytomegalic or rubella infections, intra-uterine exposure to thalidomide or valproate, chromosomal anomalies like fragile-X or Angelman syndromes, genetic disorders like inadequately treated phenylketonuria, tuberous sclerosis or Cornelia de Lange syndrome, and many others.[1,2] In the majority of cases, there is no obvious cause, although twin and sibling studies highlight the important role of genetics.[1] Inheritance is likely to be polygenic as the recurrence rate is under 10% within sibships, and as there are likely to be family members with other, but related, developmental disorders like developmental language disorders, Tourette syndrome, obsessive/compulsive disorder, or manic/depressive illness.[24] Monozygotic twins concordant for autism but not for severity of the illness suggest that epigenetic factors may play a role and that, in some cases, what is inherited may be enhanced susceptibility to some environmental factor, be it infections, immunological, or even emotional. Current research is focusing on candidate genes that may be associated with autism, for example genes on the long arm of chromosome 15 affecting the transport of the neurotransmitter serotonin,[25] but, as of this writing, many other chromosomal loci are also being considered.[26] A coherent genetic theory has yet to emerge, and prenatal diagnosis is not available unless there is a rare well-defined aetiology, such as PKU or fragile-X.

NEUROLOGICAL BASIS OF AUTISM

Consensus has not been achieved on the neurological basis of autism. Nine autopsies disclosed no cortical pathology and no evidence of infection, asphyxia, trauma, or degenerative disease of the brain. There were developmental cellular anomalies in the cerebellum and some limbic nuclei, with a suggestion of differences in children and adults that might indicate an evolution of lesions.[27] Examination of six other brains revealed similar cerebellar abnormalities in all six, with neocortical neuronal migration defects in four.[28] A handful of other case reports described a variety of similar or other developmental defects. A coherent picture of the neuropathological deficits necessary and sufficient for the emergence of autistic symptomatology has yet to emerge.

Thus far, neuroimaging has provided similarly inconsistent information. Clinical computed tomography (CT) and magnetic resonance imaging (MRI) are generally normal, or occasionally they reveal abnormalities of dubious relevance to the autism – like mild ventricular enlargement or asymmetry, thinning of the posterior corpus callosum, an arachnoidal cyst, or areas of increased or decreased density in the white matter. Reported smallness of lobules VI and VII of the cerebellar vermis[29] in some individuals with autism attracted a great deal of attention, even though not universally present. The size of the brain and head circumference are normal in the majority of individuals, with a significant minority, perhaps 10–20%, having a big brain and enlarged head circumference,[10,30] which underscores that damage to the brain is an infrequent cause of autism.

Pharmacological investigation has implicated a number of neurotransmitters and neuromodulators, including dopamine and endogenous options, in the pathophysiology of autism. Currently, serotonin is the one under most active scrutiny.[2,25] It has been known for 30 years that some 30% of individuals with autism have elevated levels of serotonin in their platelets. A recent positron emission tomography (PET) study disclosed an asymmetric decrease of serotonin in the prefrontal neocortex and thalamus with an increase in the contralateral dentate nucleus of the cerebellum in 7 sleeping boys with autism but not one girl.[31] In an uncontrolled study of 37 pre-schoolers with autism,[32] 59% were stated to have improved substantially in behaviour and language acquisition with the serotonin uptake inhibitor, fluoxetine. Based on these observations, together with the significant number of family members with major depression or manic/depressive illness, DeLong suggests that autism without a discernible cause may be a genetic disorder of serotonin metabolism.[33]

EVALUATION AND CLINICAL TESTS

Detailed family and developmental histories are key parts of the investigation of every child suspected of an autistic spectrum disorder.[10] The neurological examination[10] starts with the mental status which is evaluated by observing what the child does left to his or her own devices. Are there stereotyped behaviours such as pacing, running in circles, shaking a string, or insisting on carrying an object? Does the child fail to make demands on parents or turn around when called? What does the child do with representative toys, is it possible to engage the child in play and conversation? Depending on the language level, asking the child to point to body parts, name pictures, answer increasingly abstract questions, or tell a story or anecdote will be revealing. The child's ability to participate in an activity introduced by the examiner, for example ball playing or building with blocks, assesses joint attention and compliance, as well as gross and fine motor co-ordination. The physical examination must focus on disorders known to be associated with autism and requires undressing the child to look for cutaneous or other anomalies. The classic neurological examination, including an evaluation of tone and reflexes and measurement of the head circumference, is best left for last. This approach is efficient, as it enables an experienced clinician to detect an autistic spectrum disorder and rapidly consider some of its possible causes.

Deciding on how extensively to test a child with autism depends on whether the goal of the evaluation is research, excluding a specifically treatable condition, genetic counselling, or discussing prognosis and type of intervention.[34] With the exception of children who speak clearly in sentences, a definitive test of hearing is always indicated as there are children with autism who are also hearing impaired or deaf.[35] The test must include a physiological test, such as cochlear emissions or brain stem evoked responses, in all but fully co-operative children. What other tests to perform is driven by the clinical findings. Even in the absence of clinical seizures, a prolonged sleep-deprived sleep EEG, or even overnight EEG monitoring, is indicated in children with a history of regression, severe comprehension deficits, poorly intelligible speech, or marked language or behavioural fluctuations. Its purpose is to detect subclinical epilepsy that might respond to anti-epileptic treatment.[18] Routine imaging of the brain is not indicated, even in children with somewhat large heads, provided there is nothing to suggest tuberous sclerosis, hydrocephalus, or a structural brain lesion.[30] Without a specific indication, extensive urine and blood tests to rule out rare metabolic diseases associated with autism in single case reports are not indicated. High resolution cytogenetic chromosome examination and DNA tests for fragile-X may be indicated for genetic counselling, even in the absence of a positive family history or characteristic physical findings.[26] Consultation with a clinical geneticist expert in the identification of rare syndromes is recommended in children with unusual facies or other anomalies on physical examination.

The purpose of tests of language and neuropsychological function is to inform educators of the child's deficits and of strengths upon which to base individualized intervention.[2,36,37] In young children, IQ tests are not predictive of eventual level of cognitive ability. Psychologists who are not familiar with autism may declare a child untestable when a more experienced colleague might obtain an informative result. Questionnaires to parents like the *Vineland Adaptive Behavior Scales*[38] or *Wing Schedule of Handicaps, Behaviours and Skills*[10] provide useful functional information, which is correlated with cognitive level, but they do not replace testing of the child.

Unless a formal research protocol is being followed or surgical intervention for epilepsy considered, tests like PET and single photon emission tomography (SPECT) scans, functional MRI, event-related cortical potentials (ERP), brain electrical activity mapping (BEAM), magnetoencephalography (MEG), and other brain mapping technologies are extremely promising research tools that, currently, have little or no place in the clinical evaluation of the average child with autism.

PROGNOSIS

In the absence of a definable cause or detectable brain lesion, outcome in the individual cannot be predicted reliably in early childhood. As one might expect, earlier development of language and better intelligence and social skills are favourable indices. Because, in most cases, autism reflects atypical brain development, complete recovery is rare or non-existent, although, with optimal habilitation substantial improvement can be hoped for. In a follow-up study of 102 individuals seen in my office over a period of years, Ballaban-Gil et al.[39] found that 3 had died. Among 45 adults, 53% were living in residential placement and 44% still living at home, 16% were working in protected employment and 11% were employed in menial jobs in the open market. One was married, living independently with his non-autistic handicapped wife and was employed full-time in a low level job his parents had helped him secure. In his case, favourable outcome occurred even though seizures and behaviour problems were so severe in childhood that he had lived in a residential facility for 6 years. Whether outcome will improve with the earlier and more intensive intervention currently available to many autistic pre-schoolers remains to be seen. There is no definitive evidence to date that pharmacological intervention alters long-term prognosis, although optimal choice of drugs may make the child more amenable to educational intervention.

Table 8.3 Educational interventions for young children with autism

1. Requirements

   i   Intensive behavioural intervention

   ii Intensive language/communication intervention, including presenting language visually as well as orally if comprehension of speech is severely compromised

   iii Teaching parents appropriate behaviour management techniques

2. Potential educational settings (the choice depends on the child's changing needs; close communication with the parents is mandatory)

   i   Daily intensive one-on-one systematic behavioural conditioning approaches by an adult trainer (at home or in school. Need for temporary residential setting for intensive intervention exceptional in this age group)

   ii Daily attendance in a specialized highly structured pre-school for children with autism with a very high educator/pupil ratio

   iii Daily attendance in a preschool for handicapped children with specialized educators and an individual aide trained in management of children with autism

   iv Daily attendance in a specialized preschool with a mix of normal and handicapped children, specialized educator(s) and high educator/pupil ratio

   v   Daily attendance in a regular, well structured preschool with an individual aide trained in management of children with autism

   vi Daily attendance in a regular, well-structured pre-school with an experienced firm teacher, with/without provision of part-time individual help outside the classroom

MANAGEMENT

Physicians who dismiss children with autism and tell their parents that there is no cure and no effective treatment are ill-informed.[2,14,37,40] Although it is true that the hope for a cure is virtually always illusory, amelioration of symptoms is expected with the provision of vigorous special education (Table 8.3) and, in some children, with targeted pharmacological intervention (Table 8.4). Physicians should supply the families of children with autism with the following information:

1. Provide a clear and honest diagnosis rather than beating around the bush. A diagnosis of autism opens many doors to intensive educational intervention. If unsure of the diagnosis, tell the parents as much, but inform them that an autistic spectrum disorder is a consideration and suggest re-evaluation after a few months of intervention.

2. Discuss what is known and not known about the causes of autism, especially its genetics, pointing out the recurrence risk.

3. Discuss needed tests and referrals. Explain why extensive blind testing is unlikely to be informative and is invasive, but stress tests for which there is a clear indication.

4. Discuss the potential need for medication, emphasizing that medication is not curative and by no means always indicated. If medication is

Table 8.4 Pharmacological intervention

Class of drug	Examples	Suggested indications
Anticonvulsants	Valproate, carbamazepine; lamotrigine?	Epilepsy; subclinical epilepsy? mood stabilization
Corticosteroids	Prednisone, ACTH	Autistic regression with unequivocally epileptiform EEG?
Serotonin uptake inhibitors	Fluoxetine, sertraline	Obsessive/compulsive behaviours, perseveration, stereotypies; depression; self-injury? inadequate language?
Stimulants	Methylphenidate, amphetamine, pemoline	Attention deficit-hyperactivity disorder
Tricyclic antidepressants	Clomipramine, imipramine	Depression; obsessive/compulsive behaviours, stereotypies; self-injury?
Adrenergic antagonists	Propranolol, clonidine	Aggressivity, explosive behaviours, hyperactivity
Dopamine blockers	Thioridazine, haloperidol, pimozide, risperidone	Aggressivity, irritability, explosive behaviours; self-injury

The drugs and indications listed in this stable are provided as examples, not as specific recommendations.

The administration of medication must be based on a specific indication, as none is curative. The goal is to prescribe the smallest dose of the best tolerated and most effective drug. Potential side effects and drug interactions need to be considered. Parents must be aware that there is likely to be a good deal of trial and error, that monotherapy is desirable, that trials should be systematic and monitored, and that beneficial effects may be temporary

prescribed, explain that there is likely to be a good deal of trial and error until an effective agent is found. Unless fully familiar with psychotropic medications, refer the child to a physician with expertise in their use. Warn parents to avoid long-term administration of drugs like haloperidol and the phenothiazines with potentially irreversible side-effects like tardive dyskinesia.

5. Discuss the urgent need for intensive special education, stating that education needs to address both behavioural and communication issues. Very few physicians are equipped to provide parents with guidance regarding specific educational programmes, but they should be aware of various educational approaches for children with autism and familiar with resources in their communities to help parents select the most appropriate educational method and setting for their child. Tell parents that physicians are incompetent to make more detailed recommendations, as these are educational and not medical issues.

Key points for clinical practice

- Autism is a behaviourally-defined syndrome of highly variable severity that affects: (i) sociability; (ii) language, communication, and imaginative play; and (iii) range of interests and activities.

- The autism spectrum disorders are not rare as they affect 1–4/ 1000 individuals.

- In ICD 10 and DSM IV, pervasive developmental disorder (PDD) refers to the entire autistic spectrum. PDD-not otherwise specified (PDD-NOS) is not synonymous with PDD; it applies to individuals on the spectrum who do not fulfil criteria for any of the other subtypes of PDD.

- Genetics plays a major role among cases of undetermined aetiology, but is rarely classically Mendelian in type.

- Recurrence risk in a sibship is substantial but under 10%.

- Autism is not one disease. It has many possible aetiologies, some acquired, others genetic, so that a detailed family history and clinical evaluation are critically important.

- Extensive, blind medical investigations are rarely fruitful and are not indicated in practice.

- Autism regularly presents as inadequate language development. Hearing must be tested definitively in all young non-verbal or minimally verbal children with autism.

- Although particular aspects of cognition are characteristically impaired, mental deficiency is not universal.

- Parents of some 30% of children report an early (mean age 21 months), unexplained developmental regression or plateau involving language, but also sociability, behaviour, and play. A history of this type mandates immediate investigation.

- Prolonged EEG recordings in slow sleep to rule out subclinical epilepsy are recommended in non-verbal children and those with poor intelligibility or a history of regression, even if there are no clinical seizures.

- Epilepsy develops by adolescence in some 30% of affected individuals and is linked to the severity of mental retardation and other signs of brain dysfunction.

- There are no medications that cure autism. Selected psychotropic drugs may substantially ameliorate certain behavioural problems

- The key to management is early and vigorous intervention that addresses both behavioural and communication issues, and also teaches parents effective behavioural management strategies.

- Long-term outcome is guarded but rarely predictable in the pre-school years, so that early vigorous intervention is always indicated.

6. Make parents aware that they may need training in behaviour management techniques so that improved behaviour in school or with therapists is also evident at home.

7. Warn desperate parents willing to try anything about expensive unconventional tests, therapies, and behavioural treatments purported to improve autism dramatically, as well as miracle drugs and diets.

8. Do not attempt to provide a detailed long-term prognosis early on as it is likely to be unreliable in view of the many unknowns in the equation.

9. Refer the parents to an autism support group, which is generally a good source of information about management and educational issues and resources in the community. This group will put parents in contact with others with similar problems, reduce their sense of isolation, and may provide them with the empowerment inherent in numbers.

10. Give the parents a return appointment, unless their own physician is familiar with autism and its management.

Clearly, it is unrealistic to try to provide so much information in a brief consultation. I send a detailed consultation note to the parents which highlights my observations and what I have tried to convey, including a diagnosis, recommendations for further consultations and tests, and some general therapeutic options. Others may prefer to refer the child to a multidisciplinary team for detailed evaluation. Conveying concern and the willingness to be available, acknowledging the parents' distress but providing some realistic hope and an agenda for action will go a long way to setting them on a constructive path.

References

1 Gillberg C, Coleman M. The Biology of the Autistic Syndromes, 2nd edn. Clinics in Developmental Medicine No. 126. London: Mac Keith. 1992

2 Cohen DJ, Volkmar FR (eds) Autism and Pervasive Developmental Disorders: A Handbook, 2nd edn. New York: Wiley; 1997

3 World Health Organization. The ICD-10 Classification of Mental and Behavioural Disorders. Clinical Descriptions and Diagnostic Guidelines, 10th edn. Geneva: WHO; 1992

4 American Psychiatric Association. Diagnostic and Statistical Manual of Mental Disorders, 4th edn. Washington, DC: American Psychiatric Association; 1994

5 Lord C, Rutter M, Goode S et al. Autism diagnostic observation schedule: a standardized observation of communicative and social behavior. J Aut Dev Disord 1989; 19: 185–212

6 Lord C, Rutter M, Le Couteur A. Autism diagnostic interview – revised: a revised version of a diagnostic interview for caregivers of individuals with possible pervasive developmental disorders. J Aut Dev Disord 1994; 24: 659–685

7 Schopler E, Reichler RJ, Renner BR. The Childhood Autism Rating Scale (CARS) for Diagnostic Screening and Classification in Autism. New York: Irvington; 1986

8 Baron-Cohen S, Allen J, Gillberg C. Can autism be detected at 18 months? The needle, the haystack, and the CHAT. Br J Psychiatry 1992; 161: 839–843

9 Rapin I, Dunn M. Language disorders in children with autism. Semin Pediatr Neurol 1997; 4: 86–92

10 Rapin I (ed) Preschool Children with Inadequate Communication: Developmental Language Disorder, Autism, Low IQ. Clinics in Developmental Medicine No. 139. London: MacKeith, 1996

11 Minshew NJ, Goldstein G. Autism as a disorder of complex information processing. MRDD Res Rev 1998; 4: 129–136

12 Mundy P, Sigman M, Kasari C. The theory of mind and joint-attention deficits in autism. In: Baron-Cohen S, Tager-Flusberg H, Cohen DJ (eds) Understanding Other Minds: Perspectives from Autism. Oxford: Oxford University Press, 1993; 181–203

13 Hagberg B (ed) Rett Syndrome – Clinical and Biological Aspects. Clinics in Developmental Medicine No. 127. London: MacKeith, 1993

14 Catalano RA (ed) When Autism Strikes: Families Cope with Childhood Disintegrative Disorder. New York: Plenum, 1998

15 Tuchman RF. Acquired epileptiform aphasia. Semin Pediatr Neurol 1997; 4: 93–101

16. Frith U (ed) Autism and Asperger Syndrome. Cambridge: Cambridge University Press, 1991

17 Tuchman RF, Rapin I, Shinnar S. Autistic and dysphasic children. I: Clinical characteristics. II Epilepsy. Pediatrics 1991; 88: 1211–1225

18 Tuchman RF, Rapin I. Regression in pervasive developmental disorders: seizures and epileptiform EEG correlates. Pediatrics 1997; 99: 560–566

19 Kurita H. Infantile autism with speech loss before the age of thirty months. J Am Acad Child Adolesc Psychiatry 1985; 24: 191–196

20 Kurita H, Kita M, Miyake Y. A comparative study of development and symptoms among disintegrative psychosis and infantile autism with and without speech loss. J Aut Dev Disord 1992; 2: 175–188

21 Roulet Perez E. Syndromes of acquired epileptic aphasia and epilepsy with continuous spike-waves during sleep: models for prolonged cognitive impairment of epileptic origin. Semin Pediatr Neurol 1995; 4: 269–277

22 Rutter M, Bailey A, Bolton P, Le Couteur A. Autism and known medical conditions: myth and substance. J Child Psychol Psychiatry 1994; 2: 311–322

23 Gillberg C, Coleman M. Autism and medical disorders: a review of the literature. Dev Med Child Neurol 1996; 38: 191–202

24 DeLong GR. Children with autistic spectrum disorder and a family history of affective disorder. Dev Med Child Neurol 1994; 36: 674–688

25 Cook Jr EH, Courchesne R, Lord C et al. Evidence of linkage between the serotonin transporter and autistic disorder. Mol Psychiatry 1997; 2: 247–250

26 Gillberg C. Chromosomal disorders and autism. J Aut Dev Disord 1998; 28: 415–425

27 Kemper TL, Bauman M. Neuropathology of infantile autism. J Neuropathol Exp Neurol 1998; 57: 645–652

28 Bailey A, Luthert P, Dean A et al. A clinicopathological study of autism. Brain 1998; 121: 889–905

29 Courchesne E, Yeung-Courchesne R, Press GA et al. Hypoplasia of cerebellar vermal lobules VI and VII in autism. N Engl J Med 1988; 318: 1349–1354

30 Woodhouse W, Bailey A, Rutter M et al. Head circumference in autism and other pervasive developmental disorders. J Child Psychol Psychiatry 1996; 37: 665–671

31 Chugani DC, Muzik O, Rothermel R et al. Altered serotonin synthesis in the dentatothalamocortical pathway in autistic boys. Ann Neurol 1997; 42: 666–669

32 DeLong GR, Teague LA, McSwain Kamran M. Effects of fluoxetine treatment on language in young children with autism. Dev Med Child Neurol 1998; 40: 551–562

33 DeLong GR. Autism: new data suggest a new hypothesis. Neurology 1999; 52: 911–916

34 Rapin I. Appropriate investigations for clinical care versus research in children with autism. Brain Dev.(Tokyo) 1999; 21: 152–156

35 Jure R, Rapin I, Tuchman RF. Hearing-impaired autistic children. Dev Med Child Neurol 1991; 33: 1062–1072

36 Dunn M. Remediation of children with developmental language disorders. Semin Pediatr Neurol 1997; 4: 135–142

37 Siegel B. The World of the Autistic Child: Understanding and Treating Autistic Spectrum Disorders. New York: Oxford University, 1996

38 Sparrow SS; Balla DA; Cicchetti DV. Vineland Adaptive Behavior Scales: A Revision of the Vineland Social Maturity Scale by Edgar Doll. Circle Pines, MN: American Guidance Service; 1984

39 Ballaban-Gil K, Rapin I, Tuchman RF, Shinnar S. Longitudinal examination of the behavioral, language, and social changes in a population of adolescents and young adults with autistic disorder. Pediatr Neurol 1996; 15: 217–223

40 Wing L. The Autistic Spectrum: A Guide for Parents and Professionals. London: Constable; 1996

Thomas H. Ollendick Laura D. Seligman

CHAPTER 9

Cognitive-behaviour therapy

Cognitive-behaviour therapy (CBT) is a treatment approach that emerged from the integration of two schools of thought in experimental psychology: namely, behavioural theory and cognitive theory. The common denominator in both behavioural and cognitive theories is the insistence on rigorous standards of proof and a commitment to an experimental analysis of therapeutic processes and change. In order to fully understand the theoretical rationale behind CBT, one must first understand the conceptual underpinnings from which CBT arose.

Strict behavioural theory, first proposed by Watson in the 1920s,[1] suggests that the science of psychology must limit itself to the study of **overt** behaviour. Behaviourism can be contrasted with other theories in vogue at that time (e.g. psychoanalysis, introspectionism) which were thought by many experimentally-oriented scientists and clinicians to lead to untestable hypotheses about the causes and dynamics of human behaviour and to unsubstantiated behaviour change. More specifically, behaviourism grew in part as a reaction to these less scientific theories and in response to a movement labelled 'trained introspection',[2] the notion that individuals could be trained to objectively report on their subjective experiences.

Early behavioural theories asserted that behaviour could be acquired through classical conditioning (behaviours learned through associations between stimuli and resulting responses) and operant conditioning (responses learned when a given behaviour results in positive or negative consequences). Classical and operant conditioning models are frequently referred to as stimulus-response theories (S-R theory). In S-R theories, mediating responses

Thomas H. Ollendick PhD, Heilig-Meyers Professor of Psychology, Child Study Center, Department of Psychology, Virginia Polytechnic Institute and State University, Blacksburg, VA 24061-0355, USA (for correspondence)

Laura D. Seligman MS, Clinical Psychology Intern, The Kennedy Krieger Institute, Johns Hopkins Medical School, Baltimore, Maryland, USA emanating from within the organism (e.g. beliefs, expectations) are not regarded as causes of behaviour or, more precisely, are not viewed as proper subject matter for scientific examination. Rather, stimuli external to the organism which can be readily observed are said to determine or 'occasion' behaviour by either strengthening or weakening it.

In the 1970s, behaviourists demonstrated that people also learn relationships between stimuli and responses by observing others' experiences and imitating them,[3] as well as through their own direct experiences; this method of learning was referred to as modelling or vicarious conditioning. Behaviourists admitting vicarious learning processes into their armamentarium were labelled 'social learning theorists' because they accepted the social context as a determinant for much of behaviour. For example, a social learning theorist might suggest that a child who has a tantrum when not given a toy - or when asked to do something he/she does not wish to do – does so because he/she has seen another child rewarded for having a tantrum (e.g. by receiving the desired object, by receiving parental attention, or not having to do what he/she is asked to do). Therefore, the connection between being deprived of a desired object (the stimulus) and engaging in a tantrum (the response) is reinforced, or strengthened, because the behaviour (the tantrum) has been observed in others and rewarded.

Cognitive theories build upon social learning ones and suggest that there exists an internal mediating element, namely cognitions or thoughts, that determine how an individual will respond to any given stimulus. Therefore, an external event may produce different responses in the same individual because the stimulus is **perceived** differently. That is, it is one's perceptions of events or thoughts about events that determine behaviour, not the event itself. Therefore, paralleling the above example, a cognitive theorist might suggest the denial of the toy results in a tantrum not because of an automatic link between gratification and the tantrum but because of the child's perception or expectation that his/her desires should be gratified unqualifiedly, and immediately.

Given this brief overview of the underlying tenets of cognitive and behavioural theories, it might seem difficult to see how the two theories could be combined into one cohesive theory resulting in the integrative treatments that are known as CBT. However, over time, as the theories became more expansive, this is exactly what happened. Behaviourists shifted toward cognitive procedures and cognitive therapists adopted behavioural techniques. A bi-directional movement occurred. As the link between cognition and behaviour became more evident, therapists of both persuasions developed techniques that built upon this interface between overt and covert (e.g. thinking) processes. As the cognitive-behavioural approach emerged, it maintained an emphasis on empirical support that was critical to the behavioural and cognitive approaches, when used independently. Cognitive-behavioural theories and interventions were based upon research findings supporting the integrative role of both behaviour and cognition in affecting change. This inherent tie to empiricism is illustrated in cognitive-behavioural procedures — both the therapist and the patient are encouraged to formulate hypotheses about behaviour (what causes it, what maintains it, and what can be done to change it), perform 'experiments' (i.e. test out their hypotheses), and evaluate how effective the treatment has been (i.e., did it work?).[4,5] CBT, in its current form, is practiced by a wide array of mental health professionals including social workers, counsellors, psychologists, and psychiatrists.

THE BASICS OF COGNITIVE-BEHAVIOUR THERAPY

CBT is distinguished from other treatments in that an interaction or combination of maladaptive learning histories and erroneous or rigid perceptions of events, the self, and others is thought to be responsible for the development of psychopathology. Accordingly, the focus is on cognitions and learning as mechanisms of change as opposed to unconditional positive regard or emotional catharsis that guide the thinking of client-centred therapists and psychoanalysts, respectively. However, additional hallmarks of CBT differentiate it from other psychological treatments in other important ways; although, admittedly there is some overlap among the various treatments, especially as treatments are modified in response to current managed care demands.

First, in CBT the therapist usually plays an active and directive role, so much so that at times components of CBT are very didactic in nature. This often means parents and children can come into a session expecting the therapist will have a plan of how the session will be spent and will direct the participants to discuss a particular topic or engage them in the very behaviours (perhaps by using role-play or simulated scenarios if it is not possible to recreate the actual situations in the clinic setting) that are targeted for that particular session. In recent years, manuals that serve as guides for the treatment of diverse behavioural and emotional problems characterize the delivery of many CBT treatments. Not intended to be 'cookbooks', these manuals provide the therapist a set of guidelines for the delivery of effective interventions and assure some degree of correspondence about how the treatments are implemented by different therapists.

Second, CBT is often relatively short in duration, or at least intended to be short in duration. CBT treatment is not intended to be extended or viewed as a lifelong endeavour. However, the actual number of sessions may vary depending on the nature and severity of the presenting problems. With this caveat in mind, recent CBT treatments for children[6–8] utilise 14–20 sessions and rarely extend beyond 6 months in duration. In contrast, other psychosocial treatments may require considerably more treatment sessions, perhaps weekly or bi-weekly sessions for 1–2 year duration, as in psychoanalysis.

Third, the goals of CBT are usually 'operationalized' by defining both short and long-term goals and specifying intermediate objectives toward the accomplishment of these goals. Moreover, the goals are typically determined conjointly by the therapist and patient. Therefore, parents (and sometimes the child, depending on age and motivation) can expect to be asked to identify what they would consider acceptable goals, and how they would like to achieve those goals. Involvement of the child and his/her parents is crucial for treatment success. Termination of treatment is initiated when the goals are met and when it appears that treatment gains can be maintained without further professional intervention.

Fourth, the time that the patient spends out of session is considered much more important than that spent in session for most CBT treatments. Therefore, it is not unusual for CBT to include a 'homework' component which patients complete in their real environment (e.g. home and school) and not the therapy room. The nature of these assignments can be considerable as can be seen from the case illustrations that follow. Often, these activities are essential for treatment progress and they need to be self-initiated and require ongoing effort on the part of the patient. Even when dealing with highly motivated adults who are self-referred, compliance or adherence to the treatment regimen may be problematic. With children who are frequently referred by their teachers, ministers, parents, family physicians or paediatricians, obtaining compliance may be even more of a challenge.[9] Moreover, although parental participation is often instrumental in overcoming this obstacle, some parents may inadvertently interfere with a child's completion of homework tasks. For example, a parent may unknowingly discourage a child from completing an assigned task because of the parent's own anxiety and doubts about the child's ability to succeed. Therefore, motivation, both on the part of the child and parent, should be considered when making a referral for CBT.

Fifth, often, as alluded to above, CBT treatments for children rely on the active involvement of family members. Often, they involve parents (and occasionally siblings). Parental involvement may mean the therapist meets with the parents and child together[10] or that separate parent and child sessions will take place.[8] In the very least, cognitive-behavioural therapists will typically involve parents at the level of helping the child to complete homework assignments and take the place of the therapist outside of the therapy sessions, coaching the child to apply the skills/techniques learned in treatment.[4]

THE EFFICACY OF COGNITIVE-BEHAVIOUR THERAPY

Of course, the most important question about CBT treatments for consumers and those who refer them for treatment is whether these treatments really work. A task force was recently organised by the Section on Clinical Child Psychology (a subdivision of the Division of Clinical Psychology, American Psychological Association) to answer the more general question of whether psychosocial interventions (cognitive-behavioural and otherwise) are effective for treating children.[11] Treatments for internalising disorders (i.e. anxiety, phobias, and depression), externalising disorders (i.e. conduct disorder, attention-deficit/hyperactivity disorder) and other disorders including autism were examined.[11] Treatments whose efficacy was supported by empirical evidence were labelled either as well-established or probably efficacious. The criteria for each of these categories are presented in Tables 9.1 and 9.2.

As can be seen in Table 9.1, in order to be labelled as well-established, a psychosocial intervention needs to be shown to be superior to pill or psychological placebo (or some alternative treatment) or equivalent to an already established treatment in at least two between group design experiments or clinical trials. Moreover, it must be shown to be effective by two or more investigatory teams and the characteristics of the patient sample need to be

Table 9.1 Criteria for well-established psychosocial interventions for childhood disorders

	1. At least two well-conducted group-design studies, conducted by different investigatory teams, showing the treatment to be either:
	    a superior to pill placebo or alternative treatment, OR
	    b equivalent to an already established treatment in studies with adequate statistical power

OR	

	2. A large series of single-case design studies (i.e. $n > 9$) that both:
	    a use good experimental design AND
	    b compare the intervention to another treatment.

AND	
	3. Treatment manuals used for the intervention preferred.
AND	
	4. Sample characteristics must be clearly specified.

Table 9.2 Criteria for probably efficacious psychosocial interventions for childhood disorders

	1. Two studies showing the intervention more effective than a no-treatment control group (e.g. a waiting list comparison group).
OR	
	2. Two group-design studies meeting criteria for well-established treatment but conducted by the same investigator.
OR	
	3. A small series of single-case design experiments (i.e. $n > 3$) that otherwise meet criterion 2 for well-established treatments.
AND	
	4. Treatment manuals used for the intervention preferred.
AND	
	5. Sample characteristics must be clearly specified.

carefully specified. In the absence of between group design studies, a large series of well-controlled single case design experiments demonstrating efficacy must be conducted. In areas such as childhood depression, the small number of studies that have been conducted to date precluded the inclusion of any treatment in the well-established category.[12] However, some treatments were shown to be probably efficacious, meaning that there was empirical support for their effectiveness but results had not been replicated and/or the follow-up studies comparing the treatment to other interventions had not yet been conducted. Therefore, in our discussion we will refer more generally to empirically supported treatments; that is, those psychosocial interventions that meet criteria for either well-established or probably efficacious treatments.

In terms of treating emotional or internalising disorders, in contrast to treatments such as interpersonal therapy or supportive therapy, empirical support was found only for CBT treatments.[12,13] CBT interventions with a family or parent component were also reviewed and found to be effective; however, there was mixed evidence regarding the incremental utility of these treatments as opposed to child-focused CBT treatments alone.[12–14]

Findings regarding CBT interventions for externalising disorders were not as unequivocal. Whereas CBT interventions were among the treatments identified as empirically supported treatments for conduct disorder;[15] Pelham et al[16] concluded that CBT interventions alone have not been shown to be effective in treating attention-deficit/hyperactivity disorder (ADHD). Similarly, no empirical support was found for the use of CBT interventions in the treatment of autism.[17] However, behavioural therapies, using treatment procedures similar to or identical to those found in CBT, but without a cognitive component, were found to be the treatment of choice for autism. In the case of ADHD, behavioural therapies aimed at changing contingencies in the home and classroom were found to be effective while cognitive therapies appeared to do little to ameliorate symptoms. Similarly, although behavioural treatments for autism were found to be appropriate and easily and effectively implemented, the more cognitively focused components of CBT treatments would be difficult, if not impossible, to implement given the level of cognitive functioning often associated with autism.

In summary, the vast majority of treatments receiving empirical support were either CBT interventions or closely aligned behavioural treatments. However, it should be noted that CBT interventions are the most widely tested treatments in the majority of areas of childhood psychopathology. With increased research, it may be the case that other modes of psychosocial interventions will prove to be similarly effective; however, at the present time, with few exceptions, the empirical support for the implementation of these therapies is lacking.

In a similar development, the Society of Pediatric Psychology (another subdivision of the Society of Clinical Psychology of the American Psychological Association) has undertaken intensive study of psychosocial interventions in the treatment of both acute and chronic illnesses in children. Adjustment to a variety of illnesses including recurrent abdominal pain, diabetes, headache, and cystic fibrosis has been shown to be favourably influenced by CBT interventions. To illustrate, Janicke and Finney[18] have reviewed studies that show CBT interventions for recurrent abdominal pain to lead to reduced pain, reduced visits to their family physician or paediatrician, and increased school attendance. Similar effects for CBT have been shown with other childhood illnesses. The utility of CBT for such children is illustrated further in the sections that follow.

EXAMPLES OF COGNITIVE-BEHAVIOUR THERAPY AND ITS EFFECTIVENESS

Given that CBT has been shown to be effective in the treatment of several childhood disorders, it is important to understand what specifically takes place during the course of CBT. Rather than providing a list of the treatment methods employed by cognitive-behavioural therapists in isolation from the ways in which these methods are employed in clinical practice, below we provide a sample of CBT interventions through published experimental studies and single case studies. Treatment procedures are briefly described and the basic rationale behind them is provided. Although the treatments described are meant to address a range of childhood disorders and examples of how they have been treated, the treatment packages depicted here are intended to provide an introduction to CBT and they should not be considered an exhaustive review of the various treatments that are included under the rubric of CBT. The treatment of panic disorder and recurrent abdominal pain will be illustrated.

Cognitive-behaviour treatment of panic disorder

Panic disorder is diagnosed when an individual experiences a number of initially unexpected or 'out of the blue' panic attacks and subsequently becomes fearful of having additional attacks. A panic attack is an intense, sudden onset of anxiety that includes physiological symptoms such as chills or hot flashes, nausea, shortness of breath, and an accelerated heart rate. These physiological sensations are accompanied by cognitive symptoms as well, and may include feelings of derealisation, or the fear that one is going to die or go crazy. Panic attacks may be associated with several disorders including separation anxiety disorder (where a child experiences extreme anxiety during, or in anticipation of, separation from a primary attachment figure) or specific phobias (e.g. a fear of dogs, heights, dentists, doctors); however, panic disorder is diagnosed when the individual becomes fearful of the attacks themselves. Often, the panic attacks, which initially seem to come out of nowhere, become associated with certain places (e.g. school) or activities (e.g. attending parties) and agoraphobic avoidance, in which the child begins to avoid certain situations or restrict his/her activities, may ensue. The repeated pairing of panic attacks and the agoraphobic situations results in what is referred to as a conditioned response, in which the agoraphobic situations become a signal of danger for the child. Further, avoidance is rewarded in that the child escapes the aversive experience of anxiety; thus, the agoraphobic avoidance is operantly (negatively) reinforced. That is, the reward for the behaviour makes it more likely that the behaviour will continue. As such, avoidance may increase over time. Although the interference caused by panic disorder and agoraphobia is largely psychological in nature, owing to the physiological symptoms of panic, many times the child or his/her parents will be concerned about physical illness and, as a result, panic disorder can often be first discovered by primary care physicians and paediatricians.

Ollendick[19] reported successful results using CBT for four adolescents ranging in age from 13 to 17 years and diagnosed with panic disorder and agoraphobia. CBT treatment will be illustrated for one of the adolescents who was 16-years-old when she and her mother presented to an anxiety disorders clinic seeking treatment for her panic attacks. Reportedly, she had been experiencing the attacks since 9 or 10 years of age. In the month prior to her seeking treatment, the girl had experienced 10 attacks. She had also become fearful and avoidant of churches, malls, and parties. A thorough assessment confirmed the diagnosis of panic disorder.

Treatment was based on two behavioural and cognitive-behavioural therapies for panic disorder in adults.[20,21] The first session was largely didactic, the therapist provided information on panic disorder and anxiety and an overview of the treatment strategy. The next two sessions focused on teaching progressive muscle relaxation and cue controlled relaxation, techniques in which the patient is taught to first tense and relax muscle groups and with practice can learn to relax on cue. The rationale behind relaxation training is that relaxation and anxiety (or panic) are incompatible responses, one cannot experience both states at the same time. If the child can learn to relax, these skills can be applied when a panic attack occurs or when the child enters an agoraphobic situation. As is often the case, breathing retraining, in which the child is taught to breathe from the diaphragm, was coupled with the relaxation training. Often in cases of panic disorder, normal breathing is disrupted and the child begins to hyperventilate, adding to the feelings of panic and thus greater difficulty in breathing. Education in the use of diaphragmatic breathing can help the child to break this cycle. The girl was instructed in these techniques in session and assigned homework that entailed practice at home.

In the fourth session, various cognitive strategies were employed including assisting the girl in developing positive self-statements and coping statements that could replace the maladaptive thoughts she experienced during her attacks (e.g. thoughts that she would die). Additionally, the therapist provided the rationale for *in vivo* exposure, in which the girl would gradually approach the situations she had previously been avoiding. It was explained that if she stayed in the feared situation long enough, her anxiety would eventually dissipate and with repeated exposure, these situations would no longer be associated with anxiety. This is termed habituation. In addition, she was provided relaxation skills to reduce her anxiety while in the anxiety-provoking situation to counter the panic response. This process is referred to as counter-conditioning. Counter-conditioning is a way in which the child can unlearn the associations between the agoraphobic situations and the learned anxiety response. Additionally, the girl was instructed to use her previously acquired coping skills (e.g. positive self-statements) during the course of the *in vivo* exposures. Often, as was the case here, exposure is done in a graduated manner, with the patient starting with the least anxiety provoking situations, mastering those and then moving to increasingly more difficult situations.

Although initial exposure trials were accomplished with the assistance of the therapist, additional exposure was done outside of session with the parent assuming the role of the therapist and providing assistance. Subsequent sessions were devoted to reviewing progress, rehearsing coping strategies, and problem solving any difficulties that arose. Importantly, the girl was praised for her progress, using social approval to reinforce the girl's persistence in the exposure trials.

As explained above, the treatment goal was operationalized, in this case the criterion for termination was that the girl was to have no panic attacks for two consecutive weeks. The girl met this criterion following 10 treatment sessions. Throughout treatment, she had monitored her panic attacks (recording information including frequency and setting) and agoraphobic avoidance (using a 5-point scale ranging from 1, no avoidance or attempt to escape to 5, complete avoidance and the inability to enter the situation even when accompanied by someone who made her feel safe). Additionally, on a weekly basis, she provided ratings of her self-efficacy for approaching the agoraphobic situations; that is, the extent to which she felt capable of coping with each of the three identified agoraphobic situations, using a 5-point scale (1 representing the lowest degree of self efficacy and 5 the highest). More specifically, she identified how sure she was that she would be able to cope with: (i) being in the agoraphobic situation; (ii)

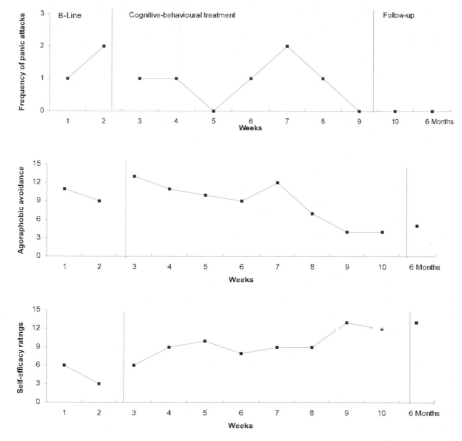

Fig. 9.1. Weekly panic attacks, agoraphobic avoidance, and self-efficacy ratings.

first noticing the signs of panic when in the agoraphobic situation; and (iii), experiencing panic symptoms while in the agoraphobic situation that increased in severity and intensity. Thus scores for each agoraphobic situation could range from a low of 3 (a 1-point response to each of the three questions) to 15 (a 5-point response to each question). Data on each of these indicators throughout treatment and at a 6 month follow-up are shown in Figure 9.1. As can be seen by examining each indicator of treatment effectiveness, the girl experienced steady improvement that was maintained in the absence of treatment for 6 months.

In this case, the therapist chose to focus on exposure to the agoraphobic situations; however, other methods of exposure have been used in treating panic disorder in youth, particularly in the absence of agoraphobic avoidance. In interoceptive exposure,[22] the symptoms of a panic attack are deliberately induced; for example, a child who experiences dizziness during a panic attack is instructed to spin in a chair or walk up and down stairs rapidly, and the focus is on having the child continue to experience the symptom until it is no longer anxiety provoking. The rationale here being that since panic disorder is a fear of panic attacks the feared stimuli that the patient attempts to avoid are the actual symptoms experienced during an attack; therefore, when there is no longer anxiety surrounding the experience of these sensations the panic attacks will dissipate.

Quite clearly, CBT treatment was found to be highly effective for this adolescent and the others treated in this study. As noted earlier, it has also been found to be effective for a variety of internalising and externalising disorders in children and adolescents. Although, the specific procedures may differ in treating these diverse children and their parents, the general tenets of CBT are followed – and enacted – in a manner similar to that illustrated here.

Cognitive-behaviour treatment of recurrent abdominal pain

Similar CBT interventions have been used in the treatment of recurrent abdominal pain. Recurrent abdominal pain is a common complaint in children with an estimated 10–15% of school-age children being affected. It is characterised by pain that is paroxysmal in nature, occurs over a period of months, and frequently interferes with daily activities and routines. For many children, the pain is characteristically resolved completely between episodes. The aetiology of recurrent abdominal pain has not been firmly established. Organic causes may be present, including constipation, peptic ulcers, metabolic disorders, and lactose intolerance among others. Although clear organic aetiology is found only in a minority of cases, evidence is increasing that subtle physiological dysfunctions may play an important role. Psychological and family factors have also been proposed to play a role. These factors include characteristics of the child (such as temperament and personality), characteristics of the parents (such as excessive anxiety, pre-occupation with heath concerns, over-protectiveness), and family conflict (such as marital discord). The disorder is probably best viewed as a psychosomatic condition that is optimally addressed by a team approach consisting of family physician, paediatrician and psychologist.[18]

Sanders and his colleagues in Australia have conducted two group design studies that illustrate a CBT intervention with this disorder.[23,24] In the first, CBT was shown to be more effective than a waiting list control group and in the second CBT was shown to be more effective than ongoing paediatric practices in Australia. Paediatric care often consists of providing reassurance to the parent and the child that there is no serious organic disease –– that many children 'grow out' of the pain –– and general advice to the parents and child about learning to cope with the pain. Such care is claimed to be effective, although controlled outcome studies are lacking.[23] In these studies, Sanders and colleagues used what they have called a CBT-based, consultative model of family intervention. The model involves conducting a comprehensive functional analysis of the child's presenting behaviour and family interactions surrounding the behaviour; discussing with the parents assessment findings that challenge maladaptive attributions or explanations of the behaviour; presenting a social learning explanation for pain; and providing active skills training by way of instructions, modelling, role-play, feedback, and homework assignments that train parents to implement change strategies in the home. Individual skills training (e.g. relaxation training, positive self-talk) is provided the children as well. Their treatment protocol has been put in manual form and has been used effectively with children between 6 and 14 years of age. Typically, treatment has consisted of six 50 min sessions. It consists of three primary components: provision of a social learning theory explanation of the pain experienced in children with recurrent abdominal pain and a detailed rationale for the pain management procedures to be enlisted, contingency management training for parents, and self-management training for children.

Session 1 involves a discussion of the assessment results and an explanation of pain and pain management procedures from a cognitive-behavioural perspective. Social learning explanations of pain in both adults and children increasingly highlight the individual's coping strategies in dealing with pain and the response of the patient's social environment to pain expression. For example, active coping responses (efforts to function despite the pain or to distract oneself from the pain) are thought to increase the child's sense of control, whereas more passive responses (depending on others for help and restricting activities) are thought to lead to withdrawal, decreased activities, and enhanced pain. Of course, a child's capacity to implement adaptive coping skills is influenced by the broader family environment. Caregivers (including parents) provide discriminative cues and selective reinforcement for behavioural expressions of pain (e.g. complaints of pain). Parental attention contingent on pain, the avoidance of non-preferred activities, and parental modelling of sick roles, in turn, affect the child's level and report of pain. Specifically, some caregiving practices (e.g. sympathy and attention, expression of concern, physical nurturance, external help seeking, or emotional reactions of anger or criticism) may serve (unexpectedly) to reinforce pain behaviours. This social learning 'conception' of pain is detailed in the first session. In session 2, parents are trained to reinforce well behaviour through contingent social attention (e.g. praise, pat on the back) and token re-enforcement in the form of happy faces or a point chart; to respond to verbal pain complaints by prompting the child to engage in competing behaviour or distracting behaviour; to ignore non-verbal pain behaviours such as grimacing and sighing; to avoid modelling sick role behaviours themselves; and to discriminate between recurrent abdominal pain symptoms and other physical complaints requiring medical attention (i.e. to respond with care and attention and to seek medical advice if the child is physically injured or suffers from pain or discomfort arising from some other illness or injury). Sessions 3, 4, and 5 are used to teach the children coping skills including relaxation and deep-breathing exercises (identical to those described above and used in the treatment of panic disorder), positive self-talk (e.g. 'be brave', 'hang in there'), distraction and engagement in competing activities, and positive imagery skills (think pleasant thoughts, imagine a 'relaxing' scene). The final and sixth session is devoted to relapse prevention training, in which children are taught problem-solving strategies for dealing with pain that might arise in future high-risk situations (e.g. when studying for examinations or participating in competitive activities). Throughout the six sessions, demonstrations and role-play activities are used to acquire and practice the learned skills and specific homework tasks are assigned. Prior to treatment, following treatment, and at 6 month and 12 month follow-up intervals, children complete pain diaries and parents complete pain observation records to monitor change.

Briefly, a pain diary was used to obtain the child's estimate of pain intensity. A 10 cm visual analogue scale, in the shape of a thermometer and representing a continuum from no pain at all to very bad pain, was used. The child was instructed to record the presence or absence of pain (by drawing a line on the thermometer) three times per day (before school, after school, and before bed). A pain intensity score was calculated by measuring the distance from the left of the child's line in millimetres. Pain ratings were calculated by summing the average daily pain intensity scores and dividing by the number of recording days. Children monitored their pain on a daily basis for 14 consecutive days at each assessment period (pretreatment, post-treatment, and 6 and 12 month follow-up). In addition, parents completed an observation record -- the Parent Observation Record – to measure their child's pain behaviour. The Parent Observation Record is a time-sampling instrument in which parents record the presence or absence of five categories of pain behaviour (complaining verbally about pain, displaying non-verbal pain behaviour, requesting medication, resting because of pain, and crying) in observation blocks of 60 min through-out the child's waking day. Data were expressed as a percentage of time intervals of pain behaviour per week (e.g. if the child exhibited any one or more of these behaviours in 10 of 50 time blocks, the resulting figure would be 20%). Such recordings were obtained for 2 weeks at the same points in time as their children completed the pain diaries.

The proportion of children pain-free at each of these intervals of time is presented in Table 9.3. As can be seen, reductions in pain were observed on both the pain diaries and the parent observation form. At post-treatment, for example, 55.6% of the children in the cognitive-behavioural family intervention reported being pain-free compared to 23.8% of children under standard paediatric care. Similarly, 70.6% of the parents receiving the cognitive-behavioural intervention reported an absence of pain behaviours in their children compared to 38.1% of the parents under standard paediatric care. The percentage of children pain-free, at least as reported by parents, continued to increase over follow-up for the CBT children (e.g. 82.4% compared to 42.1% at the 12 month follow-up). These results clearly favour CBT intervention over standard paediatric care, at least as practiced in Australia. Finney and colleagues[25] have reported similar effects in the US using child and family CBT procedures in a primary care-based

Table 9.3 Proportion of pain-free children at each phase of treatment

Measure	n	Proportion of pain-free children (%) CBFI	SPC
Pain diary			
Pretreatment	44	0.00	0.00
Post-therapy	39	55.60	23.80
6 month follow-up	39	66.70	27.80
12 month follow-up	36	58.80	36.80
Parent observation of pain behaviours			
Pretreatment	44	0.00	0.00
Post-therapy	38	70.60	38.10
6 month follow-up	38	66.70	38.90
12 month follow-up	36	82.40	42.10

CBFI = cognitive-behavioral family intervention; SPC = standard paediatric care.

paediatric psychology service in a managed care setting. They showed that 81% of parents rated their children's pain symptoms as improved or resolved after treatment. Independent outcome ratings by therapists agreed with the parent ratings.

The work of Sanders and colleagues and Finney and colleagues illustrates the efficacy of CBT interventions for children with recurrent abdominal pain. Quite clearly, not all children responded positively to these interventions. In the Finney et al study, for example, 19% of the parents rated their children's pain symptoms as unchanged or worsened. Based on the work of Sanders and colleagues, we might speculate that the children who got worse in these studies failed to learn active coping strategies to address their pain and/or their parents continued to re-inforce expressions of pain behaviour. Nonetheless, these studies show that CBT procedures are more effective than waiting list conditions (the pain does not just go away) or standard paediatric care. In addition, these studies illustrate the CBT approach to treatment: careful assessment, child and family focused interventions based in cognitive-behavioural theory, homework assignments, monitoring of treatment progress, and careful evaluation of treatment outcome.

THE ROLE OF THE PAEDIATRICIAN IN COGNITIVE BEHAVIOUR THERAPY

The examples provided above describe the use of CBT in isolation; however, it is often the case, at least for some disorders, that CBT is implemented in conjunction with medical interventions. For example, there is some suggestion that CBT used in combination with medication provides the best long-term outcomes for youth with obsessive-compulsive disorder[26] and ADHD.[16] On the other hand, there is preliminary evidence in adults that in some cases medication can actually attenuate the effectiveness of CBT.[27] Increasingly, children and their parents look to their primary care physicians or paediatricians for the medical management of psychological symptomatology; therefore, it is imperative that paediatricians are aware of the interactions between psychosocial and psychopharmacological interventions. In the same vein, given the possible benefits of medication for youth with psychiatric disorders, it is important for the practitioners of CBT to understand the impact of various drug therapies. Therefore, communication between physician and therapist serves to help each to perform their job more effectively and to better serve the patient and his or her family.[28]

Moreover, the possibilities for collaboration go beyond treatment for psychiatric disorders. In fact, CBTs have been found to be effective in treating or in aiding in the treatment of a variety of paediatric problems including recurrent abdominal pain,[23-25] as shown above, asthma,[29] headache,[30] cystic fibrosis,[31] and compliance with painful medical procedures such as bone marrow aspirations.[32,33] Given the effectiveness of such programmes, the provision of psychological interventions for medical problems in primary care settings could provide an integrated, economical, and convenient means for families to access services to augment medical interventions.[28]

REFERRING A CHILD FOR COGNITIVE-BEHAVIOURAL THERAPY

Given the history of psychology and psychiatry, psychotherapy is often perceived to be analogous with psychoanalysis, which is typically a long-term treatment focused on identifying the underlying problems which the overt symptoms are thought to symbolise. In classic psychoanalytical theory, difficulties (e.g. regressions, fixations) in the early childhood years are said to lead to problems throughout the life-span. These difficulties are often seen as the result of problematic parenting. Therefore, parents may expect that obtaining psychological treatment for their child will result in blame for their child's

Key points for clinical practice

- Cognitive behaviour therapy is based upon cognitive and behaviour theories that, in turn, are derived from principles of experimental psychology.

- Above all else, the common denominator across the various cognitive behaviour therapy procedures is an insistence on rigorous standards of proof and a commitment to the scientific process.

- Many cognitive behaviour therapy procedures have been shown to be empirically supported and are referred to as empirically supported treatments.

- Typically, cognitive behaviour therapy interventions consist of relatively short-term, directive, action-oriented, and goal-driven approaches. Moreover, they generally include homework assignments and involve members of the family in addition to the targeted child.

- For many psychiatric and medical conditions, cognitive behaviour therapy manuals specifying treatment guidelines have been developed. These manuals are intended to be used flexibly and to ensure treatment integrity.

- Cognitive behaviour therapy procedures have been found to be effective with a range of psychiatric and medical conditions, including panic disorder and recurrent abdominal pain which are illustrated in some detail in this chapter. Although all children and their families do not respond favourably to these procedures, a majority do so.

- Although cognitive behaviour therapy procedures can be used alone, and have been, we suggest that an approach which combines the knowledge, talents and skills of family practice physicians, paediatricians, and mental health professionals will prove particularly useful. However, such an integrated approach has not been rigorously examined to date and awaits empirical scrutiny and full investigation.

symptoms. This is particularly problematic because often by the time parents seek professional advice, they may feel guilty and helpless in the face of their child's symptoms. When recommending CBT for a child the physician must help reluctant or uninformed parents by providing an accurate picture of what to expect. Moreover, CBT treatments, like most psychosocial interventions, require an ongoing effort by the parents and child. Therefore, it is realistic to recommend such treatment to families who are motivated to be active participants in treatment or in cases when the physician believes this potential exists.

Although CBT interventions are becoming more commonplace, it is not safe to assume that all mental health professionals are trained to deliver such services. In the US, the Association for the Advancement of Behavior Therapy publishes a listing of behavioural and cognitive-behavioural therapists and their areas of specialisation. In other countries, similar registries are available (e.g. European Association of Cognitive and Behaviour Therapies, Australian Association of Behaviour and Cognitive Therapy). Providing a family with a proper referral is an important first step paediatricians can take to help their patients to address both the psychological and medical problems that can be treated with CBT interventions. Following referral, active collaboration with the family and mental health professional ensures the provision of integrated and optimal services across the spectrum of health-care.[28]

References

1 Watson JB. Psychology as the behaviorist views it. Psychol Rev 1913; 20: 158–177
2 Benjamin LTJ. Wilhem Wundt and the founding of the science of psychology. In: Benjamin LTJ (ed) A History of Psychology: Original Sources and Contemporary Research. New York: McGraw-Hill, 1988: 178–181
3 Bandura A. Psychological Modeling. Conflicting Theories. Chicago: Aldine-Atherton, 1971
4 Ollendick TH, Cerny JA. Clinical Behavior Therapy with Children. New York: Plenum Press, 1981
5 Krain AL, Kendall PC. Cognitive-behavioral therapy. In: Russ SW, Ollendick TH (eds.) Effective Psychotherapies with Children and their Families. New York: Plenum Press, 1999: 121–136
6 Kendall PC, Kane MT, Howard B, Siqueland L. Cognitive-behavioral Therapy for Anxious Children: Treatment Manual. Ardmore, PA: Workbooks Publishing, 1990
7 Webster-Stratton CH. Early intervention with videotape modeling: programs for families of children with oppositional defiant disorder or conduct disorder. In: Hibbs ED, Jensen PS, (eds) Child and Adolescent Disorders: Empirically Based Strategies for Clinical Practice. Washington, DC: American Psychological Association, 1996: 435–474
8 Stark KD, Kendall PC. Treating Depressed Children: Therapist Manual for 'ACTION'. Ardmore, PA: Workbooks Publishing, 1996
9 Digiuseppe R, Linscott J, Jilton R. Developing the therapeutic alliance in child-adolescent psychotherapy. Appl Prev Psychol 1996; 5: 85–100
10 Vuchinich S, Wood B, Angelelli J. Coalitions and family problem solving in the psychosocial treatment of preadolescents. In: Hibbs ED, Jensen PS (eds) Psychosocial Treatments for Child and Adolescent Disorders. Washington, DC: 1996: 497–518
11 Lonigan CJ, Elbert JC, Bennett Johnson S. Empirically supported psychosocial interventions for children: An overview. J Clin Child Psychol 1998; 27: 138–145
12 Kaslow NJ, Thompson MP. Applying the criteria for empirically supported treatments to studies of psychosocial interventions for child and adolescent depression. J Clin Child Psychol 1998; 27: 146–155
13 Ollendick TH, King NJ. Empirically supported treatments for children with phobic and anxiety disorders. J Clin Child Psychol 1998; 27: 156–167

14 Hagopian LS, Weist MD, Ollendick TH. Cognitive-behavior therapy with an 11-year-old girl fearful of AIDS infection, other diseases, and poisoning: a case study. J Anxiety Disord 1990; 4: 257–265

15 Brestan EV, Eyberg SM. Effective psychosocial treatments of conduct-disordered children and adolescents: 29 Years, 82 studies, and 5,272 kids. J Clin Child Psychol 1998; 27: 180–189

16 Pelham WE, Wheeler T, Chronis A. Empirically supported psychosocial treatments for attention-deficit hyperactivity disorder. J Clin Child Psychol 1998; 27: 190–205

17 Rogers SJ. Empirically supported comprehensive treatments for young children with autism. J Clin Child Psychol 1998; 27: 168–179

18 Janicke DM, Finney JW. Empirically supported treatments in pediatric psychology: recurrent abdominal pain. J Pediatr Psychol 1999; 24: 115–127

19 Ollendick TH. Cognitive behavioral treatment of panic disorder with agoraphobia in adolescents: a multiple baseline design analysis. Behav Ther 1995; 26: 517–531

20 Barlow DH, Craske MG, Cerny JA, Klosko JS. Behavioral treatment of panic disorder. Behav Ther 1989; 20: 261–282

21 Öst LG, Westling BE, Hellstrom K. Applied relaxation, exposure in vivo, and cognitive methods in the treatment of panic disorder with agoraphobia. Behav Res Ther 1993; 31: 383–394

22 Mattis SG. The Panic Control Treatment for Adolescents. Available from author; 1998 (unpublished)

23 Sanders MR, Rebgetz M, Morrison M et al. Cognitive-behavioral treatment of recurrent nonspecific abdominal pain in children: an analysis of generalization, maintenance, and side effects. J Consult Clin Psychol 1989; 57: 294–300

24 Sanders MR, Shepherd RW, Cleghorn G, Woolford H. The treatment of recurrent abdominal pain in children: a controlled comparison of cognitive-behavioral family intervention and standard pediatric care. J Consult Clin Psychol 1994; 62: 306–314

25 Finney JW, Lemanek KL, Cataldo MF, Katz HP, Fuqua RW. Pediatric psychology in primary health care: Brief target therapy for recurrent abdominal pain. Behav Ther 1989; 20: 283–291

26 March JS, Leonard HL, Swedo SE. Obsessive-compulsive disorder. In: March JS, (ed) Anxiety Disorders in children and Adolescents. New York: Guilford Press, 1995: 251–275

27 Woods SW, Barlow DH, Gorman JM, Shear MK. Follow-up results six months after discontinuation of all treatment. In: Barlow DH (Chair), Results from the multi-center trial on the treatment of panic disorder: cognitive behavior treatment versus imipramine versus their combination. Symposium presented at the 32nd Annual Convention of the Association for the Advancement of Behavior Therapy, Washington, DC, November 1998

28 Drotar D. Consulting with Pediatricians: Psychological Perspectives. New York: Plenum, 1997

29 Vazquez MI, Buceta JM. Effectiveness of self-management programs and relaxation training in the treatment of bronchial asthma: Relationships with trait anxiety and emotional attack triggers. J Psychosom Res 1993; 37: 71–81

30 Beames L, Sanders MR, Bor W. The role of parent training in the cognitive behavioral treatment of children's headaches. Behav Psychother 1992; 20: 167–180

31 Hains AA, Davies WB, Behrens D, Biller JA. Cognitive behavioral interventions for adolescents with cystic fibrosis. J Pediatr Psychol 1997; 22: 669–687

32 Drotar D. Psychological interventions for children with chronic physical illness and their families: toward integration of research and practice. In: Russ SW, Ollendick TH (eds) Effective Psychotherapies with Children and their Families. New York: Plenum, 1999: 447–462

33 Lemanek KL, Koontz AD. Integrated approaches to acute illness. In: Russ SW, Ollendick TH (eds) Effective Psychotherapies with Children and their Families. New York: Plenum, 1999: 463–482

Alex V. Levin

Retinal haemorrhages and child abuse

SHAKEN BABY SYNDROME

Shaken baby syndrome (SBS) is a form of child abuse in which the perpetrator violently shakes an infant resulting in brain, skeletal and/or retinal haemorrhages. Although the association of these findings had been noted by him earlier,[1] it was not until the early 1970s that John Caffey first defined the clinical symptoms and signs of shaking injuries.[2,3] However, the potential unique susceptibility of the infant brain to shaking may have been recognised in the previous century.[4] The infant and young child are particularly vulnerable because of their relatively large head, weak cervical musculature, and immature unmyelinated brain. In addition, the incompletely fused sutures and relatively increased volume of cerebrospinal fluid allow for greater movement of the brain within the cranial vault. There is a wide variability of presentation ranging from non-specific gastrointestinal symptoms or irritability to death.[5] Often, there is little or no external sign of injury.

Force required to cause injury

Although some believe that a single severe shake may be sufficient,[6,7] from the confessions of perpetrators we know that the violence which results in SBS injuries or death is extreme and usually repetitive either at the time of a single incident or over multiple episodes of shaking. The head undergoes repetitive severe anterior–posterior, side-to-side, and/or rotatory movement with repeated abrupt acceleration-deceleration.[2,3,5,8] The magnitude of acceleration–deceleration forces needed to cause these kinds of brain and eye injuries in humans and primates is extreme.[9] Despite Caffey's suggestion, in his original description of

Alex V. Levin MD FRCSC
Department of Ophthalmology, The Hospital for Sick Children, University of Toronto, 555 University Avenue, Toronto, Ontario M5G 1XB, Canada

SBS, that normal play activities such as tossing a baby playfully in the air, head banging, vigorous burping, and various playground activities could cause SBS-like injuries, it is now well recognised that this is not the case.[10] Yet, some authors still make suggestions to the contrary.[6] It appears that the amount of violence that is required to induce SBS is beyond that which any reasonable person would consider normal and in a range that even the most distraught person would recognise as injurious. A not uncommon 'explanation' offered by suspected perpetrators is that they found the child apnoeic or apparently lifeless and then shook the child to resuscitate them. Whether this type of shocking experience is enough to incapacitate one's judgement is perhaps open to speculation although I believe, from my encounters with confessed perpetrators, that the amount of violence required to cause shaking injuries is still beyond that which would be applied particularly if the caretaker still had enough contact with reality to know to call for emergency assistance. The same would hold true for those caretakers who, despite even the acknowledgement that striking a child is unacceptable, may feel that shaking is an acceptable form of punishment.[11] One group suggested that the types of injuries seen in SBS corresponded to injuries seen after motor vehicle accidents at 89 km/h.[12] Yet, remarkably creative, unique or complex stories may still create doubt and conflicting opinions amongst experts in the field.[13]

Age of victims

Infant victims are usually less than 3-years-old.[10,14] The average age of SBS victims falls between 5 and 10-months-old.[4,14–23] Most children are under 2 years of age.[14,16,18,22,24] In one study, all deaths occurred in children less than 2-years-old.[17] One author found the death rate to be higher (53% versus 14%) when the mean age of victims was 13 months as opposed to 6 months.[24] Long-term severity seems to inversely correlated with the age at presentation.[4] I have cared for a 5-year-old child with sickle cell disease who, by the admission of his teenage cousin, was beaten into unconsciousness and then shaken resulting in brain injury and retinal haemorrhages (atypical in that they were almost all preretinal overlying blood vessels suggesting vessel compromises). The child experienced anoxia induced sickling in his brain causing vascular and kidney occlusion resulting in transient renal failure. This type of unique situation, where the child is unconscious and other predisposing contributing factors such as haemoglobinopathy are present, were required to allow a child of this age to demonstrate findings, albeit atypical, of SBS. One author[7] refers to victims 'up to 15 years of age' without further information, and there is at least one case of an adult torture victim who sustained fatal shaking injuries including retinal haemorrhage although the eye findings were not further detailed.[25]

Epidemiology of abusive head trauma

Abusive head trauma is the most common type of child abuse resulting in death,[18] although it only represents 2.9–4.9% of all cases referred to child abuse teams.[15] In many areas in the US, homicide is the most common cause of child death.[18] Assault represents over half of all traumatic brain injury in the first year of life and 90% of brain injuries between 1–4 years of age.[26] The mortality rate of SBS, based on studies with more than 10 patients, is approximately 8–61%.[4,15,18,19,22,27,28] Most studies find mortality to be within the 14–25% range. Although males are more often victims of SBS than females,[22] not all studies agree[16,19] and the proportions are equal for children who die.[18] Likewise, although males are more often the perpetrator,[22] the proportions are equal for male versus female perpetrators of SBS homicide.[18] First-born children are also more likely to be victims (62–92%),[15] although this may be a reflection, in part, of separation or imprisonment of perpetrators after the first incident. Like all other forms of child abuse, no social class, religion, ethnicity, or culture are spared from SBS. Although some studies have identified low socio-economic class as a risk factor, others have found that middle class families are more often affected.[16]

Need for early recognition of abusive head trauma

The need for early recognition is underscored by the fact that 39–71% of children have a prior proven episode of abuse, neglect or shaking.[15] In one study, 4 of 6 children sent home after initial contact with the medical system, returned dead.[28] In another study, 45% of children had brain atrophy and hydrocephalus *ex vacuo* at presentation suggesting prior episode(s) of brain injury that had gone undiagnosed.[16] Centrifuged cerebrospinal fluid that is xanthrochromic may be an indicator of prior injury.[29] Although children may present dead, in neurological extremis (25–100%),[4,15] or with seizures (20–100%),[4,15] more non-specific symptoms are also well recognised. Some children may even present with no symptoms, except perhaps an increasing head circumference due to chronic subdural effusions, with or without visually insignificant retinal haemorrhages.[30] I have seen a boy with macrocephaly, marked subdural effusion, and cerebral atrophy with a single dot haemorrhage in one eye who was the victim of chronic repetitive sub-clinical shaking by a baby-sitter but presented with no subjective symptoms and a normal neurological examination. Vomiting, lethargy, irritability and/or anorexia occur in 25–100%.[4,15] Anaemia is observed in 50–100%.[15] The wide ranges of incidence statistics reflects the different populations studied (i.e. long-term survivors versus early deaths).

Perpetrators of abusive head trauma

The most common perpetrators of SBS are biological fathers and biologically unrelated boyfriends of the biological mothers.[7,16,18,22,31] Baby-sitters, females 4.4 times more often than males,[18] are the perpetrators in 4–20% of cases,[16,18,31] while biological mothers commit this crime in 5–12% of cases.[16,18,31] Baby-sitters may be less likely to confess to the act.[18] Overall, only a minority, perhaps 10–15%,[15,31] of perpetrators will confess,[10,32] although in one postmortem study, 3 of 7 (43%) perpetrators confessed.[33] In approximately 25% of cases, the perpetrator may remain unknown.[31] When a confession is not obtained, in over half of the cases, a history of minor head trauma (e.g. fall < 3 ft, bumped head on door), which does not adequately explain the injury, is offered.[31] Over 97% of those perpetrators who do confess, relate that they were present when the child became symptomatic.[18] This suggests that it is unlikely for the child to be asymptomatic for a lucid interval of sufficient time to allow transfer of care (e.g. well child dropped of at baby-sitter and later becomes symptomatic).[18]

Shaken babies are typically not physically battered and show little external evidence of trauma.[34] Accompanying sexual assault is particularly uncommon (< 0.6%).[18]

BRAIN INJURY IN SHAKEN BABY SYNDROME

Definition

Although it is beyond the scope of this paper to describe the entire range of brain injury that may occur in SBS, the most common lesion is subdural haemorrhage. In one study, this was the only brain injury that had a statistically significant correlation with death,[17] whereas other authors have found that cerebral oedema and infarction are predictors of poor outcome.[16] In the study by Green and co-workers, subdural haemorrhage was always present when any other brain injury was apparent except for the rare case when the only finding may be diffuse cerebral oedema.[17,29] This led the authors to conclude that less force was needed to generate subdural haemorrhage than for other types of SBS brain injury, such as parenchymal laceration/contusion, subarachnoid haemorrhage or parenchymal haemorrhage.

Increased intracranial pressure is common (55–85%),[15] as is bloody cerebro-spinal fluid on lumbar puncture (12–83%).[15] Brainstem lesions are uncommon (< 8%).[15] Subdural or subarachnoid blood in the posterior interhemispherical fissure may have particular diagnostic significance.[29] Late findings include cerebral atrophy, hydrocephalus *ex vacuo* , chronic subdural fluid collections, and encephalomalacia.

Incidence

One study of long-term survivors found that, at presentation, the incidence statistics were: subarachnoid haemorrhage 31%, subdural haemorrhage 23%, interhemispheric 'collection' 15%, strokes 15%, intraparenchymal haemorrhage 8%, and parenchymal tears 8%.[15] These figures are at the low end of the reported values at presentation without regard to survival: 10–72%, 10–80%, 20–100%, 25–50%, 5–30%, and 0–100%, respectively.[4,15,16,21] Subdural and subarachnoid haemorrhage, and cerebral oedema are the most consistent autopsy findings in shaken babies.[10,33,35,36] Differentiation between interhemispheric subdural versus subarachnoid blood may be difficult, but this is a very important sign which is highly correlated with non accidental as opposed to accidental injury.[10,11,36] Other findings may include chronic extra-axial fluid collections (21%)[37] and basal ganglia oedema (13%)[37] although the basal ganglia are usually spared.[10] A particularly ominous sign is the loss of grey-white differentiation and diffuse hypodensity.[10] The posterior fossa is often spared leaving it radio-dense as compared to the abnormally hypodense cerebrum, a finding called the 'reversal sign'.[10,11]

Pathogenesis

Traditionally, it has been understood that it is the shearing forces induced by shaking that result in tearing of the bridging veins, resulting in subdural haemorrhage, and diffuse axonal injury, with secondary cerebral oedema and infarction.[27,29,38,39] Although Duhaime and co-workers have suggested that impact, in addition to shaking, is necessary to create the severe injuries seen in SBS,[40] others believe that shaking alone can be sufficient.[7,11,15,17,19,21,23,29,31,33,35,36,41,42] In agreement with the possibility that shaking alone can result in death is a paper looking at autopsies done at the same location as those cited in the report from Duhaime and co-workers (Philadelphia Medical Examiner's office) just 3 years later.[43] Typically, shaken babies have no obvious evidence of blunt head injury such as skull fracture or external scalp injury.[21] However, depending on the study, 20–54% of children will have multiple ecchymoses, scars, or scalp haematoma[15] indicating that some degree of blunt trauma has occurred. Several authors have also found that, in the absence of external evidence of blunt trauma, ecchymoses may be observed on the under surface of the scalp when it is reflected off of the cranial vault at autopsy.[10,43] Some authors[18] have proposed the name 'shaken impact syndrome' or 'abusive head trauma instead of SBS to more accurately encompass the full range of aetiological mechanisms.

The model used by Duhaime[40] has been criticised because it was packed tight with wet cotton thus ignoring the relatively large cerebrospinal fluid space in infants (up to 1 cm), the stabilisation offered by the tentorium and falx, inadequate neck flexion, and the damping of brain movement by the fluid.[35,44] Others remark about the failure of the model to address the vascular insult, cerebral oedema, secondary cerebral hypoxia, and midbrain parenchymal shifts which also contribute to the brain injury after shaking.[21,45] Some authors[39] have suggested that the amount of force necessary to generate substantial brain injury is much smaller than that suggested by the findings of Duhaime and co-workers[40] and that low strain over a longer period increases the likelihood of brain injury.[38] In addition, the severity of the injury induced by shaking alone may, in part, be due to the establishment of harmonic vibration, the rotation of the neck, and/or cervical spinal cord injury.[39] Even Duhaime and her co-workers recently acknowledged that 'there is considerable controversy' concerning their original findings.[10]

Diagnosis

Although CT scan remains the procedure of choice and often the most accessible, MRI can be helpful in dating the findings and often in visualising findings that may have been missed on CT.[11,19,29,46,47] In up to 20% of cases, the initial CT scan may even be normal with abnormalities becoming apparent on repeat films taken within the first week.[19] MRI is superior at detecting cervical cord injuries that may also be found in SBS.[11]

Prognosis

A significant number of long-term survivors will experience neurological impairment. In one study, only 28% of children had normal neurological examinations at discharge from hospital.[18] In moderate length follow-up studies, 20–30% of children are normal[16,28] whereas long-term studies show that only 8–14% are normal.[4,15] Early findings include quadriplegia, diplegia, or hemiplegia with or without severe mental retardation.[4,15,16] With time, other findings may become evident including microcephaly, late hemiparesis, developmental delay, or learning disabilities.[4] These later findings may be discovered despite an interval after the injury of apparent normal neurological status that can last up to 5 years in the case of learning disabilities.[15] Children without a sign free interval and those with microcephaly have a much more dismal long-term neurological prognosis.[15] Whether these late findings are partially or completely attributed to SBS or other environmental factors is difficult to establish. Other long-term sequelae may include seizures (7–65%),[4,15,16,22,28] hydrocephalus (3–75%),[21] or psychiatric/behavioural difficulties (28–50%).[4,15] Presenting signs which are associated with a poor long-term outcome include coma, need for intubation, and the CT findings of bilateral diffuse hypodensity with loss of grey-white differentiation, or unilateral hemispherical hypodensity.[4] Seizures and/or apnoea at presentation are not correlated with severity of outcome.[4] One group of authors states that 'big black brain' (poorly perfused and oedematous parenchyma) is always associated with death or severe long-term impairment.[4]

SKELETAL INJURIES IN SHAKEN BABY SYNDROME

Three types of fracture are most common: skull, ribs, and long bone metaphysis.

Skull fracture

The incidence of skull fractures in shaken babies varies widely in the literature; from 9–31%.[15,22] In one series reporting autopsies of victims, 57% had skull fractures.[33] The parietal and occipital bones are most often affected.[15] In shaken babies, skull fractures may be linear, diastatic, depressed, single or multiple.[16] In contrast, most accidental fractures from moderate blunt trauma will be simple linear fractures, usually parietal, over the vertex, or coming from the coronal suture.[21] Fractures which are branching, stellate, crossing suture lines, bilateral, multiple, depressed in a child less than 3-years-old, more than 5 mm wide at presentation, or progressively expanding are particularly worrisome indicators for non-accidental injury in the absence of a plausible history of severe accidental injury.[21] Symptoms may be absent despite large fractures.[21]

Rib fracture

Rib fractures are the most common type of bony injury seen in SBS appearing in up to half of the cases with many children showing both old and new fractures.[31] These fractures are usually posterior–lateral as a result of direct compression from the perpetrator's hands grasping the child face-to-face by the thorax.

Long bone fracture

Injuries seen in shaken babies but rarely following accidental injury include haemorrhagic stripping of the periosteum, multiple fractures, fractures of different ages, 'corner' or 'bucket handle' fractures of the metaphyses, spiral fractures in non-mobile children, and non supracondylar humeral fracture.[21] In decreasing order of prevalence, these fractures will affect the tibia, forearm bones, femur, or humerus.[31] The fractures appear to be in large part due to shaking while the infant is held by an extremity causing the long bones to be twisted and the periosteum to be stripped. One study found the incidence of long bone fractures to be 3%.[22]

Diagnosis

Skeletal survey radiographs should be part of all SBS evaluations.[29,38]

RETINAL HAEMORRHAGES

Definition

Perhaps the most important obstacle to understanding the retinal haemorrhages seen in SBS is the failure to accurately describe them. Many papers in the literature, courtroom discussion and educational seminars refer to 'retinal haemorrhages' as if this term described all retinal findings equally. In fact, the term 'retinal haemorrhage' is perhaps no more specific as 'fracture' and one surely would not suggest that all fractures are the same in terms of pathogenesis or aetiology. Likewise, assertions that 'retinal haemorrhages' are or are not the result of non-accidental hacmorrhage must be clarified with descriptors that will offer more specificity. Retinal haemorrhages can be described in terms of where they lie topographically, the layer at which they lie, and their number or severity.

Structure of retina

The retina is a multi-layered structure that lines the inside of the eyeball and extends anteriorly to just behind the iris. The edge of the retina is called the ora serrata. If one were to place a pointer directly through the pupil along the line of sight, it would eventually touch the retina at its most posterior point: the fovea (Fig. 10.1). This is the specialised area for visual acuity and, despite being smaller than a pinhead, represents the sole part of retina used for our most acute straight ahead vision. The retina which circles the fovea within approximately 0.5 mm is called the perifoveal retina. Around this area is the macula (Fig. 10.1); additional posterior retina which extend approximately to the major arterial and venous vessels above and below (superior and inferior arcades). Just nasal to this area one can see the optic nerve entering the eyeball (Fig. 10.1). The combination of macula, optic nerve, and retina around the optic nerve (peripapillary) is called the posterior pole (Fig. 10.1).

The choroid is the vascular layer which lies underneath the retina: between the retina and the outer eyeball coat (sclera). The sclera is a tough fibrous tissue which is mostly avascular.

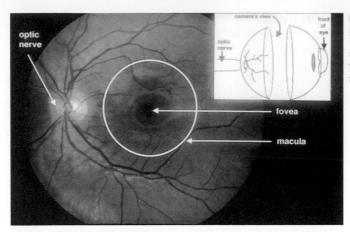

Fig. 10.1 Normal posterior pole including optic nerve, macula, and fovea with some surrounding retina.

Location of haemorrhage

As shown in Plate 10.1, Haemorrhages may lie in front of the retina (preretinal), within the layers of the retina (intraretinal) or beneath the retina (subretinal). Since retinal blood vessels run in the superficial layers of the retina, subretinal haemorrhages are easily distinguished by the presence of blood vessels **over** them. Intraretinal haemorrhages are often described as dot, blot, or flame (Plate 10.1). Dot and blot haemorrhages are usually roughly circular and lie within the deeper layers of the retina. Size distinguishes dot from blot although there are no strict objective criteria to make this distinction. Flame haemorrhages lie within the nerve fibre layer which is very superficial. The presence of blood in this layer follows the nerve fibres causing the edges to have a feathered, or flame shaped, appearance. Flame haemorrhages, and usually dot and blot haemorrhages as well, will cause blood vessel paths to 'disappear' as they run below or through the blood.

Intraretinal haemorrhages

Intraretinal haemorrhages may appear to have white centres (Plate 10.2). Although this appearance is classically associated with bacterial endocarditis (Roth spots), any condition which causes retinal haemorrhages may be associated with white centred haemorrhages either as result of central fibrin deposition, clot resolution, ischaemia, thrombotic emboli, exudate, cellular infiltrate, retinal infection, or even artefacts (light reflexes). They are also well recognised in SBS,[48] although of no specific diagnostic significance. Rather, specificity is gained more from haemorrhage distribution, extent, and other descriptors. It has been theorised that in SBS the white centre may result either from post traumatic capillary rupture with extravasation and fibrin clot formation or ischaemic foci with nerve fibre layer infarct.[48] White centring tends to be more often located in the posterior pole and affects more superficial flame and dot/blot haemorrhages.[48]

Preretinal haemorrhage

The term 'preretinal' haemorrhage is often misused in the literature and on clinical examination.[49] This can be a very important forensic distinction as it may help to distinguish traumatic retinoschisis (see below), with its diagnostic significance for SBS, from less specific forms of haemorrhage laying on top of the retina. The inner aspect of the retina is covered by a membrane called the internal limiting membrane. Technically, blood which is under the internal limiting membrane is still intraretinal as is seen in traumatic retinoschisis. Blood which is truly preretinal lies on top of the retina, in front of the internal limiting membrane. Blood in this space may also be termed subhyaloid. The eye is filled with a substance called vitreous which has a jelly like consistency. The vitreous is also known as the hyaloid body; thus the term subhyaloid. When blood extends into the potential space between retina and vitreous, then the patient has a subhyaloid haemorrhage.

Vitreous haemorrhage

If blood becomes admixed with the vitreous, this is called vitreous haemorrhage. Vitreous haemorrhage may be severe or mild. When severe, there may be an association with worse visual and neurological outcome even with vitrectomy surgery.[20] More mild vitreous haemorrhage may be visually insignificant and resolve spontaneously. All patients with vitreous haemorrhage who were less than 10-years-old in a study of over 200 patients had sustained trauma.[50] Although further details are not given, this study does demonstrate the rarity of non traumatic vitreous haemorrhage in childhood. Vitreous haemorrhage may be the result of blood breaking out of a traumatic retinoschisis cavity.[51]

Retinal haemorrhages with papilloedema

Retinal haemorrhages are often associated with and one of the distinguishing signs of papilloedema (Fig. 10.2). These haemorrhages tend to be small, few in number, flame shaped (splinter haemorrhages) and located on and radiating around the optic nerve. All or some of the other characteristic findings of papilloedema (oedema, blurry disc margins, dilated and tortuous vessels, loss of view of the vessels as they pass through the oedematous nerves) will be present. These haemorrhages are not caused by shaking *per se* and can be seen in any cause of papilloedema. It is perhaps incorrect to include these haemorrhages in the category of 'retinal haemorrhages' when discussing SBS

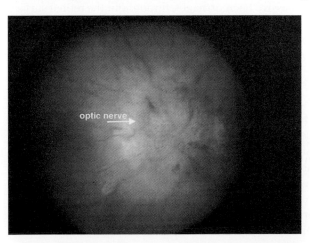

Fig. 10.2 Papilloedema. Note indistinct edges of swollen optic nerve and multiple peripapillary dot and flame haemorrhages.

optic nerve

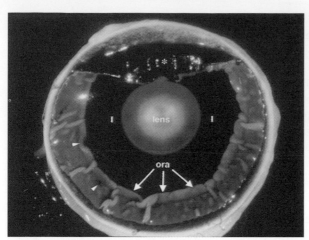

Fig. 10.3 View from inside eyeball looking out (Miyake view). The lens is seen as if the observer was standing inside the eyeball. I = back of the iris. Arrowheads indicate some of several retinal haemorrhages extending out to edge of retina (ora serrata). Superior folding over of retina (*) and all folds in retina (including fold of retina at ora) represent common fixation artefacts.

as the aetiology. However, the retinal haemorrhages associated with SBS may include haemorrhage found on the optic disc in the absence of papilloedema.[34]

Distribution of haemorrhages

The distribution of haemorrhages in the eye of a child victim of SBS may have significant diagnostic significance in some cases, particularly when haemorrhages extend out to the ora serrata (Fig. 10.3).[7,33,52] Green and co-workers showed that haemorrhages, as a group, were most likely to be found in the peripheral edges of the retinal or posterior pole in a series of 16 children who had died from SBS.[17] Gilliland and co-workers state that peripheral retinal haemorrhages are indicative of acceleration-deceleration injury although they were also observed in some cases where direct head trauma was the main cause of death.[53] They did not observe these haemorrhages in the absence of central nervous system disease and calculated that they were statistically associated with head injury. Even when observed in unrestrained rear seat passengers involved with motor vehicle accidents, they feel that acceleration-deceleration is to blame.

Certainly, the finding of massive haemorrhages, throughout the retinal surface at all layers of the retina in an infant reflects a shaking aetiology unless proven otherwise. Likewise, traumatic retinoschisis has only been reported in SBS.

Documentation

It is an integral part of the medical record which documents the presence and nature of retinal haemorrhages in cases of suspected child abuse. Unfortunately, the documentation in many cases consists only of a few words or sentences, sometimes citing only the generic presence of 'retinal haemorrhages' without further description (see above). Some examiners may use rudimentary, quickly crafted, hand-made drawings that may not adequately reflect the number, distribution, and types of retinal haemorrhages. More detailed descriptions preferably using both words and detailed drawings should be used so that all of the features of the haemorrhages may be adequately and clearly described.

One group of investigators proposed an 'eye trauma score' based on the location and type of haemorrhages, although details were not provided.[17] Other grading systems have been used for retinal haemorrhages in other settings.[54] More commonly, the examining ophthalmologist will draw a schematic diagram of the haemorrhages. The description should include an estimate of the number of haemorrhages in each eye, the distribution within the retina, the types of haemorrhages, and the presence of traumatic retinoschisis.

The forensic value of ocular photography has been recognised almost as far back as its availability.[55] It is perhaps the 'gold standard' for documenting retinal haemorrhages although this expensive equipment is not readily available in all centres and the inability to perform photography, either because of availability or lack of technical equipment or assistance, should not be considered a flaw in the medical or forensic evaluation of the child as long as the haemorrhages are well detailed by other forms of documentation. Ideally, fundus photography can be performed with a portable hand-held camera specifically designed for this purpose. However, even when available, and the operator skilled, photography of the retina in an awake child is quite difficult. Movement artefacts can be lessened with the use of a speculum and fixation of the eyeball with a forceps, cotton swab, or other ophthalmic devices, but this may not be well tolerated by the child or the parents. However, in the child who has altered state of consciousness, particularly if comatose or pharmacologically paralysed, photographs are easier to obtain and provide valuable documentation. Photography beyond the posterior pole, especially when trying to view the far edges of the retina, is still difficult. We have used wide angle contact photography with the RetCam (Massic Research Lab, Dublin, California) system and find that it gives a more 'global' view of the extent of haemorrhaging (Fig. 10.4). However, this is very expensive equipment which is not widely available and can not by done on awake infants as it requires contact of the probe with the eyeball and absence of movement.

After death, clinical examination of the eyes may be useful to help document the pattern of haemorrhages as this can be lost under the microscopic view. Sometimes, an ophthalmologist can still see through the cornea up to 72 h after death but virtually never after the eyeball has been removed. After fixation, it is essential to make a gross description of the sectioned eyeball. Photographic techniques using transillumination have been developed to best

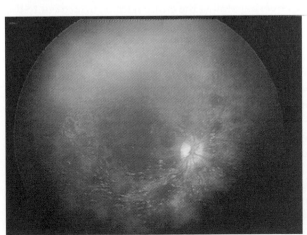

Fig. 10.4 RetCam view of retina in this shaken baby provides a wider angle view in one photograph as compared to standard retinal photography (e.g. Figs 10.1 & 10.2, Plates 10.1 & 10.2).

illustrate the haemorrhages on the gross view,[56] but routine illumination may also suffice. Alternate methods of sectioning the eyeball may allow for photographs which give a better and more understandable view of the retina, especially for lay observers such as those involved with courtroom proceedings.[57] Gross photography of the peripheral retina is also useful either from the Miyake view (Fig. 10.3) or other preparations.[57] Histological preparations should include multiple cuts, especially of the macula, and including the ora serrata. One group has proposed a grading scheme based on a 100-square grid in the eye piece of the microscope.[33] Techniques recommended for removal of the eyeball and orbital contents are described below.

Incidence of retinal haemorrhage

The incidence of retinal haemorrhage varies widely from study-to-study due to varying definitions, methods of examination, and clinical status of the child. Overall, the incidence rates vary from 30–100%.[5,10,22,40,42,58–66] A general figure of 80% might best reflect the published studies. If the study includes patients with abusive head trauma not due to shaking (i.e. entities not usually associated with retinal haemorrhages), then the SBS population is statistically diluted and a lower incidence of retinal haemorrhages will be reported.[67,68] This may be particularly true of studies which include patients seen before Caffey's original descriptions of SBS in the early 1970s.[67] If haemorrhages due to papilloedema are included the incidence will rise. If examinations are not conducted through a pharmacologically dilated pupil the incidence will fall. In a study of long-term survivors, the initial incidence of retinal haemorrhages (all inclusive) was 59%.[15] Other studies, looking at clinical examination of all patients in the presenting phase of the illness, show incidence rates ranging from 50–100%.[16,29] One study, without discerning accidental from non-accidental injury, did note that retinal haemorrhages were only found in children with other signs of head injury.[68] However, the majority of children in this study did not have retinal findings recorded.

The appearance of the retina in SBS may range from normal to just a few dot or blot haemorrhages in the posterior pole to extensive, almost confluent intraretinal haemorrhaging covering almost the entire retinal surface out to the ora serrata.[69] Traumatic retinoschisis may or may not be present. The findings in the two eyes may be mildly or dramatically asymmetric (Plate 10.1B).[33,70] Unilateral haemorrhages are less common but do occur at a rate of up to 50%.[5,16,29,33,43,61,62,70,71] Intraretinal haemorrhages are more common than pre- or subretinal blood.[7,72] Superficial intraretinal haemorrhages tend to be more common[7,70] which led one author to speculate that deeper dot and blot haemorrhages may result from extension from the more superficial layers. However, this would not explain why flame haemorrhages and dot/blot haemorrhages are usually not contiguous

Although rare, retinal haemorrhages due to SBS can occur in the absence of intracranial bleeding or cerebral oedema.[21,70] But when combined with intracranial haemorrhage, particularly subdural haemorrhage, and rib fractures, there is usually no common likely alternative explanation for the injury other than shaking.[21]

Postmortem studies

If eyes are only examined in children who have died from SBS then the incidence of retinal haemorrhages may be higher, if not 100%,[33,37,42,73] although rates as low as 49–57% have also been reported.[35,70] One study found all types of intra-ocular haemorrhages more commonly after shaking alone as opposed to shaking with impact head trauma.[43] Some findings which are clinically difficult to visualise may appear. Betz and co-workers found all layers of the retina involved and preretinal blood in each case.[33] In the study by Green and co-workers, 81% of 16 children were found to have ocular abnormalities: 75% subhyaloid haemorrhage, 75% intraretinal haemorrhage (not further specified), and 12% vitreous haemorrhage.[17] Traumatic retinoschisis was not specifically mentioned. The authors state that vitreous haemorrhage, seen only in cases with retinal detachment, may be due to blood breaking through the internal limiting membrane, a finding which very often is clinically visible in traumatic retinoschisis. Likewise, another group found blood under the internal limiting membrane in all shaken children with retinal haemorrhages although frank retinoschisis with macular folds (described as 'haemorrhagic retinal detachment') was only identified in 42 patients.[37] They also found that vitreous haemorrhage was not common,[25] although, in another study, it was seen in 27% of cases[70] and, in yet another, the incidence was 100%.[73] The second study also found that retinal haemorrhage postmortem was more common in children under 1 year of age and also found traumatic retinoschisis only in abused children.[70] This study incorporated at least some of the patients previously described by Rao.[62] One group found traumatic retinoschisis or perimacular folds in 4 of 7 abused children with severe eye findings.[73]

The most common intraretinal haemorrhages are those found in the superficial layers, such as flame haemorrhages.[37,43,62,70] Subretinal haemorrhage may be frequent in some studies[37,43] and may result in secondary disruption of the retinal pigmented epithelium.[37] Choroidal haemorrhage, which is sometimes not readily apparent clinically, can be found in 30–50% of eyes at autopsy.[17,37] It is unclear why this high incidence occurs, but this group may include particularly severe eye injury samples.

Postmortem studies are also useful in describing the distribution of the haemorrhages. One group found that there were more haemorrhages posteriorly but documents that they do indeed extend anteriorly.[17,37] Betz and co-workers demonstrated massive retinal haemorrhages at the ora serrata.[33] They found that all shaken infants had more than 20–30% of the retinal surface involved.[33]

Pathophysiology of retinal haemorrhage

It is unknown how much force it takes to create the ocular injuries seen in SBS. One group has suggested, based on incidence statistics, that relatively less force is needed to create intraretinal, subhyaloid or optic nerve sheath haemorrhage than for retinal detachment, choroidal haemorrhage or vitreous haemorrhage.[17] However, this was a study of children who had died from SBS implying that the forces were still in the severe range. There is a case report of a 9-year-old perpetrator who committed shaking of a 3-month-old which resulted in bilateral 'extensive, almost confluent intraretinal haemorrhages' extending to the ora serrata along with a femur fracture and severe brain injury.[74] This is clearly an unusual and isolated case which raises the question of whether less force is required or this child was particularly able to cause the injury or whether he is indeed the perpetrator.

With the exception of traumatic retinoschisis, for which the mechanism is well understood, there has been much debate about the exact mechanism by which retinal haemorrhages occur in SBS. In fact, different types of haemorrhages may have different causation and more than one theory may be operant in any given instance.

Terson syndrome

Terson described the association in a 60-year-old man of unspecified cerebral haemorrhage and retinal and vitreous haemorrhage.[75] The association of intracranial blood, in particular subarachnoid, with retinal haemorrhages is well recognised in adults. The retinal haemorrhage may be preretinal, intraretinal or, less commonly, subretinal.[49,76] Over the years, the syndrome has been broadened to include the association of any kind of intracranial haemorrhage with retinal haemorrhage with or without vitreous haemorrhage,[49,51,77] although some controversy may remain over the exact definition.[69,78] In adults, the most common causes are spontaneous subarachnoid haemorrhage, ruptured intracranial aneurysm, and trauma.

Subhyaloid, intraretinal, and optic nerve sheath haemorrhages are found significantly more often in subdural haemorrhage and brain trauma deaths secondary to SBS as compared to abused children with death from other causes.[17] In one study, both subdural haemorrhage and retinal haemorrhage were seen together in 60% of children.[18] In another series, all four shaken babies had subarachnoid, intra-arachnoid, and subdural optic nerve sheath haemorrhage, whereas of those with shaking plus head impact 55% had subarachnoid, 44% had intra-arachnoid, and 100% had subdural blood.[43] Haemorrhage within the optic nerve sheath is a characteristic finding of Terson syndrome and has often, but not always,[33,43,70] been described in SBS postmortem studies (Plate 10.3).[41] It is not visible to the clinician antemortem. In Terson syndrome, this appears to be an important finding the pathophysiological implications of which remain unclear. In addition, Terson syndrome can occur without optic nerve sheath haemorrhage, or haemorrhage involving only part of the length of the sheath.[49] Although significantly more common in SBS as compared to other causes of child abuse death,[17] it is also seen in many other circumstances as well. Some authors suggest that subdural optic nerve sheath haemorrhage is more characteristic of SBS whereas isolated subarachnoid optic nerve sheath haemorrhage would favour a non SBS differential diagnosis.[79] However, SBS may occur with subdural optic nerve sheath haemorrhage but no intracranial haemorrhage[55] or no retinal haemorrhage.[43]

The exact mechanism by which optic nerve sheath haemorrhage occurs is unknown. It may be due to the tracking of blood from the subarachnoid or subdural space[21,80] and/or due to sudden elevation of intracranial pressure brought on by the intracranial haemorrhage which in turn is transmitted down the optic nerve sheath causing the rupture of bridging vessels within the sheath.[63,64,76,81] Whether the optic nerve sheath blood has a role in the generation of retinal haemorrhages is also unknown. Although there was some early evidence to the contrary[82] and this may play a minor role in generating retinal haemorrhage, the current weight of evidence seems to indicate that blood in the optic nerve sheath does not directly enter the retina and the anatomy of the sheath should prevent this.[83] Some have theorised that compression or rupture of the central retinal vein may contribute[21,49,76,80,83–85] and compression of the artery might be possible. If the vein is compressed, and the thick walled artery less so, then there is a mismatch between blood entering the eye at a rate greater than it can drain. This may lead to rupture of retinal veins.[80,83] However, in SBS, the characteristic radiating pattern of superficial intraretinal haemorrhages seen in classic adult vein occlusions is usually absent. Yet, retinal ischaemia may be the cause of the uncommon observation of macular oedema.[86] At least one patient went on to develop neovascularization of the iris[86] and another neovascular glaucoma[63]: both are well recognised late complications of retinal ischaemia. I believe that orbital shaking (see below) may be a major factor in causing direct trauma to the optic nerve resulting in haemorrhage within the sheath, perhaps unrelated to the intracranial bleeding.

One postmortem study found that all children who had optic nerve sheath haemorrhage (75% of the studied SBS victims) had subdural haemorrhage with only half having subarachnoid haemorrhage.[36] Although all of the children had retinal haemorrhages, two had subdural haemorrhage and four had subarachnoid haemorrhage without optic nerve sheath haemorrhage. In one postmortem study, 83% of shaken babies with retinal haemorrhages also had cerebral oedema.[36] Another study found that, unlike retinal haemorrhages, the presence of optic nerve sheath haemorrhage is not quite statistically significant as an indicator for shaking as opposed to blunt trauma (accidental or non accidental).[35] In addition, despite a 69% incidence of optic nerve sheath haemorrhage in another postmortem study of shaken babies, using the intracranial approach to identify the entire length of the optic nerve, the authors found that blood was only found in the anterior portion of the sheath with no continuous tracking back towards the brain.[17] Others have also observed this to be the most common location.[10] Therefore, the failure to examine the entire length of optic nerve might otherwise lead to the false conclusion that the observed blood was indeed from the intracranial space.

Although Terson syndrome in adults may indeed produce a haemorrhagic retinopathy and optic nerve sheath haemorrhage that resembles the clinical picture seen in SBS, it appears to be rare in childhood in the absence of SBS and insufficient as a complete explanation for the findings in SBS. The histopathology of the retinal lesions, especially domed shaped macular haemorrhages, is quite different. In addition, we studied a consecutive series of patients with intracranial haemorrhage of any type or aetiology with the exclusion of any proven or suspected cases of SBS. We found no child with retinal haemorrhage except for those who had typical peripapillary haemorrhages due to papilloedema. Others have noted that when retinal haemorrhage is due to subarachnoid haemorrhage, the haemorrhages in the retina are usually around the optic nerve and flame shaped,[21] findings consistent with papilloedema. Our statistics allow us to predict that the maximal incidence of retinal haemorrhages not due to papilloedema in patients with intracranial haemorrhage and not due to abuse is less than 5%.

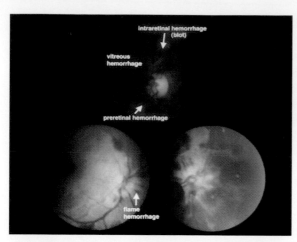

Plate 10.1 Retinal haemorrhages in shaken baby syndrome. (**A**) Upper photograph shows a variety of haemorrhages. Note that preretinal haemorrhage obscures underlying retinal blood vessel. Vitreous haemorrhage comes forward towards observer with indistinct margins. (**B**) Right (on left side) and left (on ride side) eyes of same patient. Note extreme asymmetry with left eye more affected. Left eye has many large preretinal haemorrhages.

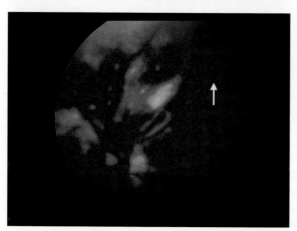

Plate 10.2 Arrow indicates one of many white centred intraretinal haemorrhages in shaken baby.

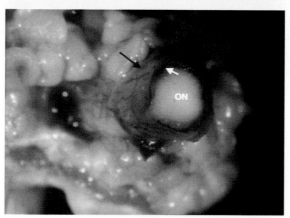

Plate 10.3 Cut section of optic nerve from a shaken baby. Black arrow indicates optic nerve sheath (dura). White arrow indicates optic nerve sheath haemorrhage. ON = optic nerve parenchyma.

This low incidence of Terson syndrome in children is also reflected in the literature on accidental head trauma, intracranial aneurysm, and arteriovenous malformations discussed below. One child was reported with a convincing story for ocular haemorrhage following subarachnoid haemorrhage although the exact cause in this ill, hospitalised infant was unknown and

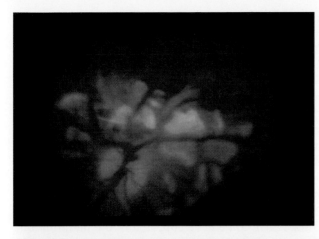

Plate 10.4 Purtscher retinopathy in shaken baby syndrome. Note large white patches in addition to retinal haemorrhages.

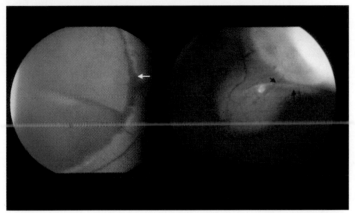

Plate 10.5 Traumatic retinoschisis and paramacular folds. Left frame shows layered blood (*) in schisis cavity. Note haemorrhagic circumferential line (white arrow) indicating edge of schisis cavity. Right frame shows another child with a hypopigmented curvilinear fold in macula (black arrow) indicating edge of schisis cavity. Arrowhead indicates retinal vessel kinking as it goes over the fold. In right frame, blood has broken out of schisis cavity diffusely into the vitreous (*).

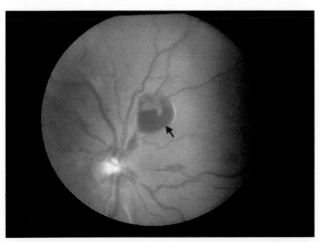

Plate 10.6 Schisis-like cavity over a blood vessel (arrow) containing a blood level. Two flame haemorrhages are also present.

may have included meningitis and/or hyponatremia.[87] The child, who had a previous normal inpatient eye examination, had bilateral subhyaloid and vitreous haemorrhage. There have also been a few cases of presumed neonatal vitreous haemorrhage attributed to Terson syndrome.[88,89] However, details are sparse, the causes are not given, the diagnosis of vitreous haemorrhage delayed, and no criteria are cited for ruling out abuse in most cases.[88]. In addition, it is unknown if these children had retinal haemorrhaging, as surgery to remove the vitreous was delayed in some so that haemorrhages, which may have been present in the retina, were not seen by the time the retina was viewable. One infant also had subretinal haemorrhage.[88] Another group reported a 5-year-old with spontaneous subarachnoid haemorrhage with a few posterior pole haemorrhages and optic nerve sheath haemorrhage.[53] In the peripheral retina, haemorrhage was microscopic only. Other occasional cases of presumed paediatric Terson syndrome have appeared in the literature but most authors agree that it is extremely rare[77] (as also evidenced by the few reports) and usually occurs with features that suggest, at the least, abusive head injury, if not shaking. For example, one case from France involved a 3-month-old with traumatic acute SDH, multiple hypodensities in the brain, and bilateral total vitreous haemorrhages.[77] No details of the history are given. This type of scenario has never been reported in any child without SBS.

Although the overwhelming majority of SBS victims with retinal haemorrhages do have intracranial haemorrhage, there are at least two reported cases of retinal haemorrhages without intracranial bleeding. One child had 'multiple dot, blot and flame-shaped haemorrhages' in both eyes.[90] This child also had profound hypothermia. Another child, in the early days of CT scanning, was found only to have diffuse cerebral oedema. We reported a case in which the intracranial haemorrhage was detected by MRI but not by CT.[46]

Increased intrathoracic pressure (Purtscher retinopathy)

Purtscher retinopathy is characterised by large white patches in the retina which may represent fat emboli, superficial retinal infarction, or exudate, following severe compressive chest trauma.[91,92] This retinal picture has been attributed to many causes, correctly or incorrectly, including head trauma and fat embolism,[92] but is rarely seen in SBS (Plate 10.4).[93,94] However, as perpetrators may compress the child's chest to a degree which causes rib fractures, there must certainly be an associated increase in intrathoracic pressure. Some authors feel that this pressure can be transmitted up to the retinal veins contributing to the formation of retinal haemorrhages.[39,91,93] Others feel the increased pressure in the thorax leads to arteriospasm with secondary endothelial damage and increased vascular permeability.[24] In addition, if retinal haemorrhages are generated by an apparent vascular malfunction, one might expect the haemorrhages to be paravascular which may or may not be observed in SBS.[21]

Occasionally a caretaker will report that they fell on the child.[13] Despite the great weight disproportion, I doubt that this type of injury would specifically result in enough compression of the chest to create retinopathy. In addition, most adults will try to brace themselves as they fall so that their complete body weight will not be felt by the child. This type of retinopathy would be more likely to require forces equivalent to a car rolling over a child's chest[13] and this is perhaps best confirmed by the **absence** of haemorrhages in some infants despite the presence of rib fractures. In addition, the presence of unilateral retinal haemorrhage in some shaken infants argues against this theory as the increased venous pressure theoretically transmitted to the eyes should be bilateral.[33]

Vitreous shaking

In children, the vitreous is particularly well attached to the retina in the posterior pole, at blood vessels, and at the peripheral retina, towards the ora serrata.[95] In fact, unlike adults, the retinal surgeon is often faced with the technical challenge of peeling the vitreous away without tearing the retina, whereas in adults the two separate with less difficulty. In children, the vitreous is also more formed and gelatinous with higher viscosity than in adults.[20,88] The retina of children is more resistant to mechanical stress.[19] That vitreous traction in children can result in histological stripping of the internal limiting membrane has been demonstrated in normal eyes at postmortem.[96] This may be a phenomenon which is unique to the childhood eye.[96]

When a child is shaken, the vitreous is also shaking, which then causes shearing forces to be applied to the retina especially at points of firm attachment. The posterior retina may be sheared at the plane of any of its 10 layers causing a cystic cavity to form which may be partially or completely filled with blood. Although, in 1991, one author[97] wrote that until 'it is unequivocally proven...it is imperative that we not equate retinal folds with child abuse', this lesion, traumatic retinoschisis (meaning 'retinal splitting'), has now been well documented in shaken babies clinically, by ultrasound, by electroretinogram, and histologically by many authors (Plate 10.5).[30,32,33,50,55,71,98] Head trauma need not be part of the shaking incident which results in retinoschisis.[41] Postmortem, the anterior-posterior shearing of the retina may be observed as a widening of any of the retinal layers and/or a stripping of just the internal limiting membrane. The vitreous may remain adherent to the affected area or, especially when blood has extended from the cavity into the vitreous, the vitreous may be detached from the retina.[51] In one interesting case, I have seen shearing at all layers of the retina including a splitting of the outer from the inner parts of the rods and cones.

In recognising traumatic retinoschisis clinically, one may observe a curvilinear edge, sometimes haemorrhagic, with or without a fold of retina or an underlying depigmentation of the retinal pigmented epithelium (the outermost (deepest) layer of retina) (Plate 10.5).[34,41,96] It is critical that this edge change be recognised since, when present, it distinguishes retinoschisis from subhyaloid haemorrhage. Particularly when the surface of the retinoschisis cavity is the internal limiting membrane, blood may break through into the subhyaloid space or vitreous. This may obscure the edge changes of the cavity which will become apparent as the blood resolves. The fold may be continuous for 360º, discontinuous, or represent just an arc.[34] It may encompass just the macula or surround the entire posterior pole including the optic nerve.[34,99] Peripheral retinoschisis cavities have also been described in SBS.[34] Both peripheral and macular traumatic retinoschisis may be associated with worse neurological injury and death although the latter was demonstrated only in a small case series.[34]

Vitreous is also well attached at superficial retinal blood vessels. At the site of blood vessel attachment vascular ruptures can occur, due to shearing injury of the vessel wall, with the accumulation of preretinal or sub-internal limiting membrane circular foci directly over the vessels (Plate 10.6).[32] This is a less specific finding as any entity which causes a focal bleed at the site of a blood vessel (e.g. leukaemia, vasculitis) can cause this small focal finding.

Although vitreous shaking with resultant shearing forces has clearly been shown to be the cause of traumatic retinoschisis both clinically and at autopsy, some authors have speculated that similar shearing forces in SBS may also be the cause of intraretinal and subhyaloid haemorrhages.[7,10,17,53] In addition, the vitreous is more firmly attached to the retina at its peripheral edges (the vitreous base). Traction at this location during shaking may be related to the observation of peripheral retinal haemorrhages in SBS.[33,42,63]

In long-term follow-up, some children with traumatic retinoschisis, particularly when only the internal limiting membrane is raised, will have no sequelae and remarkably good vision. The separated layers can be observed clinically to settle back down. Even when the internal limiting membrane remains raised, if the rest of the retina is intact, I and others have observed near normal visual recovery.[100] In other children, permanent curvilinear hypo-pigmented scars and/or retinal folds may be seen surrounding the macula or the entire posterior pole.[41] The observation of such a finding in a child with no prior history of shaking should certainly make the clinician suspect that prior SBS may have gone undiagnosed.

It should be noted that another entity which is associated with spontaneous paediatric vitreous haemorrhage (but not isolated retinal haemorrhage), juvenile X-linked retinoschisis is an entirely different disorder which is easily recognised on ophthalmic examination by an examiner familiar with this entity and would not easily be confused with SBS findings. This heritable disorder is caused by spontaneous random splitting of the superficial retinal layers due to a defect in their adherence. The gene is known and testing can be performed to confirm the diagnosis. However, the clinical appearance is entirely different than that seen in the traumatic retinoschisis of SBS. In fact, although patients with juvenile X-linked retinoschisis have 'foveal schisis' this has a diagnostic stellate or 'cartwheel' appearance and they do not get the isolated macular cysts with paramacular folds seen in SBS.

Orbital shaking

The optic nerve is longer than the distance between the apex (its entry point) of the bony orbit and the eyeball. This slack allows us to move our eyes in all directions. This may also allow for the eyeball and orbital contents to shake when the child is shaken. As the optic nerve and other intra-orbital structures (muscles, cranial nerve branches) are firmly attached both to the eyeball and the apex of the orbit (Fig. 10.5), injury may occur at these tethering locations as a result of angular, rotational or axial movements about the points of fixation. This may be one explanation for findings of optic nerve sheath haemorrhage only anteriorly (or predominantly anteriorly)[43] suggesting that the blood did not arise from communication with the intracranial space.[17] Optic nerve contusion may also occur[21] with resultant afferent pupillary defects (Marcus Gunn pupil) observed on clinical examination. Intradural optic nerve sheath

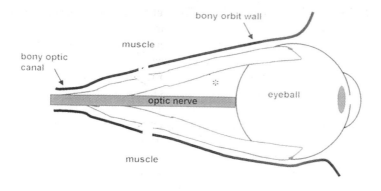

Fig. 10.5 Schematic representation of normal orbit. Note that optic nerve and muscles are fixed to bony wall at or around entrance to bony optic nerve canal. Other orbital contents including fat, other muscles, blood vessels, and cranial nerves not shown.

haemorrhage may be a sign that is characteristic of such trauma to the nerve and its sheath.[73] It occurs only rarely in adult Terson syndrome and then, only in small amounts with red bloods cells found directly contiguous with the subdural space.[80,83] In one study of shaken babies with and without blunt head impact, all had intradural haemorrhage of the optic nerve sheath [43]

The sclera is an optic nerve fixation which would, therefore, be at high risk of damage as the orbital contents are shaken.[73] Two groups have found that the presence of posterior scleral haemorrhage was statistically more likely to be seen when shaking was a component of the injury.[35,53] Intrascleral haemorrhage is seen in approximately 25% of postmortem examinations of shaken infants.[10,35] One study of adults with Terson syndrome specifically notes that the subdural and subarachnoid optic nerve sheath blood is contained in a cul-de-sac with no direct communication with or blood in the sclera.[83] Yet in a single 5-year-old with spontaneous idiopathic subarachnoid haemorrhage, intrascleral haemorrhage has been reported.[53]

Likewise, our studies using the *en bloc* technique described below, have shown laceration of the optic nerve sheath, posterior optic nerve sheath haemorrhage, posterior intradural optic nerve sheath haemorrhage, and haemorrhage within the posterior muscle and cranial nerve sheaths. Although there is some experimental evidence in cats[81] that blood in the optic nerve sheath may induce porosity of the sheath allowing blood to escape into the orbit, perhaps as a natural mechanism of decompression to protect the nerve, even this would not explain how blood could independently appear in the sheaths of other orbital nerves and the extra-ocular muscles. These cats did not have retinal or vitreous haemorrhage. In a study of human adults with optic nerve sheath haemorrhagefollowing a variety of causes of sudden increased intracranial pressure, intradural and extradural haemorrhage was observed in the majority.[46] Yet no mention is made of blood within muscle or cranial nerve sheaths, which may not have been examined. These findings may have significant diagnostic value as we also did not see them in a preterm baby with intra-ocular haemorrhage due to retinopathy or prematurity or in a child who died from severe accidental head trauma some retinal haemorrhages (see Accidental Head

Trauma below). Interestingly, the latter child did have a few microscopic red blood cells in the posterior optic nerve sheath and surrounding apical orbital fat suggesting that this single severe acceleration–deceleration injury may be a 'microcosm' of the repetitive lethal shaking seen in SBS. Even in the setting of severe accidental head trauma in adults, for example victims of motorcycle accidents who were not wearing helmets, the incidence of orbital trauma or optic nerve injury is relatively low (11% and 19%, respectively).[101] Orbital apex syndromes, as seen in our pathological specimens from abused children, are even rarer in these motorcycle accident victims (2%). However, the author does not give us information on retinal haemorrhages in this setting or on the relationship of optic nerve injury to orbital trauma or type of central nervous system injury.

Although there is no laboratory animal model for SBS and the retinal haemorrhages seen in SBS, the woodpecker does offer us some theoretical support for the concept that orbital shaking may be particularly injurious. Woodpeckers, of course, spend a lifetime of remarkable daily repetitive acceleration–deceleration with blunt impact. Yet, they do not suffer any apparent ocular injury. There are 4 ocular protective mechanisms which may prevent damage from occurring. With each impact the woodpecker closes its eyes forcibly thus tightening up the eyeball in the socket making it less able to shake. Also, with each impact, a muscle which is present in the scleral eye covering contracts, thus firming up the intra-ocular contents to make them more resistant to acceleration–deceleration. This muscle is not present in humans. In addition, the vitreous of a woodpecker is much more viscous than that of humans. Lastly, unlike humans, woodpeckers have no space between the back of the eyeball and the bony orbit. Orbital shaking can not occur.

Despite the convincing evidence that orbital shaking injury does occur, the exact mechanism by which this may induce intra-ocular haemorrhage is unclear. Perhaps disruption of autonomic nerves travelling along with the cranial nerve branches impairs retinal vascular autoregulation. Alternatively, there may be direct disruption of blood flow to and from the eye such as the ciliary circulation.[73] If the central retinal vein or artery were injured, this could lead to the same findings previously attributed to blood in the nerve sheath (see above). In addition, this mechanism may help to explain the not uncommon presence of optic atrophy seen in SBS survivors (see below).

Other contributing factors

Strangulation may be seen in association with an SBS event with retinal haemorrhages.[15,70,102] Asymmetric occlusion of the carotids may, in part, explain some of the asymmetric ocular and brain findings as well.[15,102]. The mechanism by which retinal haemorrhages may result could be due to venous stasis or retinal ischaemia. Anaemia and anoxia, although not primary independent causes of retinal haemorrhages (see below), may contribute to severity and the variable presentations between cases. Coagulopathy may be associated with abusive parenchymal brain injury particularly when the injury is fatal.[103] Severe rapid deceleration, likened by some to air pilots ejecting from their planes,[32] may play a role. Coup-contrecoup injury has been suggested to have a role by one author.[104] Retinal haemorrhages may be seen in association with central retinal vein occlusion, perhaps due to optic nerve swelling or haemorrhage within the nerve sheath. However, central retinal vein occlusion is well recognised in adults by its association with a radiating pattern of haemorrhages, usually superficial intraretinal, extending outward from the optic nerve in one or more quadrants. Central retinal artery occlusion has also been described in SBS,[1,100,105,106] however this usually results in retinal ischaemia, with or without a cherry red spot, rather than haemorrhages. In some cases, it appears that this diagnosis was actually made on late outcome findings of optic nerve atrophy and retinal vessel thinning although other mechanisms could result in similar findings.

Diagnosis of retinal haemorrhage

The non-ophthalmologist using a direct ophthalmoscope, particularly when the pupil is not dilated, is very likely to be less accurate and complete in the examination of the retina than the ophthalmologist using the binocular indirect ophthalmoscope.[107] Only with the indirect ophthalmoscope can the topography of the retinal haemorrhages be well described and the peripheral retina to the ora serrata viewed. The direct ophthalmoscope used by non ophthalmologists cannot provide these views. It is not uncommon for an initial examination done by the emergency department physician, family physician, neurologist, neurosurgeon and/or paediatrician through an undilated pupil with a direct ophthalmoscope (especially when the child is awake and non compliant) to record in the chart the absence of retinal haemorrhages. Shortly thereafter, when complete ophthalmic consultation is performed, haemorrhages may be discovered, which leads to confusion about whether or not they were present at the onset or secondary to some in-hospital event, when in fact the findings, even if extensive, were almost certainly present at the time of the first non ophthalmologist examination. Perhaps it would be advisable for the non ophthalmologist to label their examination as 'incomplete' or 'preliminary' and note the situation under which the examination was performed (e.g. undilated non compliant patient).

The many difficulties inherent in using only the direct ophthalmoscope and forensic importance of peripheral retinal haemorrhages[41] mandate that indirect ophthalmoscopy be performed by an ophthalmologist. Although some authors may have suggested a consultation protocol of lesser scope,[72] other authors and I believe it is essential for an ophthalmologist familiar with the findings in SBS, using an indirect ophthalmoscope through a pharmacologically dilated pupil to examine the entire retina to characterise the retinal haemorrhages, in all cases of possible or suspected SBS, if not all physically abused children less than 4 years-old.[17,29,39] Perhaps all children in this age group with unexplained seizures, altered mental status, hydrocephalus, cerebral atrophy, subdural effusions, or head trauma without satisfactory explanatory history should have an ophthalmology consultation. The ophthalmology examination should be conducted as early as possible in the evaluation of the patient who may be a victim of SBS.[108] Failure to perform dilated indirect ophthalmoscopy may cause positive findings to be missed.[29] In the brain dead or severely brain injured child, the pupils may be fixed and mid dilated thus obviating the need for dilating drops.

Occasionally, there may be objections or concerns about dilating the pupils if they are being used to monitor the neurological status of a severely brain injured child. Although it is rare that pupil monitoring is absolutely necessary, should such concerns arise the ophthalmologist may be given one of the following options: dilate one pupil at a time, use short acting dilating drops (phenylephrine 2.5%, tropicamide 0.5%), or conduct the examination through undilated pupils. Lenses are available which may allow the ophthalmologist a fairly wide retinal view with an undilated or poorly dilated (which sometimes occurs with the short acting drops) pupil. If using this option, the ophthalmologist should re-examine the child as soon as the clinical situation allows. Whenever possible, dilated examination is preferred. When feasible, the pupils should be examined and documented for size, shape, reactivity, and afferent defects prior to dilation (see Pupillary Abnormalities below).

After death, clinical indirect ophthalmoscopy can still be performed; sometimes for as long as 72 h, until the cornea becomes too cloudy to allow for a view. When possible, this may be useful as it adds a topographical view that may be lost to the limits of microscopic examination, particularly when limited sections of the eyeball are examined.

The eyes should be removed in all cases of sudden unexplained infant death, especially when clinical examination reveals retinal haemorrhage, there is evidence of intracranial injury, SBS is suspected, or such clinical eye examination was not performed.[108] Some have been hesitant to take this route for fear of disrupting the appearance of the corpse particularly when it may be viewed before or during the funeral. In fact, after death, the eyeballs of adults and children naturally sink into the orbit. To correct this 'sunken' appearance, it is standard procedure to place eyecaps over the eyeballs and under the lids in funeral preparation. The caps are also designed to help keep the lids from opening. Therefore, removal of the eyes in no way alters the appearance of the body. The funeral director simply fills the socket with gauze or other materials and places the very same caps.

The eyeball has traditionally been removed from an anterior (trans-conjunctival) approach as is typical for enucleation. By this technique, scissors are placed blindly behind the globe to sever the optic nerve, usually within millimetres of the eyeball. This will lead to varying segments of optic nerve at histological examination.[70] Alternatively, the eye may be removed through a combined transconjunctival and intracranial approach.[43,53] This does not induce artefact haemorrhages.[109] The latter portion of the technique begins after the brain is removed and floor of the anterior cranial fossa visible. Each orbital roof is then removed by use of saws and ronjeurs so that the orbital periosteum is visualised intact. Some authors have then incised the periosteum and carefully dissected through the orbital tissues to expose the optic nerve.[16,43,53] Although this is useful to view orbital shaking injuries and to allow for removal of a long segment of optic nerve, we prefer to remove the entire orbital contents *en bloc* with the eyeball and then fix the entire specimen together (usually for 2–3 days) before sectioning *en bloc*. It is only with these techniques that we have been able to view the orbital shaking injuries described above such as apical orbital haemorrhage and haemorrhage within the sheaths of nerves and muscles. This method is perhaps the most suitable for autopsy in the evaluation of sudden infant death where SBS is in the differential diagnosis.[16,36,57] Like standard enucleation, removal of the eyeball with the orbital contents does not mar the appearance of the corpse for funeral viewing.

Differential diagnosis

Despite the belief by some that SBS may be over diagnosed,[39] the overwhelming preponderance of medical opinion concludes that the association of characteristic brain injuries and retinal haemorrhages is diagnostic of SBS.[17,39] The Position Statement of the American Society of Neurosurgeons lists retinal haemorrhages as one of the 'cardinal findings' of non accidental injury.[110] In fact, when considering a child with the full spectrum of skeletal and brain injuries, without another compelling acceptable explanation, the presence or absence of retinal haemorrhages is not likely to raise contention with regards to the SBS diagnosis. However, although some authors feel that 'retinal haemorrhages' (using the generic non-specific terminology) are pathognomonic for child abuse,[111] a small number of intraretinal haemorrhages, in the absence of retinoschisis, confined to the posterior pole may be less specific for SBS. A pattern of multiple haemorrhages distributed throughout the retina, to the ora serrata[52,69] especially in the presence of preretinal, vitreous, or subretinal haemorrhage[21] would not be expected as a result of any of the alternate circumstances discussed below. Such a picture is virtually pathognomonic of SBS in the absence of another viable explanation. Some authors may have challenged this conclusion yet fail to provide adequate evidence to the contrary.[34] One author[97] wrote, in 1991 that 'there is no evidence that clearly establishes that retinal haemorrhages, be they intraretinal, subretinal, or subhyaloid, are indicative of nonaccidental trauma'. The text below should clearly demonstrate that this statement is absolutely false. Another author,[112] a non ophthalmologist who testified for the defence in a well-publicised case of SBS in which the perpetrator was found guilty, states that retinal haemorrhage, 'regardless of its characteristics, is at best an external marker for probable head injury'. Yes, retinal haemorrhages are most often due to head injury – that resulting from SBS. The text below will review the published evidence that shows the absolute essential need to describe the characteristics of retinal haemorrhage in assessing specificity. In addition, this author's assertions regarding other possible causes of retinal haemorrhage (ruptured vascular malformations, arachnoid cysts, central nervous system infections)[112] will be examined.

Traumatic retinoschisis has never been described in children due to any entity other than SBS so its presence is diagnostic. However, in adults, subhyaloid or sub-internal limiting membrane haemorrhages due to Terson syndrome and other disorders may appear remarkably very similar.[51,113–115] Retinal folds (sometimes referred to as paramacular folds) may even be present.[49,51,113,114,116,117] But in these adults, in all of the reported cases, the primary cause (i.e. coagulopathy, accidental head injury, intracranial aneurysm) is readily apparent and other retina findings characteristic of SBS are often absent.

In one large study of patients with Terson syndrome, there were only 5 children, all of whom were less than 1-year-old, who had subdural haemorrhage and 'haemorrhagic macular cyst' which by description (no photographs provided) sound very much like the lesion characteristic of traumatic retinoschisis.[51] Although only one child is cited as a victim of child abuse in the paper, my personal communication with the first author reveals that all five children were suspected victims of abuse (Dr F. Kuhn, personal communication). Whether or not these children were shaken in addition to sustaining impact abusive head injury is unclear.[78] The study unfortunately did not include paediatrician co-authors, so the exact circumstances of the injuries and the subsequent investigations, beyond the recognition of abuse, is not available. Dr Kuhn and co-workers believe that the presence of intracranial blood, more than a history of trauma, is the common denominator in the formation of these haemorrhagic retinal cysts,[117] yet such lesions have not been described in children other than those who are abused. In a prior publication by the same group, presumably of the same patients, one photograph is offered which shows a large bulbous mushroom-shaped subinternal limiting membrane macular haemorrhage which does not look like the traumatic retinoschisis of SBS as it lacks a demarcation fold and is larger than any lesion I have ever seen in SBS.[116] Presumably, the 4 children included in the earlier paper includes 3 of the same children from their 1998 paper and one 5-years-old.[116] If one considers just the adults in the early paper group, only 7 of 28 eyes (25%) had subinternal limiting membrane bleeding demonstrating that this is an uncommon finding in Terson syndrome. Other authors have confirmed this conclusion,[49] yet controversy remains.[117]

There are other reasons to believe that traumatic retinoschisis is different than the premacular haemorrhages seen in adults with Terson syndrome thus refuting the role of accidental head trauma in childhood haemorrhagic retinopathy similar to the picture seen in SBS. The reported lesions in adults with Terson syndrome that mimic traumatic retinoschisis seem to differ from the SBS victims in that the adult lesions may be associated with preretinal membrane formation,[51] the contraction of which may be the cause of internal limiting membrane stripping with blood accumulation. In one study of two adults with subinternal limiting membrane blood and retinal folds, the internal limiting membrane or cicatricial membrane was described as taught between the folds.[113] Both of these adults had surgery relatively late after their injury and ocular haemorrhage, so perhaps the finding was indeed cicatricial. In another study, the authors showed convincingly that the dome-shaped lesion of Terson syndrome does not involve the internal limiting membrane; but rather a membrane that forms over a preretinal haemorrhage in long standing cases.[49] This is distinctly different than the ballooning forward of the internal limiting membrane in traumatic retinoschisis. Traumatic retinoschisis has not been observed to be associated with cicatrix or internal limiting membrane contraction. In addition, optic nerve atrophy, a not uncommon long-term finding in SBS (see below) is not usually present.[51] Lastly, pigmentary changes at the edges of premacular haemorrhage in Terson syndrome, which resemble the subretinal pigmentary alterations seen at the edges of traumatic retinoschisis lesions, are probably due to breakdown products of blood rather than the shearing trauma to the retina seen in SBS.[49]

When considering the component of retinal haemorrhages in isolation, one must consider the possibility of other causes and recognize when the observed findings are more or less diagnostic of SBS. One must also remember that, with the exception of birth haemorrhages, SBS is by many orders of magnitude one of the most common causes of retinal haemorrhages in children. We must also recognize that the presence of any of the conditions listed below does not preclude the possibility (or likelihood) that the child was also shaken. It is equally as important to avoid false diagnosis of abuse as it is to avoid missing the diagnosis of abuse. Yet we must have the courage to make the correct diagnosis based on the available medical evidence, to report our appropriate suspicion as mandated by law, and to develop systems which allow minimal trauma to families even when this suspicion proves to be invalid.

The first three entities below are those which are most often suggested as a possible alternate explanation of retinal haemorrhages in an infant under suspicion as a possible victim of shaking.

Birth

Normal birth is the most common cause of retinal haemorrhages in infancy. Although retinal haemorrhages can be seen after any type of delivery,[118–123] including caesarean section,[124] they are most common after spontaneous vaginal and vacuum assisted vaginal delivery.[122–125] They have a particularly high incidence after failed vacuum extraction although there is not an increase in macular haemorrhage.[126] The exact mechanism by which these haemorrhages are caused is unknown. Theories have included direct birth or forceps trauma, increased intracranial pressure, release of extra cranial pressure, ocular or cranial compression, increased intrathoracic pressure, asphyxia, hypertension, change from maternal to new-born circulation, neck compression, and unequal pressure distributions.[122,124,127] Infants with retinal haemorrhages do not have associated brain injury.[122,124,127] There is conflicting data regarding the influence of labour length, labour severity, and maternal parity, although length of the fist stage of labour may be proportional to the incidence of haemorrhages.[54,122,124] There is some evidence that they may be due to prostaglandin release, as there is a significant increase in incidence when labour is induced with prostaglandin agents.[54] The prostaglandin effect may be mediated by changes in the blood–retinal barrier. This may also explain the lower incidence (1–12%) of retinal haemorrhage after caesarean section,[122] since amniotomy is associated with release of prostaglandins.

The incidence also depends on the time of the examination and mode of delivery. In the first 36 h of life, the aggregate incidence is approximately 2–45% with most authors citing a figure of approximately 20–30%.[118,119,121,122,124–126,128,129] By 72 h, the incidence drops to 11–15%.[119,120,122,127] The incidence of retinal haemorrhages following birth is not altered by maternal prepartum cocaine use.[130] Maternal toxaemia increases the frequency of neonatal vascular abnormalities but does not increase the number of haemorrhages.[131] Retinal haemorrhages due to birth resolve without sequelae in almost all cases.[121,122,129]

The distribution of birth-induced retinal haemorrhages can be quite widespread and may even extend to the ora serrata. Haemorrhages are found in the macula in 0–12% of cases.[125,129] Haemorrhages beyond the posterior pole and preretinal haemorrhages are uncommon.[122,123] One study found such haemorrhages in only 10% of cases.[54] Birth retinal haemorrhages are almost always limited to dot, blot, or flame haemorrhages.[122,124,131] One case of subinternal limiting membrane haemorrhage in the macula along with subhyaloid haemorrhage has been reported.[132] Subretinal haemorrhage may rarely be observed, if not clinically, then postmortem.[129] One case of choroidal haemorrhage has been reported.[121] The haemorrhages may be unilateral or bilateral although the latter is more common.[124,129] Asymmetry between the eyes can occur.[132] Haemorrhages may be more severe on the side where vacuum extraction was performed.[122,124] Vitreous haemorrhage is extremely rare, occurring in less than 2% of new-borns,[133] although in one study of surgical patients it was the cause for at least half the vitreous haemorrhages seen in the first year of life.[89] The vitreous haemorrhage, in the few reported cases, is usually unilateral unless associated with systemic disease.[89,134] It may be associated with evidence of direct ocular trauma such as hyphema in a child with face presentation.[91]

When all of the literature on this topic is taken together, we can conclude that all birth induced flame haemorrhages should be resolved by 1 week and dot/blot haemorrhages by 6 weeks. Even the case of subinternal limiting membrane haemorrhage resolved within 1 month.[132] These are actually conservative numbers in that the majority of haemorrhages, even when severe, are resolved much sooner in each category.[54] Flame haemorrhages usually resolve in 3–5 days.[118,119] I am aware of only one report where a haemorrhage, deep macular, lasted to 6-weeks-old[118] and I have seen a child with a single large (approximately 2 x 2 mm) fading peripheral birth intraretinal haemorrhage at this age. Therefore, the presence of haemorrhages of these types after the given 'deadlines', can not be attributed to birth. Likewise, retinal haemorrhages diagnosed within these timelines must be interpreted with caution when attributing them to causes other than birth. The examiner should look for signs which clearly distinguish haemorrhages as being more consistent with SBS such as traumatic retinoschisis cavities, perimacular retinal folds, severe extensive haemorrhaging, haemorrhages to the retinal periphery, subretinal haemorrhage, vitreous haemorrhage, and other systemic signs of SBS induced trauma before categorically concluding that the haemorrhages are due to SBS rather than birth. Yet there will still be cases which are left indeterminate as any haemorrhage pattern seen after birth could in fact be consistent with shaking although the converse is not true.

Accidental head trauma

The recognition of the association of traumatic intracranial haemorrhage with retinal haemorrhages in adults has led to questions regarding the possibility that intracranial haemorrhage due to accidental head injury in children might also result in Terson syndrome. This is complicated by the high frequency of caretakers offering histories of relatively minor head trauma as the cause of injuries which generated a suspicion of SBS.[10,33] One interesting study noted a disproportionately high number of deaths in children with falls of only 1–4 ft as compared to those with falls over 10 ft.[135] On further review, 71% of the children with a history of lesser falls had old fractures, bruises on their trunk or extremities, genital injury, or two impact sites. Retinal haemorrhages were seen in 71% as well. These and other[65,136,137] authors conclude that such severe injury, including retinal haemorrhage, after a minor fall should certainly raise suspicion that the history is false and the child abused. As put in a recent review, 'most investigators agree that trivial forces, such as those involving routine play, infant swings, or falls from a low height are insufficient to cause' the injuries seen in SBS.[10,138] In another review, the author writes, 'findings of retinal haemorrhage ... indicate accelerative injury'. Most authors suggest that the presence of retinal haemorrhages after an alleged short fall should cause the history to be considered suspect.[12,13,53,138] Without a history of a major-fall (> 10 ft) or high-speed motor vehicle accident, these findings typically point to shaking or shaken/impact syndrome.[137]

In fact, there is a large body of medical literature which clearly shows that accidental head trauma, especially those falls which would be considered 'household', do not adequately explain the presence of retinal haemor-rhages,[33,39,138,139] even in rare instances when unusually severe head injury, such as depressed skull fracture or intracranial haemorrhage, results from such a fall.[137,139,140] Although there are a few investigators who correctly point out that some studies use children with accidental head trauma who are too old or without sufficient intracranial haemorrhage or injury to act as sufficient comparison groups to shaken infants,[97,141] when the body of literature is taken in aggregate, it becomes clear that retinal haemorrhages are found in no greater than 3% of accidental head trauma victims and the nature of the head injury is, almost always, severe and life threatening, with an obvious mechanism that would not raise the suspicion of abuse (e.g. motor vehicle accident).[35,66,70,138,139] Even when children who die of such severe head injury are studied, less than one-third will have retinal haemorrhages unless they were abused.[35,70]

Most authors find a zero incidence of retinal haemorrhage in accidentally head injured infants less than 3 years of age even in the presence of severe brain injury, subdural and/or epidural haemorrhage.[16,33,65,111,136,138,139,142,143] Stewart looked at 37 infants less than three months of age with closed head injuries and found no retinal haemorrhages even though two had multiple skull fractures and three had intracranial haemorrhage.[142] However, we are not told if these examinations were done by ophthalmologists with pharm-acological mydriasis. Elder and others found the same zero incidence at all ages in childhood.[145] Luerssen and co-workers found a 0.6% incidence of retinal haemorrhages following accidental head trauma in a study of 811 brain trauma patients.[145] Of the 27 patients overall with retinal haemorrhages, 22 (81%) were victims of abuse. Of the five remaining children we are only told the mechanism in one: motor vehicle accident. Duhaime and coworkers reported 4 children with retinal haemorrhages (no details given) following accidental head injury: 2 motor vehicle accidents, one fall down stairs in a walker (no details given), and one fatal three-story fall.[138] The National Pediatric Trauma Registry in the US, involving 85 centres, has collected data on over 4000 cases of paediatric accidental head trauma. Only 3 had retinal haemorrhages, although it is not known how many had full dilated eye examinations (personal communication, Dr Robert Sege). Of the abusive head trauma, 27% had retinal haemorrhages.

When they do occur, haemorrhages following accidental head trauma are usually confined to the posterior pole and few in number. In a postmortem study, the children with retinal haemorrhage following head trauma included unrestrained passengers in high speed motor vehicle accidents and a child thrown from a motorcycle.[53] Although details of the haemorrhages are not given on all, at least two had peripheral retinal haemorrhage but it was felt that the cause was acceleration–deceleration rather than blunt head injury. Gilliland and Folberg showed a statistically significant greater risk for shaking as a component of injury, as opposed to blunt trauma, when retinal haemorrhage and, in particular, peripheral retinal haemorrhage, were found.[35] Some reports unfortunately only use the generic term 'retinal haemorrhages' following accidental head injury.[146] One group mentions an 8-month-old struck by a truck who sustained 'severe intracranial, optic nerve sheath, and intraocular haemorrhages identical to those seen in abused infants' but does not characterise the haemorrhages any further or indicate whether there was direct trauma to the eyeball.[43] I have seen retinal haemorrhage in one child who was thrown 50 ft from a car following a motor vehicle accident. He died within 24 h and was found to have a small number of small scattered retinal haemorrhages along the vascular arcades and in the peripapillary region along with a single haemorrhage emanating from the disc on one side. Another child was struck by a car and had bilateral scattered small (all less than 0.5 mm) dot, blot, and flame throughout the posterior pole to the equator. She survived with severe neurological sequelae. Neither child showed any of the features of SBS such as traumatic retinoschisis cavities, peripheral RH, or preretinal haemorrhage. These cases illustrate how even the most severe accidental head injuries do not often cause the extensive retinal haemorrhaging characteristic of some shaken babies.

When interpreting reports of retinal haemorrhage after accidental head trauma, one must also be sure to exclude the possibility of concomitant blunt trauma to the eyeball itself. For example, one 9-month-old child who was injured by an unusual witnessed mechanism whereby he was being swung by his legs between his father's legs and struck the back of his head hard enough to sustain significant neurological injury requiring intubation, seizures, and subdural haematoma, was described as having unilateral 'diffuse flame-shaped haemorrhages and round intraretinal haemorrhages confined predominately to the posterior pole'.[147] However, the child also had macular oedema, a finding which is unusual in a shaken baby. On further communication with the ophthalmologist who examined the child, I learned that this oedema was felt to perhaps represent Berlin oedema (commotio retina) which is the equivalent of a retinal 'bruise' due to blunt trauma.

Other studies which apparently report the occasional child with severe haemorrhages or perhaps greater than 3% incidence of children with retinal haemorrhages presumably due to accidental head trauma must be interpreted carefully. In some, the injuries occurred prior to Caffey's description of SBS thus making it possible that some children were indeed shaken but missed due to the lack of recognition of the entity.[58,85,148–153] Caffey's own 1946 paper should ironically be placed in this category.[1] In a 1944 case, before modern neuroimaging and Caffey's recognition of SBS in the 1970s, a 4-month-old child was described as having 'numerous retinal haemorrhages' bilaterally after a fall from a dressing table.[85] The child suffered significant neurological injury (which makes the history suspect) including long-term hemiparesis but is described as only having an epidural haematoma and skull fracture. The contents of the cranium beyond the dura were not investigated, so it is impossible to rule out other injuries or SBS. Often, the haemorrhages are not described[58,152] or the nature of the head injury unclear.[58,152–154] One study reported that 70% of children less than 12-years-old with abnormal eye examinations had retinal haemorrhages.[154] However, they failed to evaluate the mechanism of head injury including the differentiation of accidental versus non accidental injury.[155] Another study reporting a 12% incidence also failed to make this distinction.[156] It may be that the majority of victims in these studies who had retinal haemorrhages were actually SBS victims. This is suggested in the second study by the finding that bilateral haemorrhages were more common in infants younger than 15 months. Likewise, another early paper found an increased incidence of retinal haemorrhages (not specified further) in the SBS age range in children with acute subdural haematoma.[152] Given the early nature of the cases (1968–1973), it is impossible to know what proportion represent shaken babies.

One specific entity, the tin ear syndrome, raises the possibility that blunt ipsilateral head trauma, involving the ear could perhaps induce rotational forces severe enough to cause ocular findings similar to SBS.[9] This unique form of child abuse is readily recognised by the presence of external ear ecchymosis, ipsilateral unilateral cerebral oedema with midline shift, ipsilateral subdural and subarachnoid haemorrhage, and ipsilateral diffuse paravenous retinal haemorrhages with or without vitreous haemorrhage. However, an accidental injury of this nature has not, to my knowledge, ever been reported in a child.

There is one study, from Japan, that deserves special mention since it reports findings that are in complete disagreement with all other literature on the subject.[148] Aoki and Masuzawa report 26 children, 3–13-months-old, who sustained acute SDH following minor falls; most often (65%) simply falling backwards from a sitting or standing position onto a soft tatami mat. All but 3 had seizures. Of the 20 patients in which the information was given, all but 4 had an occipital injury site. All 26 patients had 'retinal haemorrhage and dark red semicircular preretinal haemorrhage around the' optic nerve heads. Two photographs centred on the optic nerve heads are provided which show extensive dot, blot and flame haemorrhages in one eye with a large preretinal haemorrhage in the other. There is no papilloedema. These findings are unlike any ever reported in the literature or observed by me in an accidental head trauma victim and would otherwise suggest that the babies were shaken. In fact, there are many concerns about this paper which suggest that this may indeed be the case.

The authors do not state if complete investigations were done and, to my knowledge, there were no child abuse teams formed at that time in Japan. In addition, some of the children had findings on angiography suggestive of infarction; a finding which would be inconsistent with such mild accidental trauma. The children presented between 1972 and 1983 which means that some fall into the prerecognition era (before Caffey's original description). In addition, Japan did not have reporting laws for child abuse during this period and, in fact, was in many ways behind other countries in recognition, diagnosis, and evaluation for abuse (Dr Richard Krugman, personal communication). Despite the 1993 Child Abuse Prevention Act, one author has written in 1995 that there:

> is still a lack of consensus about definitions of child abuse in Japan ... there are many
> problems confronting professional staff in using the law to protect children from

abuse. Specialists in other countries are often surprised to learn that parents who sexually abuse their children are not punished by the criminal law.[157]

Another author, also writing in 1995, states:

There is presently in Japan no legislative body dealing with child abuse, there are not enough facilities, and staff members are not suitable trained to handle such child abuse cases.[158]

This same author goes on to report a case of obvious, but missed, non accidental head injury as an example of the commonality of failed diagnosis as late as the 1990s. The first child abuse telephone hotline was not established until 1990.[157,159] At the time of writing, there are no federal statutes for mandatory reporting or criminal statutes specific to child abuse (Japanese Embassy, Ottawa, Canada, personal communication).[157] It is interesting that another paper from Japan published in 1989 and attributing chronic subdural haemorrhage to late vitamin K deficiency prior to 1980, does not even list SBS as a potential cause of SDH in their discussion of differential diagnosis.[160]

All of these factors lead to a conclusion that it is very likely that the children reported by Aoki and Masuzawa represent missed cases of SBS rather than accidental head injuries.

Cardiopulmonary resuscitation with chest compressions

The possibility that cardiopulmonary resuscitation with chest compressions (CPR-CC) might result in retinal haemorrhages came out of the recognition that Purtscher retinopathy (see above) might be an explanation of the retinal haemorrhages in SBS, particularly in view of the known compressive chest trauma that often accompanies the injury resulting in fractured ribs. In addition, many children with possible SBS arrive *in extremis* and require CPR-CC at hospital. I am aware of only one case of Purtscher retinopathy following CPR,[70] thus further challenging the possibility of a sensible pathophyiological cause and effect relationship. In this case, the child had 'damaging chest compression' following resuscitation attempts.[70] The child also had entero-colitis suggesting the possibility of concomitant sepsis that may have contributed to the retinal findings. No further details are given about the retinal findings.

Although in earlier years it had been suggested that CPR-CC could cause retinal haemorrhages,[161] several studies have now been done all of which come to the same conclusions: CPR-CC only very rarely results in retinal haemor-rhages and, when it does, the haemorrhages are few in number and confined to the posterior pole. One group[33] calls the appearance of extensive retinal haemorrhages attributed to CPR-CC as 'inconceivable' and I support this view. In discussing this topic, another author[72] writes that the child with retinal haemorrhages 'is likely to have sustained these as a result of' abuse and other authors[7] have made similar statements.

The first study on this topic, although flawed in several ways,[162] found only 6 out of 51 children with retinal haemorrhages after CPR-CC: 4 were abused, 1 was an infant who was cyanotic after a seizure of unknown aetiology followed by severe systemic hypertension, and 1 was a child pedestrian struck in a motor vehicle accident.[163] In a prospective multicentre study of 83 children (aged 1-month – 17-years, majority < 1 year) examined within 96 h of CPR-CC by paediatric ophthalmologists using full pharmacological dilation, with 55 having measured PT and PTT of which 47 were abnormally elevated, and 40 of 76 with thrombocytopenia, small punctate haemorrhages were found in the posterior pole only of 2 children (2.4%).[164] Both of these patients had elevated PT and PTT with thrombocytopenia. In another study of 45 children (aged 1-month – 15-years, 84% < 2-years-old) examined within 96 h of CPR-CC with 93% having elevated PT/PTT, 49% with thrombocytopenia, and 62% with both abnormalities, only 1 was found to have 'multiple punctate' retinal haemorrhages that were 'not consistent with' SBS.[165] This 1-month-old had elevated PTT and 60 min of CPR-CC including open heart massage which interestingly implies no increased intrathoracic pressure. This study may represent a subset of the 83 children reported by Quasney and Kerr[164] as they appear as authors on both studies. Gilliland and Luckenbach studied 169 children after death.[109] Even in the presence of disease known to be associated with retinal haemorrhages, 70 children had no retinal haemorrhages after CPR-CC. All children with retinal haemorrhages who had CPR-CC also had an underlying condition which could explain the haemorrhages, in particular, child abuse. The authors conclude that CPR-CC does not induce retinal haemorrhages. Another study reviewed the postmortem examination of 4 children with SIDS who had CPR. One had 'a few erythrocytes' under the nerve fiber layer.[43] The authors state that this would not be clinically detectable.

The definitive study would require pre- and post-CPR examinations to determine if any haemorrhages observed after CPR-CC were in fact due to the event. In an effort to get close to this ideal, but obviously unattainable, study condition, we conducted a prospective evaluation of 14 consecutive children by having the ophthalmologist carry a 'code beeper' so that eye examinations could be done with as close a proximity as possible to the event. Several of the children had their retinas examined while CPR-CC was ongoing. Retinal haemorrhages were only observed in SBS victims, one child with severe accidental head trauma, after the child (described above) had been thrown from a motor vehicle accident landing on his head resulting in death), and two children with co-existing coagulopathy (thrombocytopenia and/or disseminated intravascular coagulation resulting in a few tiny dot/blot haemorrhages in the posterior pole). Despite prolonged (cumulative 6 h over several episodes) CPR-CC in one child with thrombocytopenia, congenital heart disease, and disseminated intravascular coagulation, no haemorrhages were observed.

A pig animal model was used in an attempt to evaluate further the possibility of retinal haemorrhage following CPR-CC.[166] No retinal haemorrhages were found after 50 min of CPR-CC. However, it has been suggested that there may be problems with the pig anatomy that perhaps make it an unsuitable model.[72] In dogs, it has been shown that most of the transmission of increased intrathoracic pressure to the intracranial space is via the vertebral vascular system which is not directly involved with ocular circulation.[167]

A few isolated case reports appear in the literature suggesting a causal relationship between CPR with chest compressions and retinal haemorrhage. In a study of 20 children, Goetting and Sowa reported two children felt to have CPR induced haemorrhages.[168] Examinations were done by a non-ophthalmologist by direct ophthalmoscopy with or without pupillary dilation. Some have commented that this would lead to underestimation of the incidence.[107] One child was a 2-year-old near drowning victim with 'multiple large retinal haemorrhages bilaterally' and, therefore, probably had Valsalva retinopathy (see below) as children suffer from drowning primarily due to laryngospasm. However, the other child apparently represents a true case of retinal haemorrhage due to CPR-CC. This 6-week-old infant was admitted for near SIDS/rule out sepsis evaluation. The child had an inpatient apneic event requiring 75 min of CPR-CC. Afterwards, eye examination revealed a single approximately 0.3 mm peripapillary retinal haemorrhage. No other apparent contributing abnormalities were found at autopsy.

Weedn and coworkers reported a single child who died from severe apparently accidental hot water burns who at autopsy on microscopy was found to have 'several large patches of retinal haemorrhages situated in the nerve fiber layer in the equator and posterior pole of both eyes'.[169] There was no haemorrhage in the optic nerve sheath or central nervous system. Despite their use of the term 'large', the accompanying photographs show areas of haemorrhage that would appear punctate to an examining ophthalmologist looking at a live patient with the indirect ophthalmoscope. No further details about the haemorrhages are given. This child's clinical course was also complicated by probable sepsis, severe hypoxia and hypotension, cerebral oedema, and difficult intubation (potentially a cause of Valsalva, see below) all of which may have contributed to the haemorrhages in addition to the 45 min of CPR-CC. No coagulation study results are given although the authors comment about the absence of disseminated intravascular coagulation in choroid.

Similarly, Kramer and Goldstein reported a 17-month-old girl with fever, intractable vomiting, dehydration, and profuse watery diarrhoea felt at autopsy to be due to adenovirus.[170] The child had 'multiple scattered intraretinal and subhyaloid haemorrhages throughout the posterior poles and mid periphery bilaterally' diagnosed by a non ophthalmologist. CT scan showed diffuse cerebral oedema but no haemorrhage (confirmed postmortem). Once again there may have been many factors contributing to this child's haemorrhages including possible abuse. We are not told to what degree this was investigated. Clearly, the degree of haemorrhagic retinopathy is completely contrary to anything else every reported in the literature which would be attributable to CPR-CC.

As demonstrated by two of the reports above, occasionally, a caretaker may offer a history of vigorous attempted resuscitation at home that, due to their inexperience or lack of training, appears to be quite different from the usual CPR guidelines. Kirschner and Stein report a 3-month-old with 'retinal haemorrhages' after 'failed resuscitation', and the father's 'attempted vigorous resuscitation by chest compression'.[171] The autopsy 'confirmed the diagnosis of sudden infant death syndrome'. No other details are given. In a 1978 report, Bacon and co-workers attributed 'extensive fresh haemorrhages in the nerve–fibre layer of both fundi' and bilateral macular oedema to the mother's attempts to resuscitate by holding the 2-month-old baby to her shoulder and 'slapp[ing] him repeatedly on the back'.[161] Other similar reports from parents may include striking the child on the chest and/or back[13] or other unusual variations some of which may appear quite violent on first review. It would be difficult to study such behaviours in a scientifically controlled fashion to determine if they could indeed result in retinal haemorrhages. However, one must remember that the proper CPR routine was developed to maximize pumping pressure on the heart via directed intrathoracic pressure rises. Other unconventional methods are unlikely to be superior to CPR in raising intrathoracic pressure and, therefore, much less likely to have retinal effects.

Other causes

A variety of isolated or uncommonly reported causes of retinal haemorrhage appear in the literature and are listed below. Although paediatric ophthalmologists such as myself have collectively examined hundreds, if not thousands, of children with these problems and virtually never find a single haemorrhage, one must consider the possibility that haemorrhage might rarely occur and then attempt to understand if this could be the cause of the observed haemorrhages in a given patient based on probability, the pattern and type of haemorrhages, and the presence of associated findings recognized as SBS injuries. In addition to the entities discussed, there are a multitude of retinal disorders which are left out because of their extreme unlikeliness to be present in infants or because other concomitant findings would easily make their diagnosis recognizable on eye examination. For example, retinal haemorrhage may be associated with cytomegalovirus (CMV) retinal infection, but this only occurs in immunocompromised children or neonates with congenital CMV and is seen in the context of a characteristic pattern of yellow-white retinal necrosis.[172] Retinal haemorrhage is a not uncommon finding immediately following intra-ocular surgery (e.g. cataract, glaucoma) in children. The haemorrhages are usually intraretinal and may have white centres.[173] These haemorrhages usually resolve in 1–2 weeks, if not sooner, although I have observed preretinal and subretinal haemorrhages which lasted for approximately 4 weeks.

Once again, one must also be cautious in interpreting the literature of the 1970s and earlier. There are many examples of children, who today might obviously been recognized as victims of shaking, who had their retinal haemorrhages ascribed to other causes, as SBS was not defined at the time (e.g. case 7 of Shaw and Landers, 1975).[87]

Anaesthesia

As some children who present with severe intracranial injury require neurosurgical or other procedures under general anaesthesia, perhaps before an eye examination is conducted, it has been queried whether this could cause the subsequently discovered retinal haemorrhages. With the exception of a single reported case of an adult who sustained a single unilateral venous haemorrhage presumably due to a Valsalva manoeuvre after laparoscopic surgery in the Trendelenberg position,[174] I am unaware of such an event being reported in a child. I have observed a single subretinal haemorrhage occurring in a child who became light under anaesthesia and coughed while the eye was open for cataract surgery. Retinal haemorrhages may occur following any intra-ocular surgery in children (e.g. cataract, glaucoma) but tend to me mild intraretinal haemorrhages, occasionally preretinal, confined to the posterior pole.

Anaemia

As mentioned above, some shaken children will have anaemia. It appears that anaemia alone, even severe anaemia well beyond the levels often seen in SBS, is rarely a cause of retinal haemorrhages. Severe anaemia seems to be required before retinal haemorrhages will occasionally occur.[175] The haemorrhages are usually intraretinal. Subretinal haemorrhage has not been reported to my knowledge. The retina may appear pale or even yellowish.[176] Although the conclusions have sometimes been drawn based on populations which certainly included adults or ages are not specified, some feel that haemor-rhages alone are more likely after acute blood loss whereas exudates are more likely after severe chronic anaemia.[175] Others have pointed out that the co-existence of severe anaemia (< 8) and severe thrombocytopenia (< 50,000) significantly increases the risk for retinal haemorrhaging such that severe anaemia alone is often insufficient to cause the retinal manifestations.[177,178] In one study of 53 adults and 36 children, all patients with retinal haemorrhages had haemoglobin levels below 7.8 and none of the children had haemorrhages despite two-thirds having haemoglobin less than 7.[179] In another study, all had levels less than 5.[178] There were many causes of anaemia in these studies including iron deficiency, leukaemia (see below), malaria (see below), hereditary spherocytosis, and parasites. The first group of authors postulate that the 'striking lack of anaemic retinopathy' in children may be related to the absence of ageing effects on blood vessels.[179] This would certainly parallel the absence of vascular changes in young children with diabetes or sickle cell anaemia (see below). Of the almost 40% of adults who had haemorrhages, the majority also had cotton wool spots and exudates and all findings were confined to the posterior pole. In a review of retinal haemorrhages associated with anaemia following severe gastrointestinal haemorrhage in adults, the authors also remarked on the presence of exudates and striking resemblance to adult hypertensive retinopathy:[180] findings not seen often in SBS.

Aneurysm

Although ruptured aneurysms are a well recognized cause of retinal haemorrhages in adults,[181–184] this is a very rare occurrence in children. Fahmy found no retinal haemorrhages in individuals less than 20-years-old although the number of study children appears to be less than 5.[182] In an older study of both adults and children (numbers not given although median in fourth decade) only 19% had retinal haemorrhages and 4% had vitreous haemorrhage although many of the retinal haemorrhages appear to have been due to papilloedema.[185] When present in children, the findings are almost always confined to 1 or 2 haemorrhages on or around the optic nerve head. It is unclear whether the haemorrhages are due to the aneurysm itself or associated increased intracranial pressure. One must also be careful to distinguish primary aneurysm from traumatic aneurysm secondary to SBS.[186] In the world's literature, I am aware of only one case of 'extensive bilateral retinal haemorrhages and a large right subhyaloid haemorrhage' in a 6-week-old child with an angiography confirmed cerebral aneurysm.[187] It is also noted that there were significant psychosocial and historical risk factors for abuse. Although the CT scan was done well before the modern era of neuro-imaging and may have missed findings associated with SBS, the images provided clearly would not be consistent with typical SBS abnormalities. No investigation was conducted to prove that abuse did not play a role in the causation.

One author cites several references to support the assertion that retinal haemorrhages are non specific and can be caused by aneurysms.[112] One of the cited papers reports a single 13-month-old.[188] No retinal examination was done and there is no report or discussion or retinal haemorrhages at all. In another, an 11-month-old had 'marked papilloedema with multiple retinal haemorrhages'.[189] No further details are given. The CT scan would readily have distinguished the case from SBS. In addition, if these haemorrhages are due to the papilloedema, as implied, then this would not come into the differential diagnosis of the haemorrhagic retinopathy of SBS. The discussion section of the paper does not mention retinal haemorrhage as a feature of childhood aneurysms. Another paper only mentions a single 11-year-old with retinal haemorrhages in both eyes (no further details provided).[190] Her CT scan and age would clearly cause no confusion with SBS. The remaining paper mentions an 8-month-old with 'retinal haemorrhages bilaterally' 20 years ago before CT scanning was available.[191] The aneurysm was diagnosed by angiography and confirmed surgically. I have reviewed the medical records of the child and, although there are some inconsistencies between observers, at most the child had flame haemorrhages around the disc in one eye and 'some larger diffuse haemorrhages as well as some flame haemorrhages' in the other eye, all in the presence of papilloedema. Another non ophthalmologist observer found only 'numerous flame haemorrhages' in one eye. Once again, the majority of haemorrhages appear to be consistent with papilloedema rather than the type of haemorrhagic retinopathy characteristic of SBS. Both of these latter two papers also demonstrate, quite clearly, how readily distinguishable the neuro-imaging of paediatric intracranial aneurysm usually is from the findings of SBS.

Arachnoid cysts

Although modern neuro-imaging would readily distinguish between cysts and the findings of SBS, one author in attempting to indicate the non specificity of retinal haemorrhages, cites three references on arachnoid cysts.[112] One of the cited papers reports only one child with retinal haemorrhage: a 9-year-old with 'severe papilloedema with retinal haemorrhages bilaterally'.[192] As discussed above, haemorrhages due to papilloedema are completely non specific and not related to our discussion on the specificity of the haemorrhagic retinopathy of SBS. Nowhere in this paper is haemorrhagic retinopathy mentioned as a feature of this condition. The second paper reviewed 20 years' experience at one centre and found only 12 paediatric cases demonstrating the rarity of such a process in comparison to the more common SBS.[193] Although two children had papilloedema, retinal haemorrhages are not mentioned in any child. The last paper reports a single adult who had 'bilateral haemorrhagic papilloedema'.[193] I am not aware of any literature to support an association between arachnoid cysts and haemorrhagic retinopathy other than haemorrhages due to papilloedema.

Arteriovenous malformation

Retinal haemorrhages have been observed in adults with subarachnoid haemorrhage due to arteriovenous malformation (AVM).[184] In children, AVMs are much less common than SBS. One child who was initially thought to be a victim of SBS because of unexplained acute loss of consciousness and seizures in the presence of acute subarachnoid haemorrhage and increased intracranial pressure was found by MRI to have a large spinal cord AVM at T9–L2 with massive secondary subarachnoid haemorrhage.[194] Although the retinal haemorrhages were bilateral, no other details are given except a photograph of one eye which shows one intraretinal blot haemorrhage and a single preretinal haemorrhage over a vessel both of which are in the peripapillary area. The child also had bilateral papilloedema although these two haemorrhages do not appear to be directly related. The authors note that the brain CT scan was atypical for SBS with haemorrhage in the fourth ventricle and in the absence of more common SBS findings such as subdural haemorrhage. Focal neurological deficits of the lower extremities would also be unusual in SBS. In another case of cervical AVM with secondary subarachnoid haemorrhage in a child, bilateral retinal haemorrhages, although not great in number, did extend to the periphery in the more affected eye.[195] Once again, this diagnosis should have easily been made by neuro-imaging. Another group discusses a 7-week-old who died from a frontal lobe vascular malformation.[43] The child had unilateral subarachnoid optic nerve sheath haemorrhage but no retinal haemorrhage. In a case citing a ruptured AVM misdiagnosed as SBS, there was **no** retinal haemorrhages despite a misprint in the abstract which suggests that they were present.[79,196] In fact, the authors specifically cite the absence of retinal haemorrhage, despite the presence of optic nerve sheath haemorrhage, as reason to distinguish their case from SBS. Of course, the diagnosis of AVM is usually readily apparent to the paediatric neuroradiologist. As one author puts it: 'the diagnosis of retinal haemorrhages in patients with intracranial pathology such as malformations should not pose a diagnostic dilemma, since malformations will be obvious on radiographic examination'.[72]

Carbon monoxide poisoning

Each year, approximately 2100 deaths occur in the US due to unintentional carbon monoxide poisoning.[197] For the most part, these deaths represent inhalation due to fire or motor vehicle exhaust gases but also include other accidental exposures. Exposures may be acutely toxic or subacute with symptoms observed over longer periods.[198] Most unintentional exposures result in only one fatality although multiple victims are found in 20% of cases.[197] I am unaware of any reported cases, in which a single infant child was the only victim, perhaps because all infants should have another individual, a caretaker, in the immediate environment. In one case from 1922, a 5-year-old boy was left at home and removed the 'opening of the gas jet' then falling unconscious at the site such that 'the nature of the accident was immediately discerned'.[199] Although the child went blind from optic nerve involvement, and had anaemia, conjunctival injection, retinal venous dilation, and 'retinal cyanosis', he did not have retinal haemorrhages. The case is unusual in that symptoms persisted for 2 weeks despite removal from the carbon monoxide source suggesting that other diagnoses may have been operant. In another single case, a 6-month-old may have been affected severely whereas his older siblings had flu-like symptoms which prompted emergency room visits in the preceding week.[13] In a study of 28 affected children, only 3 were in the SBS age range.[200]

Over half of the residential exposures occur in the 'heating season': November, December, or January.[197] The most common source of CO in these cases is unvented supplemental heaters fuelled by natural gas or propane.[197,198,200,201] In one study of children with flu-like symptoms due to CO exposure, all had readily identifiable risk factors in the history with exposure either to kerosene heaters, auto exhaust, or oil heaters.[202] In another study, all affected children had identifiable exposures as well.[200]

In making the diagnosis of carbon monoxide poisoning, several key features may be helpful: season of the year, known heating system or auto exhaust environmental exposure, other affected family members from the same environment and, perhaps most importantly, clinical improvement occurring after the victim is removed from the toxic environment.[13,198,201-203] Other adults and older children in the home, as well as the immediate victim, often experience non specific flu-like symptoms including dizziness, weakness, syncope, fatigue, headache, gastrointestinal, and respiratory complaints.[13,198,204] Children with carboxyhaemoglobin levels below 15% are usually without signs or symptoms.[200] In adults, symptoms may also include skin rashes, deafness, limb oedema, or neurological abnormalities such as parasthesias, dizziness, optic nerve disease, cranial nerve palsies, cortical blindness, visual field disturbances, nystagmus, pupillary abnormalities, or coma.[198,201,204] Chronic exposures with intermittent symptoms are well recognized in adults.[204] Unlike SBS, CT changes characteristically affect the basal ganglia without intracranial haemorrhage.[13,202] Cerebral oedema may be present. Home visitation is essential to confirm and identify possible sources of exposure. In some jurisdictions, like Toronto, home carbon monoxide sensors are mandatory.

Retinal haemorrhages are a well-recognized feature of carbon monoxide poisoning in adults.[198] They are associated with carboxyhaemoglobin levels usually well above 10%.[13,203] There are very few reports of retinal examinations in affected children, particularly in the SBS age range. One 6-month-old had 'small retinal haemorrhages' although it remains unclear if this child was truly affected.[13] An 11-year-old boy was found to have disc swelling, cotton wool spots, and venous tortuosity without retinal haemorrhage.[201] After observing his retina and that of other affected family members, the authors concluded that the retinal problem was ischaemic, in keeping with the reduced oxygen carrying capacity of carboxyhaemoglobin that is the pathophysiological basis of the poisoning. Ischaemic retinopathy is characterised by these findings and often described in carbon monoxide poisoning but rarely seen in SBS. In addition to ischaemic changes including optic nerve oedema with associated peripapillary haemorrhages (as in papilloedema), one 5-year-old girl had large preretinal or superficial (subinternal limiting membrane) haemorrhages that persisted for well over 1 week.[203] However, unlike SBS, the haemorrhages did not extend to the periphery, no retinoschisis or other indicators of SBS were present, and the clinical history, including other affected family members, obviously suggested carbon monoxide toxicity. Her carboxyhaemoglobin level was 39%.

Coagulopathy

Coagulopathies rarely result in retinal haemorrhage in children. However, there are few studies in the literature specifically designed to look at this association. Conclusions can be drawn by looking at studies in which at least some patients had eye examinations (sometimes not specified). In two studies (136 children[205] and 104 children[206]) with idiopathic thrombocytopenia, none presented with visual signs suggesting an absence of significant haemorrhage in the macula. In a study of 433 children with thrombocytopenia from a wide range of causes, only 2 (< 1%) had retinal haemorrhages.[207] The haemorrhages are not described. In one case, on resolution of a vitreous haemorrhage, a single intraretinal haemorrhage at the fovea was seen.[208] In another, 'multiple dot and blot haemorrhages' were seen in conjunction with vitreous haemorrhages, although the baby was only 16-days-old thus raising the possibility that these were simply due to birth.[133] In my experience, thrombocytopenia, although uncommonly associated with retinal haemorrhages, will cause just a few intraretinal (and rarely preretinal[133]) haemorrhage in the posterior pole.

Neonatal or infantile vitreous haemorrhage may occur in the presence of disseminated intravascular coagulation (DIC)[88,133] or protein C or S deficiency.[209–214] Subretinal haemorrhage, choroidal haemorrhage, or retinal detachment may also occur.[88,209,211] However, in patients with DIC and protein C or S deficiency, the routine coagulation studies (PT, PTT, and/or platelet count) are extremely abnormal and other systemic manifestations of bleeding are present. Infants with ocular manifestations of protein S or C present in the neonatal period with multiple thromboses and purpura fulminans.[209–214] In reporting the same case twice, one group of authors has suggested that the vitreous haemorrhage may be due to retinal vessel thrombosis, perhaps occurring even before birth in some infants.[213,214] Although intracranial bleeding, such as subarachnoid haemorrhage[211] may occur, I am unaware of any cases in which this was an isolated finding or where there were retinal haemorrhages without severe vitreous haemorrhage. In addition, the parents can be tested and found to be heterozygotes.[212]

In a study of over 250 patients with vitreous haemorrhage of all ages, only 1 patient had vitreous haemorrhage on the basis of coagulopathy (thrombocytopenia).[50] The age of that patient is not given. One 4-year-old with idiopathic thrombocytopenic purpura (ITP) was reported with severe unilateral vitreous haemorrhage accompanied by subdural and intraparenchymal brain haemorrhage, petechia, and a platelet count of 7000.[208] There was no history of trauma. On examination 3 weeks prior, when the diagnosis of ITP was made and confirmed by bone marrow biopsy, the retinas were normal. In another single case, a child with ITP had a normal eye examination despite a platelet count of $1000/mm^3$ and severe cutaneous, oral, and nasal evidence of bleeding.[215] A CT scan showed a cerebellar haemorrhage very unlike that seen in SBS. The child subsequently experienced decompensation and death due to brain herniation at which time he was found to have 'bilateral retinal haemorrhages' that are not described further. We are also not told if they were simply due to papilloedema. However, these cases may be examples of the rare paediatric Terson syndrome (see above). Alternatively, the haemorrhages may be either due to thrombocytopenia or papilloedema alone. Of course, the other clinical manifestations, including the severely depressed platelet counts, of these cases would make them readily distinguishable from SBS.

In the case of spinal AVM discussed above, the PTT was slightly elevated (patient 36.3 s, control high 32 s) and not likely to have caused haemorrhaging.[194]

Coagulopathy does not cause severe extensive retinal haemorrhaging or traumatic retinoschisis and, indeed, rarely causes more than some scattered intraretinal or preretinal haemorrhages in the posterior pole. The presence of retinal haemorrhages is more likely due to SBS in the absence of another obvious explanation, than coagulopathy. Yet, all children with retinal haemorrhages without an obvious cause or in whom SBS is strongly suspected should have basic coagulation studies performed including platelet count, PT, PTT and bleeding time. This should uncover all common coagulopathies. Over half of von Willebrand patients may have normal studies.[216] Detection may require measurement of levels of Factor VIII, von Willebrand factor, or von Willebrand antigen.[216] The combination of PTT, bleeding time, and cofactor activity will successfully identify the disease 92% of the time.[217] Although a 13-year-old and a 19-year-old (who also had the heritable retinal abnormality gyrate atrophy which may have been a contributing factor) with von Willebrand disease and vitreous haemorrhage (recurrent in the patient with gyrate atrophy without retinal haemorrhage) and peripapillary retinal and subretinal haemorrhages (in the 13-year-old) have been reported.[218] I am unaware of any reports of children in the SBS age range with retinal haemorrhages due to this disorder or to any other coagulopathy in which all of these recommended studies were normal.

I am aware of one case in which a 3-day-old infant was found to have severe bilateral vitreous haemorrhages due to maternal lupus anticoagulant (personal communication, Dr Léon-Paul Noel). The mother had had a myocardial infarction previously during a pregnancy at age 31 years. Lupus anticoagulant can cross the placental barrier. However, one would not expect this to cause retinal or vitreous haemorrhages beyond the neonatal period and I am unaware of any reports of such a circumstance.

It is important to note that brain injury associated coagulopathy[103,219] has sometimes been offered as the explanation for retinal haemorrhages with the assumption, therefore, that the injury was accidental. Mild elevations of PT and PTT are not uncommon following accidental and non accidental paren-chymal brain injury but usually not in the range seen with true pre-existing coagulopathy.[219] Therefore, retinal haemorrhage would not occur on this basis alone.

Diabetes

Diabetes mellitus is perhaps one of the most common causes of retinal haemorrhage in adults. Yet, retinal involvement is extremely rare in preteen children and, to my knowledge, has never been reported in a child in the SBS age range. In a study of over 350 children, only 1 had retinal disease before 10 years of age (exact age not given) after 4 years of disease, and none at diagnosis, leading the authors to suggest that eye examinations are not necessary before 10 years.[220] In another series with 161 diabetic children, none had retinopathy before 12 years of age.[221] A study of 181 patients found no retinopathy before puberty.[222] In a large series of patients with vitreous haemorrhage, Dana and coworkers found no instance of vitreous haemorrhage due to diabetes in any patient less than 19 years of age.[50] Other studies confirm these findings and suggest that at diagnosis, and even after 3–5 years of disease, diabetes-induced retinal haemorrhages do not occur in children in the SBS age range.[221,223–225]

Extracorporeal membrane oxygenation

Although history alone would of course identify this risk factor, it is conceivable that a new-born who received extracorporeal membrane oxygenation (ECMO) could later present with retinal haemorrhages, with[226] or without intracranial haemorrhage, which might raise a question as to the possibility of shaking. This might be particularly true in that children with medical risk factors may be at higher risk of becoming child abuse victims. One difficulty in studying these patients, who often get ECMO in the first week of life, is distinguishing between normal birth haemorrhages and those due to the treatment.

The incidence of retinal haemorrhage after ECMO is 4–18%. In one study of patients who had veno-arterial ECMO, 13% of examined patients showed retinal haemorrhages all of which were few in number (< 3), visually insignificant, confined to the posterior pole, and dot or flame in character.[227] The patients were all less than 1-week-old except a 21-month-old. In another study, 2 of 11 patients examined within 3 days of ECMO discontinuation had retinal haemorrhage, each only a single intraretinal haemorrhage (one < 0.5 mm in the macula and the other approximately 2 x 4 mm in the mid peripheral zone).[228] In yet another study, the incidence of retinal haemorrhage was 4%, venous dilation 5% and venous tortuosity 1%.[229] Both preretinal and intraretinal haemorrhages were observed but further details were not given. In a study of 91 neonates examined either during bypass or within 3 weeks, 8.8% had retinal haemorrhages all of which were mild, scattered and intraretinal.[230]

The haemorrhages may appear in the eye ipsilaterally and/or contralateral to the bypass[227] although the left eye is more often affected.[228,230] Haemorrhage may or may not be associated with venous engorgement.[228] Haemorrhages may follow the major retinal vessels and are usually confined to the posterior pole.[226] Other less common evidence of bleeding may include choroidal, vitreous, or subretinal haemorrhage.[231] There appears to be no statistical correlation between retinal haemorrhage and platelet count, mortality or brain haemorrhage.[227] However, these haemorrhages are an immediate result of treatment (hyperperfusion or reperfusion) and perhaps the associated thrombocytopenia or mandatory anticoagulation that is given play a role.[231] With the exception of one case in which the haemorrhages cleared 'over ... three months',[226] no data are available, to my knowledge, on the time to resolution. But given the type of haemorrhages, it would be unlikely for them to often persist for weeks and certainly extremely unlikely that they would remain many months or years later. There is no evidence that the retina is more prone to haemorrhaging at a later date after treatment is completed.

Endocarditis, heart disease and sepsis

In 1872, Roth described white centred haemorrhages in patients with sepsis of various aetiologies including bacterial endocarditis.[48] The findings were corroborated and further defined by Litten in 1878 who coined the term 'Roth spots';[48] an eponym which has been associated with the white centred haemorrhages of bacterial endocarditis ever since.

Cyanotic congenital heart disease may also be associated with retinal haemorrhages, usually in association with retinal venous engorgement and dilation that may be more prominent unilaterally. However, extensive haemorrhage is rare. In a study of 83 children, none had retinal haemorrhages despite common evidence of a retinal vasculopathy and/or papilloedema.[232] In one reported child, who had known complex congenital heart disease, haemorrhaging was due to closure of one central retinal vein with ischaemia and secondary exudates: a clinical picture clearly different from the usual SBS victim.[233]

In addition to the vascular incompetence, vasculitis, infarction, or coagulopathy that may be associated with severe sepsis, retinal haemorrhages can rarely occur due to septic emboli in the retina. These are usually focal and few in number. In premature infants with nosocomial infection with opportunistic infection (e.g. coagulase negative staphylococci) I have seen one or two quadrants of retina having scattered small intraretinal haemorrhages that may leave tiny hypopigmented scars, usually in the mid periphery. This zonal distribution has never been noted in SBS.

Galactosaemia

As rare as galactosaemia is (approximately 1:62,000) haemorrhagic ocular complications are even rarer. In a remarkable paper reporting five cases, all had vitreous haemorrhage as well as hepatomegaly in 4 and, in all 5, clinical and/or laboratory evidence of a severe coagulopathy.[234] No child had isolated retinal haemorrhages and, in all, the vitreous haemorrhage was severe, often complicated by retinal detachment and/or subretinal haemorrhage or fibrosis. The authors note that only 4 other reports appear in the literature.

Glutaric aciduria

The reader is referred elsewhere for a more extensive review on the nature of this condition.[235] This autosomal recessive metabolic disorder is sometimes associated with subdural haemorrhage after minor or moderate head trauma.[236,237] Subdural collections may also be present after birth.[236] Macrocephaly is one of the hallmarks of the condition. It may be that the bridging veins are, therefore, 'on stretch' and more prone to shearing forces induced by minor head injury.[237] Although the disorder eventually results in serious neurological compromise, usually after an acute encephalopathic crises perhaps precipitated by a viral illness or immunisation, affected children may have normal development and tone in early childhood.[235,236] Early neurological signs are often 'subtle' and variable between examinations.[235,236] Characteristic basal ganglia disease[235] can develop even in the absence of significant changes in electrolytes or glutaric acid concentrations.[236] This area of the brain is rarely the focal location of injury in SBS. In glutaric aciduria (GA1), extreme hypotonia followed by athetosis and dystonic rigidity due to the basal ganglia involvement usually develop within 14–21 days after the initial acute presentation.[236] Temporal and frontal lobe atrophy may also be observed. Mental retardation is common.

Although more common in certain Amish and Canadian Saulteaux/Ojibway native populations, it has been described in many other ethnic groups around the world with an estimated incidence of 1/30,000 in central Europe and the

US.[235,237] The diagnosis can usually be made by testing urinary organic acids or enzyme activity in fibroblasts.[235] The gene for the enzyme which is defective, glutaryl-CoA dehydrogenase, is known and mutation analysis can be performed.[235] Details of diagnostic testing are described elsewhere.[235]

There have been several reports which unfortunately use the general term, 'retinal haemorrhages', described in association with GA1 without clear characterisation of the findings.[237] This finding, along with the possibility of subdural haemorrhage, acute encephalopathic crises, and macrocephaly in a previously well-child, has led to the consideration of GA1 as an alternative to SBS in some cases. However, after making an international search for cases, I have found only 8 cases with retinal haemorrhage and all but one have only a single dot or blot haemorrhage. Sirotnak and Greene presented one child with a small dot haemorrhage just inside the superior arcade of one eye approximately 3 mm from the optic nerve head.[238] In one of the best major reviews of GA1, retinal haemorrhages are not even listed in the Table entitled *Clinical features suggestive of glutaric aciduria type I*.[235] I am aware of only one case with 'extensive retinal haemorrhages' in both eyes. There remains much controversy about the diagnosis in that particular case as there may be shearing tears on the brain neuro-imaging as well as other possible findings which are suggestive of SBS.

Some authors and researchers have speculated that the presence of retinal haemorrhages in GA1 is not a manifestation of the disease but rather, a secondary result of increased intracranial pressure (personal communication, Dr D. Holmes Morton).[236] The described findings of only a single retinal haemorrhage would be consistent with this explanation (see Hydrocephalus below).

Haemolytic uraemic syndrome

Although patients who present with haemolytic uraemic syndrome (HUS) may have some early similarities to a child with SBS, such as lethargy, seizures or coma, the other symptoms would make the two conditions readily discernible: early gastroenteritis usually with stool culture positive for *Escherichia coli* (0157:H7), renal failure with oliguria or anuria, microcytic haemolytic anaemia, thrombocytopenia, oedema (including periocular and conjunctival), and a different pattern of brain infarcts often involving the basal ganglia. Although retinal haemorrhages have been rarely reported in affected children, they were associated with large white retinal patches the aetiology[239] of which is unclear and may represent ischaemia. One child had plasmapheresis and haemodialysis prior to eye examination.[239] Both the whitening and the haemorrhages were confined to the posterior pole. The haemorrhages were few in number and included one large (2 x 3 mm) unilateral preretinal haemorrhage, a peripapillary flame haemorrhage, and scattered dot haemorrhages. The retinal arterioles were narrowed.

Hydrocephalus, increased intracranial pressure, cerebral oedema

In the absence of intracranial bleeding (see Terson syndrome above), can isolated elevation of intracranial pressure be responsible for retinal haemorrhage in children? Although there is one case of retinal haemorrhages in a shaken baby who on CT only showed cerebral oedema (before the MRI era), another case of retinal haemorrhages with a normal CT in a shaken baby shown to have characteristic haemorrhages by MRI,[46] and rare cases with optic nerve sheath haemorrhage without intracranial haemorrhage,[57] retinal haemorrhage from elevated intracranial pressure in the absence of shaking appears to be very rare and, in my experience (having examined hundred of children with isolated hydrocephalus or cerebral oedema), when it occurs is characterised by a few intraretinal or preretinal haemorrhages in the posterior pole, particularly on or around the optic nerve. I am not aware of any case in the literature in which a child had diffuse retinal haemorrhages of multiple types, as might be more diagnostic for SBS, from isolated hydrocephalus, increased intracranial pressure, or cerebral oedema without other signs of a non SBS causative systemic disease (e.g. coagulopathy[215]) that would make the differentiation relatively easy. One must also be careful to distinguish haemorrhages that are simply due to papilloedema, which would not be uncommon in this setting, from other haemorrhages of the retina. One larger series of postmortem examinations of children concluded that 'brain oedema alone is not sufficient to cause retinal haemorrhages or other [intrascleral, optic nerve sheath] ocular haemorrhages'.[53]

Hypertension

High blood pressure is one of the most common causes of retinal haemorrhages in adults. However, this is a vary rare cause of retinal haemorrhages in young children. In a review of all children with hypertensive retinopathy presenting at Wills Eye Hospital in Philadelphia, we found that each child had an exudative retinopathy with concomitant haemorrhages as a minor feature of the clinical picture (unpublished data). All children had acute hypertension on top of chronic hypertension, usually due to renal disease, and none were in the age range for SBS. In a study of 21 hypertensive inpatient new-borns in a special care (ICU) setting, 4 (19%) had flame haemorrhages which persisted until at least 1.5-months-old (chronological age: most of the infants were premature babies) and 2 had 'blot-like' haemorrhages (one with both blot and flame).[240] Two infants also were reported to have exudates, although at least one, who also had haemorrhages, actually had cotton wool spots representing superficial retinal nerve fibre layer ischaemia rather than true exudate. One of the infants with flame haemorrhages still had this finding 10 weeks later despite control of blood pressure. However, a representative photograph shows these children to have a small number of haemorrhages, confined to the posterior pole, radiating out from the optic nerve, in association with other hypertensive vascular changes. All children with abnormal retinal findings due to hypertension (50% of the hypertensive study population) had an increase in the ratio of venous to arterial calibre either due to venous dilation or arteriolar spasm: findings not typical of SBS. In addition, hypertension was just one manifestation of other systemic disorders (e.g. sepsis, haemolytic disease) that may potentially have contributed to the retinal findings. In a study of 97 'children' (ages 6–23 years) no retinal haemorrhages were seen.[241]

Hyperviscosity/polycythemia

Although recognized in adults as a cause of retinal haemorrhages,[242] these disorders are rare in children and I am unaware of any reports of retinal haemorrhages in the SBS age group as a result.

Although polycythemia in neonates may occur, it is otherwise extraordinarily rare in the absence of leukaemia in the first 3 years of life. This would easily be detectable by an abnormal haemoglobin level. Yet, even in adults, severe elevation would be required to cause retinal haemorrhages.[176]

Hypoxia/asphyxia

The brain injuries and neurological sequelae of shaking are, in part, due to the diffuse axonal injury but also due to cerebral hypoxia.[45] This has led to concern that retinal haemorrhages may reflect hypoxia rather than shaking. Vascular tortuosity and dilation might also be expected as seen in cyanotic congenital heart disease.[232] Strangulation, with forced attempts at respiratory effort against a closed airway, might generate enough transmitted increased intra-thoracic pressure (Valsalva) to cause haemorrhages in the retina as conjunctival haemorrhages are a well recognized sequelae. This is not to be confused with the more 'passive' asphyxia seen in children with lung or vascular perfusion diseases. There is little clinical evidence to support hypoxia as a cause of retinal haemorrhage. Scores of infants with hypoxia from a variety of causes ranging from birth asphyxia to trauma have been examined by myself and other paediatric ophthalmologists without any detection of retinal haemorrhages. Yet this subject has not been studied on a specific protocol or large series. One case of retinal haemorrhages attributed to asphyxia, with no other details provided, appears in the medical literature.[17] In one study of children with cyanotic heart disease, the degree of retinal vasculopathy was correlated with the degree of hypoxia, but even in these severely hypoxic children, no retinal haemorrhages were observed.[232] A postmortem study of 19 children who died from asphyxia showed none with retinal or optic nerve sheath haemorrhages.[53]

Immunisations

I am not aware of any peer reviewed medical literature which would support a causative association between childhood immunisations and retinal haemorrhages. However, there have been court cases in which the defence has suggested such a relationship, in particular with DPT immunisation and rebleeding subdural haemorrhage.[243] In a newsletter which reviews the alleged dangers of vaccinations in children, one non physician author, referring to cases of alleged SBS that were being reviewed by her for lawyers, states: 'a close study of the history of these cases revealed something distinctly sinister: in every single case, the symptoms appeared shortly after the baby's vaccinations'.[244] Of course, given the high incidence of SBS in the very same age ranges where vaccinations are routinely given, the suggestion of a cause and effect relationship could easily be explained by chance alone. No statistical data are offered to support a true association. The author goes on to attribute retinal haemorrhages (as well as many other SBS findings and cases attributed to Munchausen syndrome by proxy) to various vaccinations. In support of this conclusion the author cites a Letter to the Editor in Lancet reporting a single case of retinal haemorrhages due to central retinal vein occlusion in a 27-year-old following hepatitis B vaccine.[245] Even if one is willing to accept this single case as a true cause and effect phenomenon, it does not in any way explain the retinal haemorrhages of SBS which rarely have the pattern of a central vein occlusion (see elsewhere herein) and have been recognized long before the introduction of hepatitis B vaccine in children. As I have discussed elsewhere in this paper, there are also great dangers in applying knowledge gained from observations of the behaviour of adult retinal vasculature to that of children (e.g. Terson syndrome, diabetes, hypertension). Lastly, this single observation regarding hepatitis B vaccine can not be applied to other vaccines such as DPT and MMR. However, another article is cited[246] in the same newsletter to support an association between pertussis vaccine and 'brain swelling and haemorrhaging of an extent similar to that caused by mechanical injuries'.[244] Clearly this paper, in which mice received direct intracerebral injection of vaccine components, has many features which preclude its use for conclusions about human intracranial haemorrhaging: the unknown validity and applicability of the animal model and procedures, the failure to perform histopathological examination of the brains (brains were weighed only; the word 'haemorrhage' does not appear in the article at all), and the failure to examine the eyes pre- or postmortem.

Incontinentia pigmentii

There is a single case report of a 6-day-old baby with 'bilateral retinal haemorrhages' (no details given).[247] The child also had classic dermatological manifestations of the disease, a positive family history for this X-linked dominant disorder, and retinal exudates. Peripheral retinal vascular abnormalities which may be associated with localised, usually temporal, peripheral retinal haemorrhages are one of the hallmarks of the disease. But the retinal appearance, along with the other systemic findings (seizures, dental abnormalities, skin lesions, developmental delay) that may be present, should quite readily allow for the diagnosis as opposed to SBS. In the reported case, the haemorrhages may have been consistent with normal birth or the usual retinal presentation for incontinentia pigmentii. Unfortunately, a misdiagnosis of SBS had been initially suggested.

Leukaemia

Leukaemia is a well-recognized cause of retinal haemorrhages, sometimes looking very similar to shaken babies in that multiple retinal layers can be involved, haemorrhages may extend to the peripheral retina, large amounts of haemorrhage may be present (both in size of individual haemorrhages and number of haemorrhages), and large preretinal collections may occur.[248] However, unlike SBS, exudates, retinal leukaemic infiltrates, iritis (or frank layering of cells in the anterior chamber), or optic nerve infiltration may be present.[248–250] In other cases, retinal haemorrhages will be the only finding.[175,248] The peripheral haemorrhages may be associated with peripheral infiltrates and are more often seen in the presence of high cellular counts in the blood stream leading to sludging in these very tiny peripheral capillaries. White centred haemorrhages are frequent; presumably due to leukaemic infiltrates causing the white centre.[176,248,250] Likewise, perivascular infiltrates ('sheathing') may be observed.[250] One study, which included adults and children (although ages not specifically given) found that the incidence of retinal haemorrhages in the acute leukaemias (as a group) was related to the degree of anaemia, degree of thrombocytopenia, and amount of circulating blast cells.[175] Other authors have also recognized the important role of concomitant thrombocytopenia and anaemia.[176,178,248] Haemorrhages are more common in the acute rather than chronic leukaemias.[176] Retinal abnormalities are more common in adults than children.[248] Of course, all children with haemorrhagic retinal findings would have an abnormal CBC indicating the presence of their leukaemic disease.[178]

Malaria

Malaria is notable for its endemic nature with 90% of the total cases each year coming from less than 20 countries. Although the highest incidence is in India, Brazil, Afghanistan, Sri Lanka, Thailand, Indonesia, Vietnam, Cambodia and China, more than 80% of cases come from sub-Saharan Africa where 5% of affected children die of the disease before 5 years of age.[251,252] The incidence in non-endemic countries may also be increasing due to immigration.[253] Most children in non-endemic populations present with less than 1 week of symptoms although over one-quarter have a symptom history of 1–4 weeks and occasionally even longer.[253] Common presenting symptoms which differ from SBS include fever (periodic or not) and chills although lethargy, anorexia, and vomiting may also be observed.[253] Almost half of affected children have splenomegaly and one-third have hepatomegaly.[253] In one study in a non-endemic area, 20% had a history of known malaria treatment.[253] All patients had a history of travel to an endemic area. Children infected with *Plasmodium vivax* present on average 6 months after exposure, whereas those infected with *P. falciparum* presented on average at 3.8 weeks.[253]

Cerebral involvement may occur and can be life threatening, particularly with *P. falciparum* infection. Cerebral disease behaves differently in children, who may show more isolated neurological disease than in adults, where it is often more systemic.[251] Ocular involvement is felt to portend a worse systemic prognosis.[254]

There have been conflicting reports regarding the ocular manifestations in children. One study found that 78% of children had retinal signs which included white centred (38%), dot/blot (25%), flame (15%), and subfoveal (10%) haemorrhages.[255] Retinal involvement is often accompanied by retinal whitening, which may infer a higher risk for cerebral involvement.[254] The whitening may be superficial or deep in the retina, and peripheral or posterior: differences that may in part be due to severity.[254,255,256] Retinal vessels may also appear to have white or orange 'sheathing', although it is not clear whether this represents true inflammatory sheathing or abnormalities in flow of the parasitised intravascular red cells.[254–256] Lewallen and others report that retinal haemorrhages, although more often seen in cerebral malaria, do not have prognostic significance.[254,255] Several causes of the haemorrhages have been postulated including the contributing factors of anaemia, hypoxia, increased vascular permeability, and microvascular occlusion.[255]

Diagnosis is best made by the use of both thick and thin smears of peripheral blood.[252] Quantitative buffy coat analysis with acridine orange staining may also be useful. Acridine orange can also be used to stain tissue biopsies. A diagnostic dilemma may occur in endemic areas where parasitemia alone is insufficient to make a clinical diagnosis of malaria. However, the presence of retinal whitening and other ocular and systemic manifestations of the infection would make confusion with SBS unlikely.

Meningitis

Despite occasionally being listed in the differential diagnosis of retinal haemorrhages, meningitis is actually an extremely rare cause. A 12-year-old girl with meningococcal meningitis was found to have a single large unilateral subretinal and vitreous haemorrhage first diagnosed with the onset of visual loss 6 days into her illness while on antibiotic treatment.[257] The CT scan was normal. The authors state that they are unaware of any prior reports of haemorrhage due to bacterial meningitis. Although no data is given, meningococcus is a well recognized cause of coagulopathy which could have been the inciting factor. Another paper, written before Caffey's recognition of SBS and CT neuro-imaging, mentions that retinal haemorrhages were seen in a group of 116 patients with subdural haematoma and effusion of which 5% were attributed to meningitis.[151] However, the authors do not say if any of the retinal haemorrhages were observed in the meningitis patients specifically. A 3-week-old with meningitis and 'necrotizing encephalitis' was reported to have posterior pole haemorrhages and in the peripheral retina, subclinical microscopic haemorrhage.[53] These may have been normal birth haemorrhages, however.

I have observed one extraordinary case of severe bilateral panretinal haemorrhage due to meningitis. The haemorrhages were all radiating out from the disc in a linear fashion characteristic of a central retinal vein occlusion. In addition, the retinal arteries seemed to be non perfused and there was severe ischaemia and oedema of the maculae characteristic of a central retinal artery occlusion. Indeed, this retinal picture which is distinctly different from that seen in SBS, proved to be due to compression of the artery and vein along their course within the optic nerve as a result of complete filling of the optic nerve sheath with frank pus discovered at autopsy. In fact, the entire cerebrospinal fluid spaces were replaced by frank pus. This case would have caused no confusion with SBS. Likewise, another child with meningitis and unilateral haemorrhages due to retinal vein thrombosis has been reported (no further details given).[53]

Menkes disease

This X-linked recessive disorder, also known as Menkes kinky hair syndrome, is caused by a deficiency in a copper binding ATP-ase. As a result, there is a failure of copper transport with copper deficiency in serum, liver and brain. The earliest systemic manifestations include neonatal hypothermia, failure to thrive, seizures, and developmental regression. The characteristic hair is also noted in infancy. Untreated patients rarely survive beyond 3 years. Although aberrant eyelashes and anterior iris stromal hypoplasia have been reported in one paper,[258] structural malformations of the eye are not common. However, visual function is usually impaired early in infancy and deteriorates with disease progression. Nystagmus may be present.[258] I am aware of one case in which retinal haemorrhages were part of the disease complex.[259] This patient had other classic signs of Menkes disease including typical hair quality and, at autopsy, cerebral vessel abnormalities. There were retinal haemorrhages in the peripheral retina predominantly including some hyaloid haemorrhage. This is a very unusual distribution not commonly seen even in SBS. The retinal haemorrhages presumably occurred due to abnormalities of the retinal vessels. There was a clinically apparent retinal arteriopathy that should have been visible had the child been examined by an ophthalmologist before death. This finding, along with the other characteristic historical, physical, and laboratory findings should allow for differentiation from SBS.

Munchausen syndrome by proxy, suffocation

Munchausen syndrome by proxy (MBP), or factitious illness by proxy, is a form of child abuse in which the caretaker, usually the mother, creates the appearance of illness in their child either by direct physical injury (e.g. smothering), falsification of physical findings, falsification of history, or manipulation of laboratory tests. One child was found to have retinal haemorrhages which were not further described, in association with mild papilloedema.[260] CT scan and postmortem examination showed cerebral oedema. On history, the mother admitted to shaking the infant on more than one occasion. The cause of death was suspected to be suffocation which is the most common form of MBP. Suffocation induces an extreme Valsalva manoeuvre which is a well recognized cause of retinal haemorrhages in adults.

Prematurity

Retinopathy of prematurity (ROP) is associated with retinal haemorrhages. However, the haemorrhages occur at the peripheral circumferential demarcation between the vascularized and avascular retina that characterises the disease. Although this demarcation may occasionally arise in the posterior pole (zone I ROP), the haemorrhages would be associated with the obvious ROP abnormalities, in particular neovascularization (stage 3 ROP) and a raised ridge at the demarcation, rather than being randomly scattered. In addition, haemorrhages would be associated with active disease which is easily diagnosed in the premature infant at risk. Occasionally, a vascular tuft in the active zone, may bleed allowing preretinal blood to flow posteriorly onto the posterior pole. This may be more likely to occur after ophthalmic examination or treatment.

One study (see details above) of hypertensive neonates, in which the average birth age was before term, showed some retinal haemorrhages that would not be expected in older children.[240] However, we are not told if there was a relationship between susceptibility to retinal vascular abnormalities and gestational age. Late haemorrhage, especially vitreous haemorrhage, could occur following ROP in the presence of cicatricial changes such as retinal detachment. However, to my knowledge, there is no medical literature to otherwise support a particular predisposition for the premature retina to develop retinal haemorrhages at other times late in infancy in retina that is otherwise grossly normal in appearance.

Rocky Mountain spotted fever

Rocky Mountain spotted fever (RMSF) has been rarely associated with retinal haemorrhages. Retinal oedema, exudates, and venous engorgement are common accompanying findings,[261,262] that would help to distinguish RMSF from SBS. One 13-year-old boy, with typical manifestations of the disease had a haemorrhagic retinopathy noted on autopsy.[263] In a series of 6 children, all > 5-years-old, two had retinal haemorrhages.[262] The haemorrhages were very few in one case and flame shaped. In the other, they were white centred. In both cases, the clinical history was diagnostic and the children also had retinal exudates which in one photograph readily distinguish the retina from SBS. The same is true of another report in a 7-year-old.[261] I am unaware of any similarly affected children in the SBS age range. In addition, the characteristic petechial rash, oedema, hepatospenomegaly and positive serology and, when available, history of tick exposure, should distinguish RMSF from SBS.

Seizures

Many child victims of SBS present with seizures which may lead to a question about their role in the genesis of observed retinal haemorrhage particularly since they may increase intrathoracic pressure or be associated with a Valsalva manoeuvre. Despite unreferenced statements which suggest that retinal haemorrhages could 'possibly' result from 'prolonged' seizures,[21] this has never been adequately documented. One study of 33 non-abused children with seizures, ranging in age from 4 months to 14 years (mean and median less than 4 years), found no retinal haemorrhages for a predicted maximal possible incidence of < 1%.[264] Three children had status epilepticus, 7 (22%) had at least one bout of vomiting, two children also had CPR-CC, one had accidental head trauma, and many had accompanying neurological disorders. All children were examined within 48 h of a seizure. Although one 23-day-old child, examined after study enrolment was closed, had two single fading haemorrhages, these are most likely birth induced haemorrhages. The same group conducted another study of 32 children under 2 years of age to more closely approximate the SBS victim age range.[265] The patients included one child with 'spontaneous' brain haemorrhage, one with hydrocephalus, and 15.6% with vomiting. Once again, no seizures were found representing a 95% upper confidence limit of 10% incidence. Although both studies would have been strengthened by excluding children with focal, absence, or myoclonic seizures, the findings of these authors certainly conforms with my empiric conclusions reached after having examined hundreds of children with seizures, without ever observing a case of seizure induced retinal haemorrhage.

Sickle cell disease, haemoglobinopathies

Retinal haemorrhages do not occur in infants or toddlers due to sickle cell disease or other haemoglobinopathies although peripheral retinal neovascularization has been described in a 7-year-old child.[266] In Dana's large series of patients with vitreous haemorrhage no instance of vitreous haemorrhage due to sickle cell disease occurred in any patient less than 19-years-old.[50]

Sudden infant death syndrome (crib death, cot death, acute life threatening events)

Sudden infant death syndrome (SIDS) is the most common cause of death between 1 and 12 months of age.[267] Children who die from SIDS may share several features in common with those who are the victims of SBS including the absence of an explanatory history and the possibility of 'prodromal symptoms' such as gastrointestinal complaints.[15,29,267] However, SIDS victims have some distinguishing features as well: younger average age (2–4 months), specific family and environmental risk factors, and no evidence of trauma by history, clinical examination or autopsy. SIDS victims are by definition less than 1-year-old.[267] As stated by the American Academy of Pediatrics: 'it is uncommon for death due to child abuse to be confused with SIDS'.[267]

Although no formal study has been conducted to examine the antemortem or postmortem ocular findings of children who die of SIDS or survive a 'near-miss' SIDS episode, there still remains no report to my knowledge of retinal haemorrhages despite the fact that thousands of children have been examined. Two infants thought to have SIDS had retinal haemorrhages attributed to CPR-CC (see above).[168,171] One study looked at 10 SIDS victims postmortem and found no retinal haemorrhages.[33] Another study examined the postmortem of 6 infants and found only one with 'a few erythrocytes' under the nerve fibre layer at autopsy.[43] One study found no retinal, optic nerve sheath, or intrascleral haemorrhage in 13 SIDS victims postmortem.[53] One infant with a diagnosis of 'SIDS' who had a few posterior pole haemorrhages also had a coagulopathy.[259]

The American Academy of Pediatrics position statement lists retinal haemorrhages as an exclusion factor for SIDS: if present, then the infant is **not** a SIDS victim.[267]. The statement also re-inforces the importance of a complete autopsy, skeletal survey, and death scene investigation before making the diagnosis of SIDS, which is by definition a diagnosis that is made only after the exclusion of other diagnoses. Although not specifically addressed in the statement, perhaps, eyeball removal and examination, using the combined intracranial-transconjunctival approach as discussed above, should be part of the complete autopsy required in the investigation of any unexplained sudden infant death.

Valsalva

Increased intrathoracic pressure via Valsava manoeuvre is a well-recognized cause of retinal haemorrhage in adults.[91,268] The classic retinal picture is a single 'boat-shaped' preretinal haemorrhage over the macula presumably due to a ruptured superficial retinal vessel, but diffuse intraretinal haemorrhaging can uncommonly occur as can optic nerve sheath haemorrhage or Purtscher retinopathy.[91,268] I am unaware of any specific reports in children other than a 10-year-old with a single macular haemorrhage,[268] although the haemorrhagic retinopathy noted in a child after near drowning (although attributed to CPR)[168] may be a good example, as drowning deaths are precipitated by laryngeal spasm. Valsalva retinopathy is unlikely to play a role in SBS as children are usually either too young or obtunded to a degree that they are unable to generate a Valsalva manoeuvre independently.

Vasculitis

Although vasculitic disease can cause retinal haemorrhage in children, the haemorrhages are usually intraretinal, paravenous or pararterial, and often associated with retinal oedema and/or exudates. Vascular tortuosity may also be seen. Other signs of the systemic disease, such as systemic lupus erythematosis, are usually present. These disorders are exceedingly uncommon in the SBS age range.

Vitamin K deficiency (haemorrhagic disease of the newborn)

Haemorrhagic disease due to vitamin K deficiency in new-borns may occur at three different times: (i) on the first day of life due to prenatal ingestion by the mother of certain drugs (phenobarbital, phenytoin, rifampin, isoniazid, phenylbutazone, or anticoagulants);[269] (ii) between days 2–5 (classic form); or (iii) beyond the second week (late form). The late form is particularly associated with intracranial bleeding. It usually occurs at 1–3 months of age and is more commonly seen in breast fed babies.[269,270] However, late cases may occur as early as 10-days-old.[271] One paper reported infants between 4–7-months-old with chronic subdural haematoma and retinal haemorrhages attributed to the late form of vitamin K deficiency prior to 1980,[160] although on retrospective review, I wonder if these may have been shaken babies (see above).

The classic form of haemorrhagic disease is most often characterised by gastrointestinal, umbilical stump, or intracranial bleeding along with multiple ecchymoses. The first symptoms and signs of the late form include sudden pallor, irritability, decreased appetite, poor sucking, and/or high pitched crying in many infants.[271] Approximately half show readily apparent clinical signs of a bleeding disorder.[271] At admission, almost all will show altered consciousness that may range from mild to coma and seizures.[271] Almost half have eye movement or pupil disorders.[271] Intracranial findings include herniation, ventricle compression, arterial infarction, and subarachnoid, subdural, intraventricular, or intraparenchymal haemorrhage.[271]

The retinal haemorrhages may be difficult to distinguish from normal birth haemorrhages (within the timelines given above). I have seen one child whose haemorrhages were strictly paravenous. One group described the findings as 'papillary stasis'.[269] Although this is not clarified, this terminology also suggests a venous change. One child with the late form, had multiple flame, dot, blot, and possibly small preretinal haemorrhages radiating out from the optic nerve throughout the posterior pole in the published photograph.[272] In addition, the child had diffuse cerebral oedema and subdural blood. This clinical picture would be difficult to distinguish from a shaken baby. However, the child had obvious and fatal intramuscular bleeding, rectal bleeding, severe anaemia (haemoglobin 3.0 g/dl), and elevated PT and PTT along with a history of exclusive breast feeding and no vitamin K in the neonatal period.

Since the 1970s, in most countries, all children receive either injectable or oral vitamin K in the neonatal period to prevent primary deficiency disorders. Vitamin K does decrease the frequency of neonatal birth retinal haemorrhages.[127] Haemorrhagic disorders due to vitamin K deficiency may also occur in association with diseases that compromise vitamin K supply, such as chronic diarrhoea and liver disease. Children less than 6-months-old who have perinatal complications, are receiving antibiotics, and are breast fed are at greatest risk.[103] All forms of the disorder are characterised by a coagulopathy easily recognized by marked elevation of routine clotting studies, in particular, the PTT. In one study, all PT values except one were over 60 and PTT values were greater than 120.[271] However, other severely affected infants have been reported with less dramatically elevated results although still clearly in the abnormal range.[272] Correction of the coagulopathy after the administration of vitamin K confirms the diagnosis.

Timing of retinal haemorrhage

There is wide spread variability in the time it takes for retinal haemorrhages of all types to disappear. The haemorrhages may resolve within the first few days following injury or they may remain for several months.[63,72,93,98,100,273] Macular haemorrhages, preretinal haemorrhages, and haemorrhage within schisis cavities, tend to resolve more slowly.[98] Some authors and I have observed remarkable rapid clearing of 'extensive' intraretinal and preretinal haemorrhages within 6 weeks, if not sooner, yet other cases which proceed to macular scarring, vitreous organisation, and retinal traction may also occur.[46,61,98] As a result, retinal haemorrhages in living children can **not** be used to time and date the injury except at the extreme outliers: fading haemorrhages are unlikely to have occurred within the last few hours and widespread intraretinal haemorrhages are unlikely to last more than 6 months. Nashelsky and Dix reviewed the literature in an attempt to collect data that would aid in the time interval between lethal shaking and the onset of symptoms.[27] They showed that there was no adequate published evidence to allow for such conclusions. They did not specifically address the issue of retinal haemorrhages.

There is some evidence to support a delay of 1–2 days between injury and the presence of vitreous haemorrhage.[7,84,100] This has been my clinical experience, although severe retinal injury, particularly when associated with retinal detachment, at the time of shaking can result in immediate vitreous haemorrhage as well. Delayed vitreous haemorrhage has also been suggested by postmortem study.[70] Vitreous blood in SBS appears to be blood that ruptures through areas of traumatic retinoschisis or subyhyaloid collections into the vitreous. Once blood is in the vitreous, it can take many months for it to resorb. Surgery may be required if spontaneous resolution does not proceed at a satisfactory pace.

It is not uncommonly suggested, particularly in courtroom debates, that a child with retinal haemorrhages should show signs of visual dysfunction. The American Academy of Pediatrics position statement on SBS even lists 'unable to follow movement' as a 'typical' sign found at presentation.[29] Others have found that a lack of visual response at presentation correlates with poor outcome and death.[34] Although this is true for the 'convulsing or comatose' child being discussed in the relevant paragraph of the AAP statement, children who have been shaken but do not lose consciousness may show remarkably normal vision despite large haemorrhage involving and obscuring the fovea. This may be due to several reasons. Firstly, a child with unilateral sparing of the fovea will appear to function normally even if the other eye is acutely blind. This is a result of the unique wiring of the childhood developing visual system that allows the brain to instantaneously 'turn off' (suppression) the central vision in the affected eye. Unfortunately, this is also the mechanism by which the more affected eye may also develop amblyopia from lack of use. Secondly, infants and young children actually require very poor visual acuity to maintain apparently normal visual function in their activities of daily living. A child who is legally blind (vision of 20/200 or worse) may still be able to follow and play with the large toys that make up their objects of interest. Even with poor vision, the use of other senses, will allow them to recognize individuals and stare at the face of their feeding caretaker as if their was no visual impairment at all. Lastly, although the fovea is our critical area for visual acuity, the surrounding areas of retina in the macula do indeed see, albeit with a blurrier image. Combined with the decreased visual demands of childhood, non-foveal vision may allow normal functioning. Although some astute observers may be able to sense a lesser abnormality, only the infant with extremely severe bilateral visual disruption (e.g. bilateral total retinal detachment or dense vitreous haemorrhage) is likely to be identified clearly by their caretakers as having a visual deficit.

Postmortem histology may identify the presence of intraretinal hemosiderin-laden macrophages suggesting an older injury.[37,73] Iron staining may, therefore, be useful.[43,70] However, dating may still be imprecise and some infants will show no iron staining or hemosiderin.[43,52,62]

Other clinical signs of prior injury would include depigmented circular posterior pole line or retinal folds corresponding to the edges of prior retinoschisis cavities.[99,100] Other late findings include optic atrophy or peripheral retinal scars. However, when such chronic lesions are found clinically, one can not date the exact onset of injury.

Treatment of retinal haemorrhage

Although no treatment is necessary for retinal haemorrhages, if the fovea is obscured for a prolonged period of time, especially when the contralateral fovea is not involved, then amblyopia may result. In these cases, patching of the better eye, may be used to prevent and treat amblyopia. Surgical intervention to remove vitreous blood or blood within a traumatic retinoschisis cavity is controversial,[69,78] but may be helpful in some cases.[51] As both will resolve with time, it is up to the ophthalmologist's judgement to choose between waiting for spontaneous resolution (with the risk of amblyopia, near-sightedness, pigmentary retinopathy, retinal detachment, strabismus)[88,89] or surgical intervention (with the risks of surgery such as cataract, surgical sacrifice of the lens, and retinal tears).[20,88] In my experience, blood within a retinoschisis cavity can take weeks or months to resolve but may layer within the cavity thus exposing the fovea. As the schisis cavity often flattens spontaneously with a good visual prognosis, I am aware of no reports of surgical intervention. One group of authors reported their results of vitrectomy in 5 babies.[20] Although the blood was successfully removed, three of the children, all of whom had severe dense haemorrhages, were found to have retinal holes, macular holes, or retinal ischaemia once the retina was viewed after removal of the blood. They also had poor neurological outcome contributing to the dismal visual results. However, 2 children with less dense vitreous haemorrhages and no underlying retinal injury did better.[20]

Prognosis of retinal haemorrhage

Severe visual impairment or blindness are a well-recognized sequelae of SBS that are usually recognized in the early recovery period.[15] In one study, no child who had a sign-free interval after the SBS incident was later discovered to have visual impairment.[15] Another study found that even in the 'good outcome' group, 10% had impaired vision.[14] The incidence of blindness in long-term survivors is 15–28%,[4,28] with an additional 15% experiencing other forms of visual impairment.[15] Taking all forms of visual impairment together, one survey reported adverse visual outcomes in 67%.[22] In addition to visual loss, patients may experience visual field loss, colour vision impairment, decreased contrast sensitivity, decreased binocularity (e.g. strabismus, unequal vision), and superimposed secondary amblyopia. The presence of retinal haemorrhages correlates with the severity of acute neurological presentation[274] and may be a predictor of poor long-term neurological sequelae.[15]

However, retinal haemorrhages, and even macular retinoschisis do not seem to be the major cause of visual loss. Although some chronic retinal pigmentary changes or chronic irregularity of the internal limiting membrane may be seen,[98] visual acuity may even be normal after traumatic retinoschisis in the absence of other brain or ocular sequelae, although patching treatment for amblyopia may be needed to achieve this result.[34] The internal limiting membrane does not appear to be necessary for good vision from the macula.[116]

Cortical visual impairment and optic nerve atrophy are the main causes of long-term visual impairment in survivors of SBS. Retinal haemorrhages or retinoschisis are usually an insufficient explanation for optic atrophy. Even papilloedema does not adequately explain this phenomenon. Rather, I believe that it is direct injury to the optic nerve, as illustrated in our postmortem studies (see above), which is responsible. This again underscores the importance of these findings and this technique.

OTHER OCULAR INJURIES

The full scope of ocular injuries due to child abuse is beyond the scope of this paper and reviewed elsewhere.[275] However, it is important to recognize that SBS may be associated with eye abnormalities in addition to retinal haemorrhages.

Retinal detachment

In severe shaking, focal or complete detachment of the retina may occur. The mechanism is most likely related to shearing stresses from the shaking vitreous which is firmly attached, particularly in the peripheral retina, where most detachments originate,[17] although haemorrhagic detachment may also be rarely observed.[21,37] In addition, the possibility of direct ocular trauma associated with battering must also be considered especially when there is other evidence of blunt eye trauma.[276] Eyes with detachment may be found to have vitreous haemorrhage as well, although many other studies have shown vitreous haemorrhage in the absence of detachment. Certainly, vitreous haemorrhage may also occur before detachment.[86] Detachment may occur due to fibrous organisation of the vitreous following vitreous haemorrhage resulting in blindness.[24] Retinal detachment is an uncommon finding in most studies although one postmortem study reported detachment in 10 of 16 eyes[17] and a few studies from before the recognition of SBS (with evidence of direct eye trauma as well) report detachment also.[61,63,277] Detachment is significantly associated with SBS as compared to other causes of abuse deaths. Detachment is significantly associated with a higher incidence of all types of intraocular and optic nerve sheath haemorrhages as well as subdural haemorrhage but not with other SBS induced brain injuries.

Other authors have reported giant retinal tears although in at least one case, this may have been a result of vitrectomy surgery for vitreous haemorrhage.[20]

Macular oedema

Although clinically uncommon, one postmortem study found macular oedema, primarily involving the outer plexiform layer, in all cases of traumatic retinoschisis with macular folds.[37] These children were also described as having 'haemorrhagic retinal detachment'. I have observed similar findings on histology postmortem and believe that the shearing of this layer of the retina gives a false impression of oedema. Other authors have suggested the presence of 'exudate'[21, 94] or cotton wool spots[86]. One must be careful to distinguish this from the white patches consistent with Purtscher retinopathy (see above). Yet, macular oedema may be detected on occasion.[86] Diffuse retinal oedema with or without macular involvement has been described in one child.[86] Retinal vascular incompetence following haemorrhage may be the source of oedema.[11] One author has suggested the occasional presence of severe peripheral exudation ('snow banks') although this was before the recognition of SBS and may have included inflammatory responses to direct blunt ocular trauma.[94]

Subretinal fibrosis

This late finding represents scar tissue formation after the initial injury.[86] It may result from subretinal haemorrhage, retinal detachment, or traumatic retinoschisis. Other forms of retinal scarring may also occur.[24]

Corneal abnormalities

Corneal abrasion has been reported in a surprisingly high 10% of shaken infants in one study,[15] although it is rarely noted in other studies.

Cataract

Although one study reported a 10% incidence,[16] cataract is generally considered an uncommon manifestation of SBS that usually occurs only in severely disrupted eyes with only a few reports from before the recognition of SBS[63,277] and even fewer thereafter. Although such severe disruption of the eye contents might result in cataract, blunt trauma to the globe should also be considered. The same applies to the rare finding of ectopia lentis.[21]

Subconjunctival haemorrhage

Although reported rarely in shaken babies,[106] subconjunctival haemorrhage may occur following covert suffocation or secondary to Valsalva. Birth is also a well recognized cause with 0.5–13% of new-borns affected.[119,120]

Hyphema

Although uncommon, hyphema (blood in the anterior chamber of the eye between the cornea and iris) may escape detection until the autopsy. One study identified red blood cells in the anterior chamber (no quantification given) in 17% of victims at autopsy.[37]

Cranial nerve palsy

Cranial nerves III, IV, V, VI, and VII may all be affected although uncommonly (≤ 5%).[16] Gaze abnormalities (e.g. eye deviation) may also occur as a result of central brain injury.[86]

Ptosis

Reports of ptosis[186] may be due to involvement of cranial nerve III or direct blunt trauma to the periorbita.

Optic nerve atrophy

This is one of the most common causes of visual loss following SBS being present in up to 45% of survivors.[60–63,99,100,105,106,186,278] Compression of neural fibres by haemorrhage in the nerve sheath may play a role.[62,186] Yet it can not be explained by the retinal injury except perhaps in cases of total retinal detachment. Rather, I suspect that the direct optic nerve injury sustained as a result of orbital shaking (*vide supra*) is the cause. One of our cases was found to have a posterior optic nerve sheath laceration as well. Papilloedema (see below) may also have a role in the generation of optic atrophy but this is uncommon unless the optic nerve swelling is chronic or severe.[69]

Visual evoked potentials can be helpful in demonstrating damage to the anterior visual pathways.[20] Afferent pupillary defect (Marcus Gunn pupil) may be observed if the optic nerve injury is worse on one side.[20]

Papilloedema

Swelling of the optic nerve may or may not be present in SBS. Acute papilloedema is mentioned infrequently,[52,61,73,94,99,105,278–280] especially when considered in view of the more frequently noted optic atrophy. Yet one study found 7 of 13 victims with optic disc swelling postmortem.[43] This may not have been clinically evident in all cases. The low incidence in survivors supports a conclusion that papilloedema is not the cause of optic atrophy. Alternative explanations, such as orbital shaking, retrograde transynaptic degeneration from cortical injury to the visual pathways, or alternations in CSF dynamics may be important. The low incidence of papilloedema may reflect protection to the effects of increased intracranial pressure from the unfused sutures of younger infants. In addition, obscuration of the optic nerve from clinical view due to overlying retinal or vitreous haemorrhage may lead to under recognition. When present, papilloedema may be a poor prognostic indicator. In one study, autopsy study, the incidence was 40%.[62] In one postmortem study, the incidence was only 17%.[37] Both of these cases also showed optic nerve infarction.

Pupillary abnormalities

Abnormalities of pupillary size or reactivity, including anisocoria or non reactive pupils (e.g. bilateral fixed and dilated), may be secondary to brain injury.[21,34,86,186] In one small study, anisocoria had an intermediate correlation with fatal outcome.[34] Pupillary abnormalities may also be caused by direct blunt eye trauma. An afferent pupillary defect (Marcus Gunn pupil) may be caused by optic nerve injury (see Orbital shaking above) or extremely severe retinal disease such as complete detachment.

Cortical injury

Injury to the occipital cortex is perhaps the most common cause of visual loss which may leave the survivor blind and/or severely visually handicapped. This may occur as the result of infarction, contusion, shearing/laceration, diffuse axonal injury, intraparenchymal haemorrhage, cerebral oedema, increased intracranial pressure, venous thrombosis, or contre-coup injury.[8,20,24,59,60] Acute occipital infarcts or oedema were seen in 6 (28%) of Zimmerman's 21 abused patients under the age of 2 years.[59] An additional 3 patients (14%) had occipital pathology on follow-up CAT scans.[59] However, it is not clear whether all of the infants in this study were shaken. Another group, found that MRI revealed focal occipital lesions in one of four patients.[281] Unfortunately, CT and MRI findings during the acute phase following injury do not necessarily predict long-term visual outcome.

One study found that 35% of 23 children without retinal injury had visual loss.[149] In another paper, 2 of 11 SBS victims were blind bilaterally, 3 blind unilaterally, and 6 with other levels of cortical or visual pathway injury induced visual diminishment.[61] Although this study was published well before the recognition of SBS, the patient population was almost certainly made up predominately by SBS victims. Although visual field loss may also occur due to stroke or injury within the visual pathways,[59] this is less common. One study found that 50% of survivors had gaze disorders due to central nervous system injury.[5]

Peri-ocular ecchymosis

It was actually Caffey who first reported peri-orbital ecchymosis in what we would now recognize as a shaken infant.[1] However, external ecchymosis is uncommon in shaken babies and the presence of peri-orbital bruising would suggest the possibility of direct eye or facial trauma as part of the injury.

References

1 Caffey J. Multiple fractures in the long bones of infants suffering from chronic subdural haematoma. Am J Roentgenol Radium Ther 1946; 56: 163–173
2 Caffey J. On the theory and practice of shaking infants. Am J Dis Child 1972; 124: 161–169
3 Caffey J. The whiplash shaken infant syndrome: manual shaking by the extremities with whip-lash-induced intracranial and intraocular bleedings, linked with residual permanent brain damage and mental retardation. Pediatrics 1974; 54: 396–403
4 Duhaime A et al. Long-term outcome in infants with the shaking-impact syndrome. Pediatr Neurosurg 1996; 24: 292–298
5 Ludwig S, Warman M. Shaken baby syndrome: a review of 20 cases. Ann Emerg Med 1984; 13: 51–54
6 Taff M, Boglioli L, DeFelice J. Commentary on controversies in shaken baby syndrome and on Gilliland MGF, Folberg R. Shaken babies – some have no impact injuries, (J Forensic Sci 1996; 41:114–116). J Forensic Sci 1996; 41: 729–730

7 Lancon J, Haines D, Parent A. Anatomy of the shaken baby syndrome. Anat Rec 1998; 253: 13–18

8 Dykes L. The whiplash shaken infant syndrome: what have we learned? Child Abuse Negl 1986; 10: 211–221

9 Hanigan W, Peterson R, Njus G. Tin ear syndrome: rotational acceleration in pediatric head injuries. Pediatrics 1987; 80: 618–622

10 Duhaime A et al. Nonaccidental head injury in infants – the 'shaken-baby syndrome' N Engl J Med 1998; 338: 1822–1829

11 Cox L. The shaken baby syndrome: diagnosis using CT and MRI. Radiol Technol 1996; 67: 513–520

12 Gilliland M, Folberg R. Author's response. J Forensic Sci 1996; 41: 730

13 Rosenberg N et al. Retinal hemorrhage. Pediatr Emerg Care 1994; 10: 303–305

14 Swenson J, Levitt C. Shaken baby syndrome: diagnosis and prevention. Minn Med 1997; 80: 41–44

15 Bonnier C, Nassogne M, Errard P. Outcome and prognosis of whiplash shaken infant syndrome; late consequences after a symptom-free interval. Dev Med Child Neurol 1995; 37: 943–956

16 Ewing-Cobbs L et al. Neuroimaging, physical, and developmental findings after inflicted and noninflicted traumatic brain injury in young children. Pediatrics 1998; 102: 300–307

17 Green M et al. Ocular and cerebral trauma in non-accidental injury in infancy: underlying mechanisms and implications for paediatric practice. Br J Ophthalmol 1996; 80: 282–287

18 Starling S, Holden J, Jenny C. Abusive head trauma: the relationship of perpetrators to their victims. Pediatrics 1995; 95: 259–262

19 Feldman K, Brewer D, Shaw D. Evolution of the cranial computed tomography scan in child abuse. Child Abuse Negl 1995; 19: 307–314

20 Matthews G, Das A. Dense vitreous hemorrhages predict poor visual and neurological prognosis in infants with shaken baby syndrome. J Pediatr Ophthalmol Strabismus 1996; 33: 260–265

21 Brown J, Minns R. Non-accidental head injury, with particular reference to whiplash shaking injury and medico-legal aspects. Dev Med Child Neurol 1993; 35: 849–869

22 Child Abuse Prevention Center. Research project on the incidence and risk factors of shaken baby syndrome in the State of Utah. 1998

23 Alexander R et al. Incidence of impact trauma with cranial injuries ascribed to shaking. Am J Dis Child 1990; 144: 724–726

24 Jacobi G. Schadensmuster schwerer mißhandlungen mit und ohne todesfolge. Monatsschr Kinderheilkd 1986; 134: 307–315

25 Pounder D. Shaken adult syndrome. Am J Forensic Med Pathol 1997; 18: 321–324

26 Kraus J, Rock A, Hemyari M. Brain injuries among infants, children, adolescents, and young adults. Am J Dis Child 1990; 144: 684–691

27 Nashelsky M, Dix J. The time interval between lethal infant shaking and the onset of symptoms: a review of the shaken baby syndrome literature. Am J Forensic Med Pathol 1995; 6: 154–157

28 Fischer H, Allasio D. Permanently damaged: long-term follow-up of shaken babies. Clin Pediatr 1994; 33: 696–698

29 American Academy of Pediatrics Committee on Child Abuse and Neglect. Shaken baby syndrome: inflicted cerebral trauma. Pediatrics 1993; 92: 872–875

30 Weinberg H, Tunnessen W. Megacephaly: heeding the head. Contemp Pediatr 1996; 13: 169, 172, 175

31 Lazoritz S, Baldwin S, Kini N. The whiplash shaken infant syndrome: has Caffey's syndrome changed or have we changed his syndrome? Child Abuse Negl 1997; 21: 1009–1014

32 Andrews A. Ocular manifestations of child abuse. Penn Med 1996; 99S: 71–75

33 Betz M et al. Morphometrical analysis of retinal hemorrhages in the shaken baby syndrome. Forensic Sci Int 1996; 78: 71–80

34 Mills M. Funduscopic lesions associated with mortality in shaken baby syndrome. J Am Assoc Pediatr Opthalmol Strabismus 1998; 2: 67–71

35 Gilliland M, Folberg R. Shaken babies – some have no impact injuries. J Forensic Sci 1996; 41: 114–116

36 Munger C et al. Ocular and associated neuropathologic observations in suspected whiplash shaken infant syndrome: a retrospective study of 12 cases. Am J Forensic Med Pathol 1993; 14: 193–200

37 Hymel K et al. Comparison of intracranial computed tomographic (CT) findings in pediatric abusive and accidental head trauma. Pediatr Radiol 1997; 27: 743–747

38 Ellis M. The pathology of fatal child abuse. Pathology 1997; 29: 113–121

39 Wilkins B. Head injury – abuse or accident? Arch Dis Child 1997; 76: 393–396

40 Duhaime A et al. The shaken baby syndrome: a clinical, pathological, and biomechanical study. J Neurosurg 1987; 66: 409–415

41 Massicotte S et al. Vitreoretinal traction and perimacular retinal folds in the eyes of deliberately traumatized children. Ophthalmology 1991; 98: 1124–1127

42 Hadley M et al. The infant whiplash-shake injury syndrome: a clinical and pathological study. Neurosurgery 1989; 24: 536–540

43 Budenz D et al. Ocular and optic nerve hemorrhages in abused infants with intracranial injuries. Ophthalmology 1994; 101: 559–565

44 Sunderland R. Commentary. Arch Dis Child 1997; 76: 396–397.

45 Geddes J. What's new in the diagnosis of head injury? J Clin Pathol 1997; 50: 271–274

46 Levin A et al. Shaken baby syndrome diagnosed by magnetic resonance imaging. Pediatr Emerg Care 1989; 5: 181–186

47 Sato Y et al. Head injury in child abuse: evaluation with MR imaging. Radiology 1989; 173: 653–657

48 Kapoor S et al. The significance of white-centered retinal hemorrhages in the shaken baby syndrome. Pediatr Emerg Care 1997; 3: 183–185

49 Weingeist T et al. Terson's syndrome: clinicopathologic correlations. Ophthalmology 1986; 93: 1435–1442

50 Dana M et al. Spontaneous and traumatic vitreous hemorrhage. Ophthalmology 1993; 100: 1377–1383

51 Kuhn F et al. Terson syndrome: results of vitrectomy and the significance of vitreous hemorrhage in patients with subarachnoid hemorrhage. Ophthalmology 1998; 105: 472–477

52 Lambert S, Johnson T, Hoyt C. Optic nerve sheath hemorrhages associated with the shaken baby syndrome. Arch Ophthalmol 1986; 104: 1509–1512

53 Gilliland M, Luckenbach M, Chenier T. Systemic and ocular findings in 169 prospectively studied child deaths: retinal hemorrhages usually mean child abuse. Forensic Sci Int 1994; 68: 117–132

54 Schoenfeld A et al. Retinal hemorrhages in the newborn following labor induced by oxytocin or dinoprostone. Arch Ophthalmol 1985; 103: 932–934

55 Bedell A. The importance of ophthalmoscopic photographs in forensic medicine: Kodachromes. Trans Am Ophthalmol Soc 1955; 53: 63–73

56 Nolte K. Transillumination enhances photographs of retinal hemorrhages. J Forensic Sci 1997; 42: 935–936

57 Gilliland M, Folberg R. Retinal hemorrhages: replicating the clinician's view of the eye. Forensic Sci Int 1992; 56: 77–80

58 Howard M, Bell B, Uttley D. The pathophysiology of infant subdural haematoma. Br J Neurosurg 1993; 7: 355–365

59 Zimmerman R et al, Computed tomography of craniocerebral injury in the abused child. Radiology 1979; 130: 687–690

60 Frank Y, Zimmerman R, Leeds N. Neurological manifestations in abused children who have been shaken. Dev Med Child Neurol 1985; 27: 312–316

61 Harcourt B, Hopkins D. Ophthalmic manifestations of the battered-baby syndrome. BMJ 1971; 3: 398–401

62 Rao N et al. Autopsy findings in the eyes of fourteen fatally abused children. Forensic Sci Int 1988; 39: 293–299

63 Mushin A. Ocular damage in the battered-baby syndrome. BMJ 1971; 3: 402–404

64 Miziara C et al. Sindrome da crianca espancada: aspectos neurologicos em 7 casos (The battered child syndrome: neurologic aspects in 7 cases). Arq Neuropsiquiatr 1988; 46: 359

65 Billmire M, Myers M. Serious head injury in infants: accident or abuse? Pediatrics 1985;
    75: 340–342

66 Johnson D, Braun D, Friendly D. Accidental head trauma and retinal hemorrhage.
    Neurosurgery 1993; 33: 231–235

67 Kahn Y et al. Traumatic mechanisms of head injury in child abuse. Childs Brain 1983;
    10: 229–241

68 Greenes D, Schutzman S. Occult intracranial injury in infants. Ann Emerg Med 1998; 32:
    680–686

69 Mills M. Terson syndrome. Ophthalmology 1998; 105: 2161–2162

70 Riffenburgh R, Sathyavagiswaran L. Ocular findings at autopsy of child abuse victims.
    Ophthalmology 1991; 98: 1519–1524

71 Tyagi A, Willshaw H, Ainsworth J. Unilateral retinal hemorrhages in non-accidental
    injury. Lancet 1997; 349: 1224

72 Gayle M et al. Retinal hemorrhage in the young child: a review of etiology, predisposed
    conditions, and clinical implications. J Emerg Med 1995; 13: 233–239

73 Elner S et al. Ocular and associated systemic findings in suspected child abuse: a
    necropsy study. Arch Ophthalmol 1990; 108: 1094–1101

74 Coats D, Paysse E. Dolls and shaken baby syndrome. J Am Assoc Pediatr Opthalmol
    Strabismus 1998; 2: 65

75 Terson A. De l'hémorrhagie dans le corps vitré au cours de l'hémorrhagia cérébrale.
    Clin Ophthalmol 1900; 6: 309–312

76 Muller P, Deck J. Intraocular and optic nerve sheath hemorrhage in cases of sudden
    intracranial hypertension. J Neurosurg 1974; 41: 160–166

77 Billotte C et al. A propos de syndrome de Terson et d'un cas post-traumatique chez le
    nourrisson. Bull Soc Opthal Fr 1988; 88: 111–114

78 Kuhn F et al. Author's reply. Ophthalmology 1998; 105: 2162–2163

79 Weissgold D et al. Ruptured vascular malformation masquerading as battered/shaken
    baby syndrome: a nearly tragic mistake. Surv Ophthalmol 1995; 39: 509–512

80 Manschot W. Subarachnoid hemorrhage: intraocular symptoms and their pathogenesis.
    Am J Ophthalmol 1954; 38: 501–505

81 Brinker T et al. Breakdown of the meningeal barrier surrounding the intraorbital optic
    nerve after experimental subarachnoid hemorrhage. Am J Ophthalmol 1997; 124:
    373–380

82 Paton L. VII. Diseases of the nervous system: 1. Ocular symptoms in subarachnoid
    haemorrhage. Trans Ophthalmol Soc UK 1924; 110–124

83 McDonald A. Ocular lesions caused by intracranial hemorrhage. Trans Am Ophthalmol
    Soc 1931; 29: 418–432

84 Vanderlinden R, Chisolm L. Vitreous hemorrhages and sudden increased intracranial
    pressure. J Neurosurg 1974; 41: 167–176

85 Manschot W. The fundus oculi in subarachnoid haemorrhage. Acta Ophthalmol 1944;
    33: 281–299

86 Wong J, Wong P, Yeoh R. Ocular manifestations in shaken baby syndrome. Singapore
    Med J 1995; 36: 391–392

87 Shaw H, Lander M. Vitreous hemorrhage after intracranial hemorrhage. Am J
    Ophthalmol 1975; 80: 207–213

88 Ferrone P, de Juan E. Vitreous hemorrhage in infants. Arch Ophthalmol 1994; 112:
    1185–1189

89 Miller-Weeks M et al. Myopia induced by vitreous hemorrhage. Am J Ophthalmol 1990;
    109: 199–203

90 Wahl N, Woodall B. Hypothermia in shaken infant syndrome. J Pediatr Emerg Care
    1995; 1: 233–234

91 Duane T. Valsalva hemorrhagic retinopathy. Trans Am Ophthalmol Soc 1972; 70:
    298–313

92 Marr W, Marr E. Some observations on Purtscher's disease: traumatic retinal
    angiopathy. Am J Ophthalmol 1962; 54: 693–705

93 Tomasi L, Rosman P. Purtscher retinopathy in the battered child syndrome. Am J Dis
    Child 1986; 93: 1335–1337

94 Gilkes M. Fundi of battered babies. Lancet 1967; 2: 468–469

95 Hogan MJ. The vitreous, its structure, and relation to the cilliary body and retina. Invest Ophthalmol 1963; 2: 418–445

96 Sebag J. Age-related differences in the human vitreoretinal interface. Arch Ophthalmol 1991; 109: 966–971

97 Tongue A. The ophthalmologist's role in diagnosing child abuse. Ophthalmology 1991; 98: 1009–1010

98 Spaide R et al. Shaken baby syndrome. American Family Physician 1990; 41: 1145–1152

99 Gaynon M et al. Retinal folds in the shaken baby syndrome. Am J Ophthalmol 1988; 106: 423–425

100 Greenwald M et al. Traumatic retinoschisis in battered babies. Ophthalmology 1986; 93: 618–625

101 Keane J. Neurologic eye signs following motorcycle accidents. Arch Neurol 1989; 46: 761–762

102 Bird C et al. Strangulation in child abuse: CT diagnosis. Radiology 1987; 163: 373–375

103 Hymel K et al. Coagulopathy in pediatric abusive head trauma. Pediatrics 1997; 99: 371–375

104 Wolter J. Coup-contrecoup mechanism of ocular injuries. Am J Ophthalmol 1975; 56: 785–796

105 Jensen A, Smith R, Olson M. Ocular clues to child abuse. J Pediatr Ophthalmol 1971; 8: 270–272

106 Roussey M et al. L'ophtalmologiste et les victimes de sevices. J Fr Ophtalmol 1987; 10: 201–205

107 Hertle R, Quinn G, Duhaime A. Retinal hemorrhage after cardiopulmonary resuscitation. Pediatrics 1990; 86: 649–650

108 Snodgrass G. The eye and the brain in non-accidental injury involving young children. Br J Ophthalmol 1996; 80: 275

109 Gilliland M, Luckenbach M. Are retinal hemorrhages found after resuscitation attempts? A study of the eyes of 169 children. Am J Forensic Med Pathol 1993; 14: 187–192

110 Luerssen TG, Bruce DA, Humphreys RP. Position statement on identifying the infant with nonaccidental central nervous system injury (the whiplash-shake syndrome). Pediatr Neurosurg 1993; 19: 170

111 Eisenbrey A. Retinal hemorrhage in the battered child. Child Brain 1979; 5: 40–44

112 Plunkett J. Shaken baby syndrome and the death of Matthew Eappen: a forensic pathologist's response. Am J Forensic Med Pathol 1999; 20: 17–21

113 Keithahn M et al. Retinal folds in Terson syndrome. Ophthalmology 1993; 100: 1187–1190

114 Ulbig M et al. Long-term results after drainage of premacular subhyaloid hemorrhage into the vitreous with a pulsed Nd:YAG laser. Arch Ophthalmol 1998; 116: 1465–1469

115 Toosi S, Malton M. Terson's syndrome – significance of ocular findings. Ann Ophthalmol 1987; 19: 7–12

114 Morris R et al. Hemorrhagic macular cysts in Terson's syndrome and its implications for macular surgery. Dev Ophthalmol 1997; 29: 44–54

117 Morris R, Kuhn F, Witherspoon C. Hemorrhagic macular cysts. Ophthalmology 1994; 101: 1

118 Sezen F. Retinal haemorrhage in newborn infants. Br J Ophthalmol 1970; 55: 248–253

119 Baum J, Bulpitt C. Retinal and conjunctival haemorrhage in newborn. Arch Dis Child 1970; 45: 344–349

120 Jain I et al. Ocular hazards during birth. J Pediatr Ophthalmol Strabismus 1980; 171: 14–16

121 Planten J, Schaaf P. Retinal haemorrhage in the newborn. Ophthalmologica 1971; 162: 213–222.

122 Schenker J, Gombos G. Retinal hemorrhage in the newborn. Obstet Gynecol 1966; 27: 521–523

123 Egge K, Lyng G, Maltau J. Effect of instrumental delivery on the frequency and severity of retinal hemorrhages in the newborn. Acta Obstet Gynecol Scand 1981; 60: 153–155.

124 Levin S et al. Diagnostic and prognostic value of retinal hemorrhages in the neonate. Obstet Gynecol 1980; 155: 309–314

125 Berkus M et al. Cohort study of silastic obstetric vacuum cup deliveries: I. Safety of the instrument. Obstet Gynecol 1985; 66: 503–509

126 Berkus M et al. Cohort study of silastic obstetric vacuum cup deliveries: II. Unsuccessful vacuum extractions. Obstet Gynecol 1986; 68: 662–666

127 Maumenee A, Hellman L, Shettles L. Factors influencing plasma prothrombin in the newborn infant. Bull Johns Hopkins Hosp 1941; 68: 158–168

128 Smith W et al. Magnetic resonance imaging evaluation of neonates with retinal hemorrhages. Pediatrics 1992; 89: 332–333

129 von Noorden G, Khodadoust A. Retinal hemorrhage in newborns and organic amblyopia. Arch Ophthalmol 1973; 89: 91–93

130 Stafford J et al. Prenatal cocaine exposure and the development of the human eye. Ophthalmology 1994; 101: 301–308

131 Sihota R, Bose S, Paul A. The neonatal fundus in maternal toxemia. J Pediatr Ophthalmol Strabismus 1989; 26: 281–284

132 Paris C et al. Neonatal macular hemorrhage. Int Ophthalmol 1991; 15: 153–155

133 Wiznia R, Price J. Vitreous hemorrhages and disseminated intravascular coagulation in the newborn. Am J Ophthalmol 1976; 82: 222–226

134 Paciuc M, Garcia-Alonso P, Moragrega E. Hyphema and vitreous hemorrhage in a newborn. J Pediatr Ophthalmol Strabismus 1988; 19: 680

135 Chadwick D et al. Deaths from falls in children: how far is fatal? J Trauma 1991; 31: 1353–1355

136 Shugerman R et al. Epidural hemorrhage: is it abuse? Pediatrics 1996; 97: 664–668

137 Reiber G. Fatal falls in childhood: how far must children fall to sustain fatal head injury? Report of cases and review of the literature. Am J Forensic Med Pathol 1993; 14: 201–207

138 Duhaime A et al. Head injury in very young children: mechanism, injury types, and ophthalmologic findings in 100 hospitalized patients younger than 2 years of age. Pediatrics 1992; 90: 179–185

139 Buys Y et al. Retinal findings after head trauma in infants and young children. Ophthalmology 1992; 99: 1718–1723

140 Wheeler D, Shope T. Depressed skull fracture in a 7-month-old who fell from bed. Pediatrics 1997; 100: 1033–1034

141 James D, Leadbetter S. Letter to the Editor. Forensic Sci Int 1996; 82: 255

142 Stewart G. [Letter]. Pediatr Emerg Care 1994; 10: 62

143 Alario A et al. Do retinal hemorrhages occur with accidental head trauma in young children? Am J Dis Child 1990; 144: 445

144 Elder J, Taylor R, Klug G. Retinal hemorrhage in accidental head trauma in childhood. J Paediatr Child Health 1991; 27: 286–289

145 Luerssen T et al. Retinal hemorrhages, seizures, and intracranial hemorrhages: relationships and outcomes in children suffering traumatic brain injury. Concepts Pediatr Neurosurg 1991; 11: 87–94

146 Humphreys R, Hendrick E, Hoffman H. The head-injured child who 'talks and dies': a report of 4 cases. Childs Nerv Syst 1990; 6: 139–142

147 Duhaime A et al. Disappearing subdural hematomas in children. Pediatr Neurosurg 1996; 25: 116–122

148 Aoki N, Masuzawa H. Infantile acute subdural hematoma. J Neurosurg 1984; 61: 273–280

149 Hollenhorst R, Stein H. Ocular signs and prognosis in subdural and subarachnoid bleeding in young children. Arch Ophthalmol 1958; 60: 187–192

150 Phelps C. The association of pale-centered retinal hemorrhages with intracranial bleeding in infancy. Am J Ophthalmol 1971; 72: 348–350

151 Till K. Subdural haematoma and effusion in infancy. BMJ 1968; 3: 400–402

152 Gutierrez F, Raimondi A. Acute subdural hematoma in anfancy and childhood. Childs Brain 1975; 1: 269–290

153 Sparacio R, Khatib R, Cook A. Acute subdural hematoma in infancy. NY State J Med 1971; 71: 212–213

154 Cantani A, Bamonte G. Epidemiology of ocular complications of childhood head trauma. Pediatr Emerg Care 1990; 6: 271-274

155 Levin A. Ocular complications of head trauma in children. Pediatr Emerg Care 1991; 7: 129–130

156 Raimondi A, Hirschauer J. Head injury in the infant and toddler. Coma scoring and outcome scale. Childs Brain 1984; 11: 12–35

157 Ikeda Y. Child abuse and child abuse studies in Japan. Acta Paediatr Jpn 1995; 37: 240–247

158 Saito S. Early intervention in case of child abuse: co-operation between the hot-line and local facilities. Acta Paediatr Jpn 1995; 37: 262–271

159 Kobayashi M et al. Child abuse viewed through the hot-line in Osaka, Japan. Acta Paediatr Jpn 1995; 37: 272–278

160 Matsuzaka T et al. Incidence and causes of intracranial hemorrhage in infancy: a prospective surveillance study after vitamin K prophylaxis. Brain Dev 1989; 11: 384–348

161 Bacon C. Sayer G, Howe J. Extensive retinal haemorrhages in infancy-an innocent cause. BMJ 1978; 1: 281

162 Levin A. Retinal hemorrhages after cardiopulmonary resuscitation: literature review and commentary. Pediatr Emerg Care 1986; 2: 269

163 Kanter R. Retinal hemorrhage after cardiopulmonary resuscitation or child abuse. J Pediatr 1986; 180: 430–432

164 Quasney M, Kerr N. Do retinal hemorrhages occur after CPR in children? A prospective, multi-institutional study [abstract]. The Second National Conference on Shaken Baby Syndrome, Salt Lake City, Utah, September 15, 1998

165 Odom A. et al. Prevalence of retinal hemorrhages in pediatric patients after in-hospital cardiopulmonary resuscitation: a prospective study. Pediatrics 1997; 99: E3

166 Fackler J, Berkowitz I, Green R. Retinal hemorrhage in newborn piglets following cardiopulmonary resuscitation. Am J Dis Child 1992; 146: 1294–1296

167 Guerci A et al. Transmission of intrathoracic pressure to the intracranial space during cardiopulmonary resuscitation in dogs. Circ Res 1905, 56. 20–30

168 Goetting M, Sowa B. Retinal haemorrhage after cardiopulmonary resuscitation in children: an etiologic evaluation. Pediatrics 1990; 85: 585–588

169 Weedn V, Mansour A, Nichols M. Retinal hemorrhage in an infant after cardiopulmonary resuscitation. Am J Forensic Med Pathol 1990; 11: 79 82

170 Kramer K,Goldstein B. Retinal hemorrhages following cardiopulmonary resuscitation. Clin Pediatr 1993; 32: 366–368

171 Kirschner R, Stein R. The mistaken diagnosis of child abuse. Am J Dis Child 1985; 139: 873–875

172 Baumal C et al. Screening for pediatric cytomegalovirus retinitis. Arch Pediatr Adolesc Med 1996; 150: 1186–1192

173 Fechtner R et al. Complications of glaucoma surgery: ocular decompression retinopathy. Arch Ophthalmol 1992; 110: 965–968

174 Bolder P, Norton M. Retinal hemorrhage following anesthesia. Anesthesiology 1984; 61: 595–597

175 Holt J, Gordon-Smith E. Retinal abnormalities in diseases of the blood. Br J Ophthalmol 1969; 53: 145–160

176 Kearns T, Changes in the ocular fundus in blood diseases. Med Clin North Am, 1959; 40: 1209–1216

177 Rubenstein R, Yanoff M, Albert D. Thrombocytopenia, anemia, and retinal hemorrhage. Am J Ophthalmol 1968; 65: 435–439

178 Marshall R. Review of lesions in the optic fundus in various diseases of the blood. Blood 1959; 14: 882–891

179 Merin S, Freund M. Retinopathy of severe anemia. Am J Ophthalmol 1968; 66: 1102–1106

180 Pears M, Pickering G. Changes in the fundus oculi after haemorrhage. Quart J Med 1960; 29: 153–178

181 Keane J. Retinal hemorrhages: Its significance in 100 patients with acute encephalopathy of unknown cause. Arch Neurol 1979; 36: 691–694

182 Fahmy J. Fundal haemorrhages in ruptured intracranial aneurysms. I. Material, frequency and morphology. Acta Ophthalmol 1973; 51: 289–298

183 Rácz, Bobest M, Szilvássy I. Significance of fundal hemorrhage in predicting the state of the patient with ruptured intracranial aneurysm. Ophthalmologica 1977; 175: 61–66

184 Shaw H, Landers M, Sydnor C. The significance of intraocular hemorrhages due to subarachnoid hemorrhage. Ann Ophthalmol 1977; 9: 1403–1405

185 Timberlake W, Kubik C. Follow-up report with clinical and anatomical notes on 280 patients with subarachnoid hemorrhage. Trans Am Neurol Assoc 1952; 77: 26–30

186 Lam C et al. Traumatic aneurysm from shaken baby syndrome. Neurosurgery 1996; 39: 1252–1255

187 McLellan N, Prasad R, Punt J. Spontaneous subhyaloid and retinal haemorrhages in an infant. Arch Dis Child 1986; 61: 1130–1132

188 Nishio A et al. Anterior communicating artery aneurysm in early childhood: report of a case. Surg Neurol 1991; 35: 224–229

189 Crisostomo E, Leaton E, Rosenblum E. Features of intracranial aneurysms in infants and report of a case. Dev Med Child Neurol 1986; 28: 62–76

190 Kanaan I, Lasjaunias P, Coates R. The spectrum od intracranial aneurysms in pediatrics. Minim Invasive Neurosurg 1995; 38: 1–9

191 Tekkök IH, Ventureyra EC. Spontaneous intracranial hemorrhae of structural origin during the first year of life. Childs Nerv Syst 1997; 13: 154–165

192 Smith R, Smith W. Arachnoid cysts of the middle cranial fossa. Surg Neurol 1976; 5: 246–252

193 Aicardi J, Bauman F. Supratentorial extracerebral cysts in infants and children. J Neurol Neurosurg Psychiatry 1975; 38: 57–68

194 Clark R et al. Retinal hemorrhages associated with spinal cord arteriovenous malformation. Clin Pediatr 1995; 34: 281–283

195 Smith C, Jay V. Postmortem study of intraocular hemorrhage associated with natural disease. The National Conference on Shaken Baby Syndrome, Salt Lake City, Utah, November 1996

196 Levin A. Pediatric ophthalmology. Can J Ophthalmol 1996; 31: 141

197 Yoon SS, Macdonald SC, Parrish G. Deaths from unintentional carbon monoxide poisoning and potential for prevention with carbon monoxide detectors. JAMA 1998; 279: 685–687

198 Kelley J, Sophocleus G. Retinal hemorrhages in subacute carbon monoxide poisoning. JAMA 1978; 239: 1515–1517

199 Abt I, Witt D. A case of carbon monoxide poisoning in a child. Med Clin North Am 1922; 5: 1645–1651

200 Crocker P, Walker J. Pediatric carbon monoxide toxicity. J Emerg Med 1985; 3: 443–448

201 Bilchik R, Muller-Bergh H, Freshman M. Ischemic retinopathy due to carbon monoxide poisoning. Arch Ophthalmol 1971; 86: 142–144

202 Baker M, Henretig F, Ludwig S. Carboxyhemoglobin levels in children with nonspecific flu-like symptoms. J Pediatr 1988; 113: 504

203 Ferguson L, Burke M, Choromokos E. Carbon monoxide retinopathy. Arch Ophthalmol 1985; 103: 66–67

204 Breysse P. Chronic carbon monoxide poisoning. Industr Med Surg 1961; 312: 20–22

205 Hoyle C, Darbyshire P, Eden O. Idiopathic thrombocytopenia in childhood: Edinburgh experience 1962–1982. Scott Med J 1986; 31: 174–179

206 Simons S et al. Idiopathic thrombocytopenic purpura in children. J Pediatr 1975; 87: 16–22

207 Cohn J. Thrombocytopenia in childhood: an evaluation of 433 patients. Scand J Haematol 1976; 16: 226–240

208 Frankel C, Pastore D. Idiopathic thrombocytopenic purpura with intracranial hemorrhage and vitreous hemorrhage. Clin Pediatr 1990; 29: 725–728

209 Pegelow C et al. Severe protein S deficiency in a newborn. Pediatrics 1992; 89: 674–676

210 Peters C et al. Homozygous protein C deficiency: observations on the nature of the molecular abnormality and the effectiveness of Warfarin therapy. Pediatrics 1988; 81: 272–276

211 Pulido J et al. Protein C deficiency associated with vitreous hemorrhage in a neonate. Am J Ophthalmol 1987; 104: 546–547

212 Estellés A et al. Severe inherited 'homozygous' protein C deficiency in a newborn infant. Thromb Haemostas 1984; 52: 53–56

213 Mahasandana C et al. Neonatal purpura fulminans associated with homozygous protein S deficiency. Lancet 1990; 335: 61–62

214 Mahasandana C et al. Homozygous protein S deficiency in an infant with purpura fulminans. J Pediatr 1990; 117: 750–753

215 Woerner S, Abildgaard C, French B. Intracranial hemorrhage in children with idiopathic thrombocytopenic purpura. Pediatrics 1981; 67: 453–460

216 Harley J. Disorders of coagulation misdiagnosed as nonaccidental bruising. Pediatr Emerg Care 1997; 13: 347–349

217 Werner E et al. Relative value of diagnostic studies for von Willebrand disease. Pediatrics 1992; 121: 34–38

218 Shiono T et al. Vitreous, retinal and subretinal hemorrhages associated with von Willebrand's syndrome. Graefe's Arch Clin Exp Ophthalmol 1992; 230: 496–497

219 Hymel K et al. Coagulopathy in pediatric abusive head trauma. Pediatrics 1997; 99: 371–375

220 Klein R et al. Incidence of retinopathy and associated risk factors from time of diagnosis of insulin-dependent diabetes. Arch Ophthalmol 1997; 115: 351–356

221 Verougstraete C et al. First microangiographic abnormalities in childhood diabetes – types of lesions. Graefe's Arch Clin Exp Ophthalmol 1991; 229: 24–32

222 Jackson, R et al. Retinopathy in adolescents and young adults with onset of insulin-dependent diabetes in childhood. Ophthalmology 1982; 89: 7–13

223 Palmberg P et al. The natural history of retinopathy in insulin-dependent juvenile-onset diabetes. Ophthalmology 1981; 88: 613–618

224 Frank R et al. Retinopathy in juvenile-onset diabetes of short duration. Ophthalmology 1980; 87: 1–9

225 Klein R et al. The Wisconsin epidemiologic study of diabetic retinopathy: II. Prevalence and risk of diabetic retinopathy when age at diagnosis is less than 30 years. Arch Ophthalmol 1984; 102: 520–526

226 Sethi S. Retinal hemorrhages after extra corporeal membranous oxygenation. North Carolina Med J 1990; 51: 246

227 Pollack J, Tychsen L. Prevalence of retinal hemorrhages in infants after extracorporeal membrane oxygenation. Am J Ophthalmol 1996; 121: 297–303

228 Patrias M, Rabinowicz I, Klein M. Ocular findings in infants treated with extracorporeal membrane oxygenator support. Pediatrics 1988; 82: 560–564

229 Varn M et al. Retinal examinations in infants after extracorporeal membrane oxygenation. J Pediatr Ophthalmol Strabismus 1997; 34: 182–185

230 Young T et al. Extracorporeal membrane oxygenation causing asymmetric vasculopathy in neonatal infants. J Am Assoc Pediatr Opthalmol Strabismus 1997; 1: 235–240

231 Carney M, Wortham E, Al-Mateen K. Vitreous hemorrhage and extracorporeal membrane oxygenation. Am J Ophthalmol 1993; 115: 391–393

232 Peterson R, Rosenthal A. Retinopathy and papilledema in cyanotic congenital heart disease. Pediatrics 1972; 49: 243–249

233 VanderVeen D, Pasquale L, Fulton A. Central retinal vein occlusion in a young child with cyanotic heart disease. Arch Ophthalmol 1997; 115: 1077

234 Levy H et al. Vitreous hemorrhage as an ophthalmic complication of galactosemia. J Pediatr 1996; 129: 922–925

235 Baric I et al. Diagnosis and management of glutaric aciduria type I. J Inherit Metab Dis 1998; 21: 326–340

236 Morton D. GA1 must be part of megacephaly differential. Contemp Pediatr 1996; 14: 158

237 Kohler M, Hoffmann G. Subdural haematoma in a child with glutaric aciduria type 1. Pediatr Radiol 1998; 28: 582

238 Sirotnak A, Greene C. Evaluation of abusive head trauma and GA-1 (glutaric aciduria type I) [abstract]. The Second National Conference on Shaken Baby Syndrome, Salt Lake City, Utah, September 14, 1998

239 Lauer A et al. Hemolytic uremic syndrome associated with Purtscher-like retinopathy. Arch Ophthalmol 1998; 116: 1119–1120

240 Skalina M et al. Hypertensive retinopathy in the newborn infant. J Pediatr 1983; 103: 781–786

241 Daniels S et al. The prevalence of retinal vascular abnormalities in children and adolescents with essential hypertension. Am J Ophthalmol 1991; 111: 205–208

242 Carr R, Henkind P. Retinal findings associated with serum hyperviscosity.Am J Ophthalmol 1963; 57: 23–31

243 Hanchette J, Kaplan S. Vaccination nation: children on the frontline. Families claim vaccine damage followed by unfair prosecution. Gannet News Service, August 31, 1998

244 Scheibner V. Shaken baby syndrome: the vaccination link. Nexus 1998; 35–38, 87

245 Devin F et al. Occlusion of central retinal vein after hepatitis B vaccination. Lancet 1996; 347: 1626

246 Iwasa S, Ishida S, Kiyoto A. Swelling of the brain of mice caused by pertussis vaccine – its quantitative determination and the responsible factors in the vaccine. Jpn J Med Sci Biol 1985; 38: 53–65

247 Ciarallo L. Two cases of incontinentia pigmentii simulating child abuse. Pediatrics 1997; 100: E6

248 Guyer D et al. Leukemic retinopathy: relationship between fundus lesions and hematolgic parameters at diagnosis. Ophthalmology 1989; 96: 860–864

249 Clarke W. Leukemic infiltrates in the optic nerve in acute lymphoblastic leukemia. Can Ophthal Case Consult 1998; 2: 24–25

250 Rosenthal A. Ocular manifestations of leukemia: a review. Ophthalmology 1983; 90: 899–905

251 Lewallen S. Ocular malaria. Ophthalmology 1997; 104: 564

252 Biswas J et al. Ocular malaria: a clinical and histopathologic study. Ophthalmology 1997; 103: 1471–1475

253 Pender E, Newman J. Malaria in children. Pediatr Emerg Care 1990; 6: 40–42

254 Lewalen S. The fundus in severe malaria. Arch Ophthalmol 1998; 116: 542

255 Hero M et al. Photographic and angiographic characterization of the retina of Kenyan children with severe malaria. Arch Ophthalmol 1997; 115: 997–1003

256 Harding S, Hero M, Winstanley P. The fundus in severe malaria. Arch Ophthalmol 1998; 116: 542–543

257 Fraser S, Horgan S, Bardavio J. Retinal haemorrhage in meningitis. Eye 1995; 9: 659–660

258 Ferreira R et al. Menkes disease: new ocular and electroretinographic findings. Ophthalmology 1998; 105: 1076–1078

259 Smith C, Jay V. Postmortem study of intraocular hemorrhage associated with natural disease. The National Conference on Shaken Baby Syndrome, Salt Lake City, Utah, November 1996

260 Valentine J et al. Clinical and toxicological findings in two young siblings and autopsy findings in one sibling with multiple hospital admissions resulting in death. Am J Forensic Med Pathol 1997; 18: 276–281

261 Raab E, Leopold I, Hodes H. Retinopathy in Rocky Mountain spotted fever. Am J Ophthalmol 1969; 68: 42–46

262 Presley G. Fundus changes in Rocky Mountain spotted fever. Am J Ophthalmol 1969; 67: 263–267

263 Sulewski M, Green R. Ocular histopathologic features of a presumed case of Rocky Mountain spotted fever. Retina 1986; 6: 125–130

264 Sandramouli S et al. Retinal haemorrhages and convulsions. Arch Dis Child 1997; 6: 449–451

265 Tyagi A et al. Can convulsions alone cause retinal haemorrhages in infants? Br J Ophthalmol 1998; 82: 659–660

266 Jacobson M et al. A randomized clinical trial of feeder vessel photocoagulation of sickle cell retinopathy: a long-term follow-up. Ophthalmology 1991; 98: 581–585

267 American Academy of Pediatrics Committee on Child Abuse and Neglect. Distinguishing sudden infant death syndrome from child abuse fatalities. Pediatrics 1994; 94: 124–126

268 Schipper I. Valsalvamonöver: nicht immer gutartig [Valsalva's maneuver: not always benign]. Kiln Mbl Augenheilk 1991; 198: 457–459

269 Soylu H et al. Intracerebral hemorrhage: a rare late manifestation of vitamin-K deficiency in a breastfed infant. Turk J Pediatr 1997; 39: 265–269

270 Motohara K et al. Severe vitamin K deficiency in breast-fed infants. J Pediatr 1984; 105: 943–945

271 Chaou W, Chou M, Eitzman D. Intracranial hemorrhage and vitamin K deficiency in early infancy. J Pediatr 1984; 105: 880–884

272 Wetzel R, Slater A, Dover G. Fatal intramuscular bleeding misdiagnosed as suspected nonaccidental injury. Pediatrics 1995; 95: 771–773

273 Giangiacomo J, Barkett K. Ophthalmoscopic findings in occult child abuse. J Pediatr Ophthalmol Strabismus 1985; 22: 234–237

274 Wilkinson W et al. Retinal hemorrhage predicts neurologic injury in the shaken baby syndrome. Arch Ophthalmol 1989; 107: 1472–1474

275 Levin A. Ocular manifestations of child abuse. Ophthalmol Clin North Am 1990; 3: 249–264

276 Weidenthal D, Levin D. Retinal detachment in a battered infant. Am J Ophthalmol 1976; 81: 725–727

277 Kiffney G. The eye of the 'battered child'. Arch Ophthalmol 1964; 72: 231–233

278 Friendly D. Ocular manifestations of physical child abuse. Trans Am Acad Ophthalmol Otolaryngol 1971; 75: 318–332

279 Smith S, Hanson R. 134 battered children: a medical and psychological study. BMJ 1974; 3: 666–670

280 Ober R. Hemorrhagic retinopathy in infancy: a clinicopathologic report. J Pediatr Ophthalmol Strabismus 1980; 17: 17–20

281 Alexander R, Scor D, Smith W. Magnetic resonance imaging of intracranial injuries from child abuse. J Pediatr 1986; 109: 975–979

Retinal haemorrhage and child abuse

T.J. David

Paediatric literature review – 1998

ALLERGY AND IMMUNOLOGY

Immunology

Novembre E, Cianferoni A, Bernardini R et al. Anaphylaxis in children: clinical and allergologic features. Pediatrics 1998; 101: e8. *Prevention is almost impossible.*

Ponsonby AL, Couper D, Dwyer T et al. Cross sectional study of the relation between sibling number and asthma, hay fever, and eczema. Arch Dis Child 1998; 79: 328–333. *The protective effect of sibling number is not understood.*

CARDIOVASCULAR

Craig JE, Scholz TA, Vanderhooft SL et al. Fat necrosis after ice application for supraventricular tachycardia termination. J Pediatr 1998; 133: 727. *Report of a case at 14 days of age.*

McConnell ME, Hannon DW, Steed RD et al. Fatal obliterative coronary vasculitis in Kawasaki disease. J Pediatr 1998; 133: 259–261. *Sudden death was due to obliteration of the coronary artery. See also pp. 177-179, pp. 254-258 and Pediatrics 1998; 101: 108–112.*

Mendelsohn AM, Shim D. Inroads in transcatheter therapy for congenital heart disease. J Pediatr 1998; 133: 324–333. *Review.*

Professor T.J.David MD PhD FRCP FRCPCH DCH, Booth Hall Children's Hospital, Charlestown Road, Blackley, Manchester M9 7AA, UK

Nakamura Y, Yanagawa H, Ojima T et al. Cardiac sequelae of Kawasaki disease among recurrent cases. Arch Dis Child 1998; 78: 163–165. *Sequelae are more likely in this group.*

Pelech AN. The cardiac murmur. When to refer? Pediatr Clin North Am 1998; 45: 107–122. *Review.*

Quinlivan RM, Robinson RO, Maisey MN. Positron emission tomography in paediatric cardiology. Arch Dis Child 1998; 79: 520–522. *Review.*

Reller MD, Morris CD. Is Down syndrome a risk factor for poor outcome after repair of congenital heart defects? J Pediatr 1998; 132: 738–741. *Only complete atrioventricular septal defect was associated with significantly higher mortality.*

Skinner JR. Echocardiography on the neonatal unit: a job for the neonatologist or the cardiologist? Arch Dis Child 1998; 78: 401–407. *Both can do it.*

Sullivan ID. Parent arterial duct: when should it be closed? Arch Dis Child 1998; 78: 285–287. *Review.*

COMMUNITY

Bannon MJ, Ross EM. Administration of medicines in school: who is responsible? BMJ 1998; 316: 1591–1593. *There is no easy solution.*

Barlow J, Stewart-Brown S, Fletcher J. Systematic review of the school entry medical examination. Arch Dis Child 1998; 78: 301–311. *Data on the effectiveness are not available.*

Billingham K, Hall D. Turbulent future for school nursing and health visiting. BMJ 1998; 316: 406–407. *Change the bathwater – but hang on to the baby.*

Davis JA. Masculinism disguised as feminism. Arch Dis Child 1998; 78: 497–499. *We should be making it possible for women who choose to devote themselves to child rearing to do so without the opprobrium of others or the sacrifice of their own aspirations.*

DiGuiseppi C, Roberts I, Li L et al. Determinants of car travel on daily journeys to school: cross sectional survey of primary school children. BMJ 1998; 316: 1426–1428. *The strongest predictors of car travel to school were car ownership, greater distance to school, attendance at an independent school, and parental worry about abduction.*

Fleming DM, Charlton JRH. Morbidity and healthcare utilisation of children in households with one adult: comparative observational study. BMJ 1998; 316: 1572–1576. *Children in single parent families should be targeted for immunisation and accident prevention.*

Friman PC, Handwerk ML, Swearer SM et al. Do children with primary nocturnal enuresis have clinically significant behavior problems? Arch Pediatr Adolesc Med 1998; 152: 537–539. *Primary nocturnal enuresis does not present with significant behavioural comorbidity in most cases.*

McKenzie S. Can I have a letter for the housing, doctor? Arch Dis Child 1998; 78: 505–507. *Annotation and commentary.*

Schwartz RH. Adolescent heroin use: a review. Pediatrics 1998; 102: 1461–1466. *Review. See also Arch Pediatr Adolesc Med 1998; 152: 952–960.*

Scott S. Intensive interventions to improve parenting. Arch Dis Child 1998; 79: 90–93. *Review. See also Arch Dis Child 1998; 78: 293–300.*

Shaywitz SE. Dyslexia. N Engl J Med 1998; 338: 307–312. *Review.*

Tripp JH, Cockett M. Parents, parenting, and family breakdown. Arch Dis Child 1998; 78: 104–108. *Review.*

Webb E. Children and the inverse care law. BMJ 1998; 316: 1588–1591. *If Britain is to change its attitudes to children fundamentally, a children's rights commissioner must be appointed.*

Wright CM, Callum J, Birks E et al. Effect of community based management in failure to thrive: randomised controlled trial. BMJ 1998; 317: 571–574. *Health visitor intervention, with limited specialist support, can significantly improve growth.*

Accidents

Bernard PA, Johnston C, Curtis SE et al. Toppled television sets cause significant pediatric morbidity and mortality. Pediatrics 1998; 102: e32. *Report of 73 cases (28 deaths). For dangers of trampolines see Arch Pediatr Adolesc Med 1998; 152: 694–699.*

Clamp M, Kendrick D. A randomised controlled trial of general practitioner safety advice for families with children under 5 years. BMJ 1998; 316: 1576–1579. *General practitioner advice, coupled with access to low cost equipment increased use of safety equipment and other safe practices.*

Curfman GD. Fatal impact   concussion of the heart. N Engl J Med 1998; 338: 1841–1843. *Sudden death can occur when a hard ball strikes the chest just before the peak of the T wave. See also pp 1805–1811.*

Fergusson E, Li J, Taylor B. Grandmothers' role in preventing unnecessary accident and emergency attendances: cohort study. BMJ 1998; 317: 1685. *Children who have a grandmother involved in their care are less likely to present to accident and emergency with minor or trivial conditions.*

Hergenroeder AC. Prevention of sports injuries. Pediatrics 1998; 101: 1057–1063. *Review.*

Jennett B. Epidemiology of head injury. Arch Dis Child 1998; 78: 403–405. *Review.*

Mucklow ES, Evans G. Stress fractures in a hyperactive 3 year old girl. Lancet 1998; 349: 854. *Fractures of tibia and fibula.*

Osberg JS, Schneps SE, DiScala C et al. Skateboarding. Arch Pediatr Adolesc Med 1998; 152: 985–991. *More dangerous than roller skating or in-line skating. For bicycle handlebar injury see Pediatrics 1998; 102: 596–601.*

Saffle JR. Predicting outcomes of burns. N Engl J Med 1998; 338: 387–388. *Review. See also pp. 362-366.*

Stallard P, Velleman R, Baldwin S. Prospective study of post-traumatic stress disorder in children involved in road traffic accidents. BMJ 1998; 317: 1619–1623. *One in three children was found to suffer from post-traumatic stress disorder when assessed 6 weeks after their accident.*

Cerebral palsy

Collins M, Paneth N. Preeclampsia and cerebral palsy: are they related? Dev Med Child Neurol 1998; 40: 207–211. *Detailed discussion – no clear answer is available yet. For perinatal correlates; see Pediatrics 1998; 102: 315–322.*

Pharoah POD, Cooke T, Johnson MA et al. Epidemiology of cerebral palsy in England and Scotland, 1984–1989. Arch Dis Child 1998; 79: F21–F25. *No significant time trend in prevalence of cerebral palsy in any of the birthweight groups.*

Strauss D, Shavelle R. Life expectancy of adults with cerebral palsy. Dev Med Child Neurol 1998; 40: 375. *The key predictors were lack of basic functional skills: mobility and feeding.*

Williams K, Alberman E. Survival in cerebral palsy: the role of severity and diagnostic labels. Dev Med Child Neurol 1998; 40: 376–379. *Quadriplegic children with severe functional disability are likely to experience a life-threatening event before they reach adolescence. See also pp. 182-185.*

Wright FV, Sheil EMH, Drake JM et al. Evaluation of selective dorsal rhizotomy for the reduction of spasticity in cerebral palsy: a randomized controlled trial. Dev Med Child Neurol 1998; 40: 239–247. *Led to significantly greater motor impairment. See also pp. 219-238.*

Child abuse

David TJ, Hershman DA, McFarland AE. Pretrial liaison between doctors in alleged child abuse. Arch Dis Child 1998; 79: 205–206. *Explanation of role of experts meetings.*

Davis P, McClure RJ, Rolfe K et al. Procedures, placement, and risks of further abuse after Munchausen syndrome by proxy, non-accidental poisoning, and non-accidental suffocation. Arch Dis Child 1998; 78: 217–221. *Report of a national study of 119 cases.*

Duhaime AC, Christian CW, Rorke LB et al. Nonaccidental head injury in infants – the 'shaken baby syndrome'. N Engl J Med 1998; 338: 1822–1829. *Whether shaking alone can cause the constellation of findings associated with the syndrome is still debated.*

Kini N, Lazoritz S. Evaluation for possible physical or sexual abuse. Pediatr Clin North Am 1998; 45: 205–219. *Review.*

Lloyd B. Subdural haemorrhages in infants. BMJ 1998; 317: 1538–1539. *Almost all are due to abuse but abuse is often not recognised. See also pp. 1558-1561. See also Lancet 1998; 352: 335.*

Mathew MO, Ramarnohan N, Bennet GC. Importance of bruising associated with paediatric fractures: prospective observational study. BMJ 1998; 317: 1117–1118. *Most fractures are not associated with bruising.*

Meadow R. Munchausen syndrome by proxy abuse perpetrated by men. Arch Dis Child 1998; 78: 210–216. *Report of 15 cases.*

Infant feeding

Lucassen PLBJ, Assendelft WJJ, Gubbels JW et al. Effectiveness of treatments for infantile colic: systematic review. BMJ 1998; 316: 1563–1569. *Recommends a one week trial of a hypoallergenic formula milk.*

Willatts P, Forsyth JS, DiMondugno MK et al. Effect of long-chain polyunsaturated fatty acids in infant formula on problem solving at 10 months of age. Lancet 1998; 352: 688–691. *Supplementation appears to lead to higher problem solving scores.*

Wilson AC, Forsyth JS, Greene SA et al. Relation of infant diet to childhood health: seven year follow up of cohort of children in Dundee infant feeding study. BMJ 1998; 316: 21–25. *Breast feeding and the late introduction of solids may have a beneficial effect on childhood health and subsequent adult disease.*

Handicap

Badawi N, Watson L, Petterson B et al. What constitutes cerebral palsy? Dev Med Child Neurol 1998; 40: 520–527. *Review.*

Carr LJ, Cosgrove AP, Gringras P et al. Position paper on the use of botulinum toxin in cerebral palsy. Arch Dis Child 1998; 79: 271–273. *Review.*

Pueschel SM. Should children with Down syndrome be screened for atlantoaxial instability? Arch Pediatr Adolesc Med 1998; 152: 123–125. *Review. See also pp. 119-122.*

Reddihough DS, King J, Coleman G et al. Efficacy of programmes based on conductive education for young children with cerebral palsy. Dev Med Child Neurol 1998; 40: 763–770. *Similar progress to those involved in traditional programmes.*

Immunisation

American Academy of Pediatrics. Committee on Infectious Diseases. Age for routine administration of the second dose of measles-mumps-rubella vaccine. Pediatrics 1998; 101: 129–133. *Review.*

Banatvala JE. Rubella – could do better. Lancet 1998; 351: 849–850. *Review.*

Belshe RB, Mendelman PM, Treanor J et al. The efficacy of live attenuated, cold-adapted, trivalent, intranasal influenza virus vaccine in children. N Engl J Med 1998; 338: 1405–1412. *Safe, immunogenic, and effective. See also pp. 1459-1461.*

Cutts FT, Steinglass R. Should measles be eradicated? BMJ 1998; 316: 765–767. *Review.*

Fairchok MP, Trementozzi DP, Carter PS et al. Effect of prednisone on response to influenza virus vaccine in asthmatic children. Arch Pediatr Adolesc Med 1998; 152: 1191–1195. *Children can be effectively vaccinated while they are receiving prednisone therapy.*

Finn A, Bell F. Polio vaccine: is it time for a change? Arch Dis Child 1998; 78: 571–574. *Review.*

Gershon A. Varicella: to vaccinate or not to vaccinate? Arch Dis Child 1998; 79: 470–471. *Review. See also pp. 472-480.*

Goldblatt D, Miller E, McCloskey N et al. Immunological response to conjugate vaccines in infants: follow up study. BMJ 1998; 316: 1570–1571. *May provide long-term protection even when circulating antibody titres are low.*

Hawe P, McKenzie N, Scurry R. Randomised controlled trial of the use of a modified postal reminder card on the uptake of measles vaccination. Arch Dis Child 1998; 79: 136–140. *A modest but important improvement. See also BMJ 1998; 316: 1569–1570.*

Lagos R, Valenzuela MT, Levine OS et al. Economisation of vaccination against *Haemophilus influenzae* type b: a randomised trial of immunogenicity of fractional-dose and two-dose regimens. Lancet 1998; 351: 1472–1476. *These alternative regimens could bring the cost of Hib vaccines within reach of countries that currently cannot afford them. See also pp. 1446-1447.*

Leask JA, Chapman S. An attempt to swindle nature: press anti-immunisation reportage 1993-1997. Aust N Z J Public Health 1998; 22: 17–26. *The anti-immunisation lobby exacerbates parental doubts.*

Lewindon PJ, Harkness L, Lewindon N. Randomised controlled trial of sucrose by mouth for the relief of infant crying after immunisation. Arch Dis Child 1998; 78: 453–456. *Sucrose solution at a high concentration reduces infant distress.*

Metcalf J. Is measles infection associated with Crohn's disease? BMJ 1998; 316: 166. *The current evidence does not prove a causal link.*

Miller E. Collapse reactions after whole cell pertussis vaccination. BMJ 1998; 316: 876–877. *The so-called hypotonic-hyporesponsive episode, remains a contra-indication to further doses. See also pp. 902-903.*

Nicoll A, Elliman D, Ross E. MMR vaccination and autism 1998. BMJ 1998; 316: 715–716. *Heavily criticised claim of damage from MMR. See also Lancet 1998; 351: 905–909.*

Nilsson L, Kjellman NIM, Bjorksten B. A randomized controlled trial of the effect of pertussis vaccines on atopic disease. Arch Pediatr Adolesc Med 1998; 152: 734–738. *No increase in atopy after vaccination.*

Peltola H, Patja A, Leinikki P et al. No evidence for measles, mumps, and rubella vaccine-associated inflammatory bowel disease or autism in a 14-year prospective study. Lancet 1998; 351: 1327–1328. *Important negative study. See also p.955 and pp. 1355-1358.*

Salisbury DM. Association between oral poliovaccine and Guillain-Barre syndrome? Lancet 1998; 351: 79–80. *Review.*

Screening/surveillance

Mazzocco MMM, Myers GF, Hamner JL et al. The prevalence of the FMR1 and FMR2 mutations among preschool children with language delay. J Pediatr 1998; 132: 795–801. *Screening is warranted, particularly when there is a family history of mental retardation. See also pp. 762-764.*

Richardson MP, Williamson TJ, Reid A et al. Otoacoustic emissions as a screening test for hearing impairment in children recovering from acute bacterial meningitis. Pediatrics 1998; 102: 1364–1368. *Feasible and effective.*

Stewart-Brown S, Snowdon SK. Evidence-based dilemmas in pre-school vision screening. Arch Dis Child 1998; 78: 406–407. *Review.*

Stevens JC, Hall DMB, Davis A et al. The costs of early hearing screening in England and Wales. Arch Dis Child 1998; 78: 14–19. *Universal neonatal screening is the most cost effective approach. See also Lancet 1998; 352: 1957–1964.*

Sudden infant death syndrome (SIDS)

Douglas AS, Helms PJ, Jolliffe IT. Seasonality of sudden infant death syndrome in mainland Britain and Ireland 1985-95. Arch Dis Child 1998; 79: 269–270. *Seasonality remains an aetiological clue. For risk factors in The Netherlands, see pp. 386-393.*

Ford RPK, Schluter PJ, Mitchell EA et al. Heavy caffeine intake in pregnancy and sudden infant death syndrome. Arch Dis Child 1998; 78: 9–13. *There is an association.*

Hodgman JE. Apnea of prematurity and risk for SIDS. Pediatrics 1998; 102: 969–971. *Review.*

Kohlendorfer U, Kiechl S, Sperl W. Living at high altitude and risk of sudden infant death syndrome. Arch Dis Child 1998; 79: 506–509. *Altitude of residence is a significant risk predictor of SIDS.*

Ledwidge M, Fox G, Matthews T. Neurocardiogenic syncope: a model for SIDS. Arch Dis Child 1998; 78: 481–483. *Hypothesis based on observations of a case occurring in hospital.*

Milerad J, Vege A, Opdal SH et al. Objective measurements of nicotine exposure in victims of sudden infant death syndrome and in other unexpected child deaths. J Pediatr 1998; 133: 232–236. *92% had significant exposure and 25% had levels of nicotine only found in habitual smokers.*

Mitchell EA, Thompson JMD, Ford RPK et al. Sheepskin bedding and the sudden infant death syndrome. J Pediatr 1998; 133: 701–704. *If an infant needs to be placed prone a sheepskin should not be used as underbedding.*

Ponsonby AL, Dwyer T, Couper D et al. Association between use of a quilt and sudden infant death syndrome: case-control study. BMJ 1998; 316: 195–196. *Increased the risk particularly among older infants who sleep supine or on their side.*

Rees K, Wright A, Keeling JW et al. Facial structure in the sudden infant death syndrome: case-control study. BMJ 1998; 317: 179–180. *Backset maxillae and mandibles could predispose to narrowing and occlusion of upper airways.*

Schwartz PJ, Stramba-Badiale M, Segantini A et al. Prolongation of the QT interval and the sudden infant death syndrome. N Engl J Med 1998; 338: 1709–1714. *Claims there is an association. See also pp. 1760-1761.*

Skadberg BT, Morild I, Markestad T. Abandoning prone sleeping; effect on the risk of sudden infant death syndrome. J Pediatr 1998; 132: 340–343. *SIDS is rare when prone sleeping is avoided.*

DERMATOLOGY

Anonymous. Treating head louse infections. Drug Ther Bull 1998; 36: 45–46. *Review.*

Burns DA. Infestations in schoolchildren. Prescribers J 1998; 38: 80–86. *Review.*

Ladhani S, Evans RW. Staphylococcal scalded skin syndrome. Arch Dis Child 1998; 78: 85–88. *Review.*

Pomeranz AJ, Fairley JA. The systematic evaluation of the skin in children. Pediatr Clin North Am 1998; 45: 49–63. *Review.*

ENDOCRINOLOGY

Baylis PH, Cheetham T. Diabetes insipidus. Arch Dis Child 1998; 79: 84–89. *Review.*

Cheetham TD, Hughes IA, Barnes ND et al. Treatment of hyperthyroidism in young people. Arch Dis Child 1998; 178: 207–209. *Review.*

Clayton PE, Tillmann V. Advances in endocrinology. Arch Dis Child 1998; 78: 278–284. *Review.*

DeVroede M, Beukering R, Spit M et al. Rectal hydrocortisone during stress in patients with adrenal insufficiency. Arch Dis Child 1998; 78: 544–547. *A potentially safe alternative to parenteral administration.*

Gnanalingham MG, Newland P, Smith CP. Accuracy and reproducibility of low dose insulin administration using pen-injectors and syringes. Arch Dis Child 1998; 79: 59–62. *All three devices are unacceptably inaccurate when delivering 1 unit doses.*

Hughes IA. Congenital adrenal hyperplasia – a continuum of disorders. Lancet 1998; 352: 752–754. *Review. For high mortality in Indian girls see J Pediatr 1998; 133: 516–520.*

Karlsson B, Gustafsson J, Hedow G et al. Thyroid dysfunction in Down's syndrome: relation to age and thyroid autoimmunity. Arch Dis Child 1998; 79: 242–245. *Autoimmune thyroid disease is common after 8 years of age.*

Diabetes

Baumer JH, Hunt LP, Shield JPH. Social disadvantage, family composition, and diabetes mellitus: prevalence and outcome. Arch Dis Child 1998; 79: 427–430. *Family structure and parental diabetes have adverse effects.*

Davis EA, Keating B, Byrne GC et al. Impact of improved glycaemic control on rates of hypoglycaemia in insulin dependent diabetes mellitus. Arch Dis Child 1998; 78: 111–115. *An increase in moderate and severe hypoglycaemia as the mean HbA1c of the group decreased.*

Shield JPH, Baum JD. Advances in childhood onset diabetes. Arch Dis Child 1998; 78: 391–394. *Review.*

Growth

Brook CGD, De Vries BBA. Skeletal dysplasias. Arch Dis Child 1998; 79: 285–289. *Review.*

Cole T. Growing interest in overgrowth. Arch Dis Child 1998; 78: 200–204. *Review.*

Doull IJM, Campbell MJ, Holgate ST. Duration of growth suppressive effects of regular inhaled corticosteroids. Arch Dis Child 1998; 78: 172–173. *Most suppression occurred during the initial 18 weeks. See also BMJ 1998; 316: 668–672, J Pediatr 1998; 132: 472–477 and 381–382.*

Khadilkar VV, Frazer FL, Skuse DH et al. Metaphyseal growth arrest lines in psychosocial short stature. Arch Dis Child 1998; 79: 260–262. *Multiple growth arrest lines in the distal end of the radius or vertebrae should alert clinicians to an alternative diagnosis in a child with growth hormone insufficiency.*

McCaughey ES, Mulligan J, Voss LD et al. Randomised trial of growth hormone in short normal girls. Lancet 1998; 351: 940–944. *Effectively increased height SD score with no untoward effect on pubertal progression.*

Prentice AM. Body mass index standards for children. BMJ 1998; 317: 1401–1402. *Are useful for clinicians but not yet for epidemiologists.*

EAR, NOSE AND THROAT

Findlay CA, Macdonald JF, Wallace AM et al. Childhood Cushing's syndrome induced by betamethasone nose drops, and repeat prescriptions. BMJ 1998; 317: 739–740. *Report of 2 cases.*

Luxon LM. Toys and games: poorly recognised hearing hazards? BMJ 1998; 316: 1473. *Hearing loss from noisy toys.*

McCracken GH. Treatment of acute otitis media in an era of increasing microbial resistance. Pediatr Infect Dis J 1998; 17: 576–579. *Review. See also pp. 565-570 and 571–575.*

Pitkaranta A, Virolainen A, Jero J et al. Detection of rhinovirus, respiratory syncytial virus, and coronavirus infections in acute otitis media by reverse transcriptase polymerase chain reaction. Pediatrics 1998; 102: 291–295. *Both viruses are important causes. See also pp.400–401.*

Uhari M, Kontiokari T, Niemela M. A novel use of xylitol sugar in preventing acute otitis media. Pediatrics 1998; 102: 879–884. *Xylitol sugar, when given as a syrup or chewing gum was effective and decreased the need for antimicrobials. See also pp.974–975.*

GASTROENTEROLOGY

Aggarwal V, Williams MD, Beath SV. Gastrointestinal problems in the immunosuppressed patient. Arch Dis Child 1998; 5: 5–8. *Review.*

Carlsson A, Axelsson I, Borulf S et al. Prevalence of IgA-antigliadin antibodies and IgA-antiendomysium antibodies related to celiac disease in children with Down syndrome. Pediatrics 1998; 101: 272–275. *Screening is justified in patients with Down syndrome.*

Ghosh S, Drummond HE, Ferguson A. Neglect of growth and development in the clinical monitoring of children and teenagers with inflammatory bowel disease: review of case records. BMJ 1998; 317: 120–121. *Growth is often not monitored.*

Hoekstra JH. Toddler diarrhoea: more a nutritional disorder than a disease. Arch Dis Child 1998; 79: 2–5. *Review.*

Mahajan L, Wyllie R, Olivia L et al. Reproducibility of 24 hour intraesophageal pH monitoring in pediatric patients. Pediatrics 1998; 101: 260–263. *The investigation should be extended or repeated if the result does not correlate with the patient's clinical history.*

Wakefield AJ, Murch SH, Anthony A et al. Ileal-lymphoid-nodular hyperplasia, non-specific colitis, and pervasive developmental disorder in children. Lancet 1998; 351: 637–641. *Preliminary uncontrolled observations in a high selected sample.*

Walker LS, Guite JW, Duke M et al. Recurrent abdominal pain: a potential precursor of irritable bowel syndrome in adolescents and young adults. J Pediatr 1998; 132: 1010–1015. *Female patients with a history of recurrent abdominal pain may be at increased risk of IBS during adolescence and young adulthood.*

GENETICS AND MALFORMAIONS

Malformations

McGuaghran JM, Kuna P, Das V. Audiological abnormalities in the Klippel-Feil syndrome. Arch Dis Child 1998; 79: 352–355. *35 of 44 patients had audiological abnormalities.*

Stoler JM, Huntington KS, Peterson CM et al. The prenatal detection of significant alcohol exposure with maternal blood markers. J Pediatr 1998; 133: 346–352. *The presence of positive markers was more predictive of infant outcome than any self-reporting measure. See also pp. 316–318.*

Genetics

Cnossen MH, de Goede-Bolder A, van den Broek KM et al. A prospective 10 year follow up study of patients with neurofibromatosis type 1. Arch Dis Child 1998; 78: 408–412. *In 62 of 150 children (41.3%) complications were present.*

Woods CG. DNA repair disorders. Arch Dis Child 1998; 78: 178–184. *Review.*

HAEMATOLOGY

Adams RJ, McKie VC, Hsu L et al. Prevention of a first stroke by transfusion in children with sickle cell anemia and abnormal results on transcranial Doppler ultrasonography. N Engl J Med 1998; 339: 5–11. *Transfusion greatly reduces the risk. See also pp. 42-44.*

Andrew M, Michelson AD, Bovill E et al. Guidelines for antithrombotic therapy in pediatric patients. J Pediatr 1998; 132: 575–588. *Review.*

Calpin C, Dick P, Poon A et al. Is bone marrow aspiration needed in acute childhood idiopathic thrombocytopenic purpura to rule out leukemia? Arch Pediatr Adolesc Med 1998; 152: 345–347. *Not for typical ITP.*

Medeiros D, Buchanan GR. Major hemorrhage in children with idiopathic thrombocytopenic purpura: immediate response to therapy and long-term outcome. J Pediatr 1998; 133: 334–339. *17% of children with ITP had major hemorrhage. See also pp 313-314.*

Miller K, Buchanan GR, Zappa S et al. Implantable venous access devices in children with hemophilia: a report of low infection rates. J Pediatr 1998; 132: 934–938. *Low complication rate.*

Olivieri NF, Brittenham GM, McLaren CE et al. Long-term safety and effectiveness of iron-chelation therapy with deferiprone for thalassemia major. N Engl J Med 1998; 339: 417–423. *Deferiprone does not adequately control body iron burden in patients with thalassemia and may worsen hepatic fibrosis. See also pp. 468-469.*

Rothenberg ME. Eosinophilia. N Engl J Med 1998; 338: 1592–1600. *Review.*

Tripp JH, McNinch AW. The vitamin K debacle: cut the Gordian knot but first do no harm. Arch Dis Child 1998; 79: 295–297. *Review. See also pp.300–305 and BMJ 1998; 316: 161–162, 173–193 and 230.*

Weatherall DJ. Hemoglobin Eβ-thalassemia: an increasingly common disease with some diagnostic pitfalls. J Pediatr 1998; 132: 765–767. *Review.*

INFECTIOUS DISEASE

American Academy of Pediatrics. Committee on Infectious Diseases. Severe invasive group A streptococcal infections: a subject review. Pediatrics 1998; 101: 136–140. *Review.*

American Academy of Pediatrics. Committee on Infectious Diseases. Prevention of rotavirus disease: guidelines for use of rotavirus vaccine. Pediatrics 1998; 102: 1483–1491. *80% efficacy for prevention of severe illness.*

Arditi M, Mason EO, Bradley JS et al. Three-year multicenter surveillance of pneumococcal meningitis in children: clinical characteristics, and outcome related to penicillin susceptibility and dexamethasone use. Pediatrics 1998; 102: 1087–1097. *Neither penicillin susceptibility or dexamethasone use affected outcome.*

Friedman CR, Torigian C, Shillam PJ et al. An outbreak of salmonellosis among children attending a reptile exhibit at a zoo. J Pediatr 1998; 132: 802–807. *Washing hands was highly protective.*

Granier S, Owen P, Pill R et al. Recognising meningococcal disease in primary care: qualitative study of how general practitioners process clinical and contextual information. BMJ 1998; 316: 276–279. *Doctors should not be deterred from diagnosing meningococcal disease and starting antibiotic treatment if the child is otherwise well, if the rash has an unusual or scanty distribution, or if the rash is non-haemorrhagic. For lumbar puncture debate see pp. 1015–1016.*

Klein JL, Millman GC. Prospective, hospital based study of fever in children in the United Kingdom who had recently spent time in the tropics. BMJ 1998; 316: 1425–1426. *Malaria, dengue, dysentery, typhoid and hepatitis were all seen.*

Kristiansen BE, Tveten Y, Jenkins A. Which contacts of patients with meningococcal disease carry the pathogenic strain of *Neisseria meningitidis*? A population based study. BMJ 1998; 317: 621–625. *High rate of carriage in household members and kissing contacts.*

Mathew V, Alfaham M, Evans MR et al. Management of tuberculosis in Wales: 1986–1992. Arch Dis Child 1998; 78: 349–353. *Only 10% completed treatment, in 37% treatment was inadequate, and in the remainder either the choice of drugs or the duration of treatment was inappropriate.*

Murphy MS. Guidelines for managing acute gastroenteritis based on a systematic review of published research. Arch Dis Child 1998; 79: 279–284. *Review.*

Nadelman RB, Wormser GP. Lyme borreliosis. Lancet 1998; 352: 557–565. *Review.*

Petursson G, Helgason S, Gudmundsson S et al. Herpes zoster in children and adolescents. Pediatr Infect Dis J 1998; 17: 905–908. *No patient developed postherpetic neuralgia.*

Richardson S, Grimwood K, Gorrell R et al. Extended excretion of rotavirus after severe diarrhoea in young children. Lancet 1998; 351: 1844–1848. *Extended excretion could explain some cases of the postgastroenteritis syndrome.*

Sokal EM, Melchoir M, Cornu C et al. Acute parvovirus B19 infection associated with fulminant hepatitis of favourable prognosis in young children. Lancet 1998; 352: 1739–1741. *Parvovirus was found in 4 of 21 patients.*

AIDS

Kaplan J. 1997 USPHS/IDSA report on the prevention of opportunistic infections in patients infected with human immunodeficiency virus. Pediatrics 1998; 102: 1064–1085. *Review.*

Leroy V, Newell ML, Dabis F et al. International multicentre pooled analysis of late postnatal mother-to-child transmission of HIV-1 infection. Lancet 1998; 352: 597–600. *Risk of late postnatal transmission should be balanced against the effect of early weaning on infant mortality and morbidity and maternal fertility. See also BMJ 1998; 316: 268–270.*

Oleske J. Antiretroviral therapy and medical management of pediatric HIV infection. Pediatrics 1998; 102: 1005–1062. *Review.*

Richardson MP, Sharland M. Late diagnosis of paediatric HIV infection in south west London. BMJ 1998; 316: 271–272. *The mother's HIV infection had been detected by antenatal testing in only one (6%) of the 17 children born in London.*

METABOLIC

Chesney RW. A new form of rickets during infancy. Arch Pediatr Adolesc Med 1998; 152: 1168–1169. *Editorial review.*

Clayton PT. Disorders of cholesterol biosynthesis. Arch Dis Child 1998; 78: 185–189. *Review.*

Freeze HH. Disorders in protein glycosylation and potential therapy; tip of an iceberg? J Pediatr 1998; 133: 593–600. *Review.*

Guffon N, Souillet G, Maire I et al. Follow-up of nine patients with Hurler syndrome after bone marrow transplantation. J Pediatr 1998; 133: 119–125. *There was a beneficial effect of bone marrow transplantation on visceral features but dysostosis multiplex worsened. See also pp.7–9.*

Pfitzner MA, Thacher TD, Pettifor JM et al. Absence of vitamin D deficiency in young Nigerian children. J Pediatr 1998; 133: 740–744. *Dietary calcium insufficiency, without pre-existing vitamin D deficiency, accounts for the development of clinical rickets in Nigerian children.*

MISCELLANEOUS

Kumar P, Taxy J, Angst DB et al. Autopsies in children. Are they still useful? Arch Pediatr Adolesc Med 1998; 152: 558–563. *Autopsy can provide additional information in more than one-third of paediatric deaths.*

MacFaul R, Stewart M, Werneke U et al. Parental and professional perception of need for emergency admission to hospital: prospective questionnaire based study. Arch Dis Child 1998; 79: 213–218. *Medical professionals and parents differ in their views about admission for acute illnesses. See also pp. 219–224.*

Platt MJ. Child health statistics review, 1998. Arch Dis Child 1998; 79: 523–527. *Recent trends.*

Prazar GE. The aural infrared thermometer: a practitioner's perspective. J Pediatr 1998; 133: 471–472. *Review.*

Stovroff M, Teague WG. Intravenous access in infants and children. Pediatr Clin North Am 1998; 45: 1373–1393. *Review.*

Whybrew K, Murray M, Morley C. Diagnosing fever by touch: observational study. BMJ 1998; 317: 321. *Touch will seriously overestimate the incidence of fever, but with touch, fever will rarely be missed. A patient who does not feel hot is very likely not to have fever.*

NEONATOLOGY

Ahn MO, Korst LM, Phelan JP et al. Does the onset of neonatal seizures correlate with the timing of fetal neurologic injury? Clin Pediatr 1998; 37: 673–676. *Not a reliable indicator. For injury prevention strategies see J Pediatr 1998; 132: S30–S34.*

American Academy of Pediatrics. Committee on Drugs. Neonatal drug withdrawal. Pediatrics 1998; 101: 1079–1088. *Review.*

Anonymous. Which vitamin K preparation for the newborn? Drug Ther Bull 1998; 36: 17–24. *Review.*

Avon Premature Infant Project. Randomised trial of parental support for families with very preterm children. Arch Dis Child 1998; 79: F4–F11. *No developmental benefit.*

Badawi N, Kurinczuk JJ, Keogh JM et al. Antepartum risk factors for newborn encephalopathy: the Western Australian case-control study. BMJ 1998; 317: 1549–1553. *Many of the causal pathways start before birth. See also pp. 1554–1558.*

Barr RG. Reflections on measuring pain in infants: dissociation in responsive systems and 'honest signalling'. Arch Dis Child 1998; 79: F152–F156. *Review.*

Bhuta T, Ohlsson A. Systematic review and meta-analysis of early postnatal dexamethasone for prevention of chronic lung disease. Arch Dis Child 1998; 79: F26–F33. *Significant reduction in risk of chronic lung disease. See also Lancet 1998; 352: 835–836.*

Bloomfield FH, Teele RL, Voss M et al. The role of neonatal chest physiotherapy in preventing postextubation atelectasis. J Pediatr 1998; 133: 269–271. *Physiotherapy is ineffective.*

Carter BS, McNabb F, Merenstein GB. Prospective validation of a scoring system for predicting neonatal morbidity after acute perinatal asphyxia. J Pediatr 1998; 132: 619–623. *Useful for rapidly identifying the term and near-term newborn at risk for multiple organ system morbidity.*

Casuals DM, Marlow N, Speidel BD. Outcome of resuscitation following unexpected apparent stillbirth. Arch Dis Child 1998; 78: F112–F115. *36% survived apparently intact.*

Dammann O, Leviton A. Is some white matter damage in preterm neonates induced by a human pestvirus? Arch Dis Child 1998; 78: F230–F231. *Some forms of white matter damage might be caused by transplacental viral infection.*

Demissie K, Marcella SW, Breckenridge MB et al. Maternal asthma and transient tachypnea of the newborn. Pediatrics 1998; 102: 84–90. *Maternal asthma is a risk factor.*

Doron MW, Venesse-Meehan KA, Margolis LH et al. Delivery room resuscitation decisions for extremely premature infants. Pediatrics 1998; 102: 574–582. *Resuscitation at delivery usually postponed death by only a few days, decreasing prognostic uncertainty and honouring what physicians perceived were parents' wishes for care, without substantially contributing to overtreatment.*

Drack AV. Preventing blindness in premature infants. N Engl J Med 1998; 338: 1620–1621. *Review. See also pp. 1572-1576.*

Edwards AD, Nelson KB. Neonatal encephalopathies. BMJ 1998; 317: 1537–1538. *It is time to reconsider the cause of encephalopathies.*

Edwards AD, Wyatt JS, Thoresen M. Treatment of hypoxic-ischaemic brain damage by moderate hypothermia. Arch Dis Child 1998; 78: F85–F91. *Review. See also pp. F88-F91 and Pediatrics 1998; 102: 885–892. For MRI predictors of outcome see pp.323–328.*

Emsley HCA, Wardle SP, Sims DG et al. Increased survival and deteriorating developmental outcome in 23 to 25 week old gestation infants, 1990–4 compared with 1984–9. Arch Dis Child 1998; 78: F99–F104. *The rise in disability with improved survival was due to blindness, myopia, and squint.*

Fowlie PW, Schmidt B. Diagnostic tests for bacterial infection from birth to 90 days – a systematic review. Arch Dis Child 1998; 78: F92–F98. *Existing studies are unsatisfactory.*

Gospe SM. Current perspectives on pyridoxine-dependent seizures. J Pediatr 1998; 132: 919–923. *Review.*

Hall RT, Hall FK, Daily DK. High-dose phenobarbital therapy in term newborn infants with severe perinatal asphyxia: a randomized, prospective study with three-year follow-up. J Pediatr 1998; 132: 345–348. *Associated with a 27% reduction in the incidence of seizures and a significant improvement in neurological outcome at 3 years of age.*

Hegyi T, Carbone T, Anwar M et al. The apgar score and its components in the preterm infant. Pediatrics 1998; 101: 77–81. *Remains the best tool for the identification of infants in need of resuscitation.*

International PHVD Drug Trial Group. International randomised controlled trial of acetazolamide and furosemide in posthaemorrhagic ventricular dilation in infancy. Lancet 1998; 352: 433–440. *Treatment is associated with a higher rate of shunt placement and increased neurological morbidity.*

Isaacs D. Prevention of early onset group B streptococcal infection: screen, treat, or observe? Arch Dis Child 1998; 79: F81–F82. *Review.*

Lucas A, Morley R, Cole TJ. Randomised trial of early diet in preterm babies and later intelligence quotient. BMJ 1998; 317: 1481–1487. *Suboptimal nutritional management during a critical period of rapid brain growth could be harmful.*

Marlow N. High frequency ventilation and respiratory distress syndrome: do we have an answer? Arch Dis Child 1998; 78: F1–F2. *Review.*

Mercuri E, Dubowitz L, Brown SP et al. Incidence of cranial ultrasound abnormalities in apparently well neonates on a postnatal ward: correlation with antenatal and perinatal factors and neurological status. Arch Dis Child 1998; 79: F185–F189. *Ultrasound abnormalities are common.*

Modi N. Hyponatraemia in the newborn. Arch Dis Child 1998; 78: F81–F84. *Review.*

Papile LA, Tyson JE, Stoll BJ et al. A multicenter trial of two dexamethasone regimens in ventilator-dependent premature infants. N Engl J Med 1998; 338: 1112–1118. *Treatment at two weeks is more hazardous and no more beneficial than treatment at four weeks of age.*

Parry GJ, Gould CR, McCabe CJ et al. Annual league tables of mortality in neonatal intensive care units: longitudinal study. BMJ 1998; 316: 1931–1935. *Annual league tables are not reliable indicators of performance or best practice.*

Pietrantoni M, Stewart DL, Ssemakula N et al. Mortality conference: twin-to-twin transfusion. J Pediatr 1998; 132: 1071–1076. *Case presentation. Prenatal ultrasonography has changed the operational definition of this disorder.*

Seri I, Abbasi S, Wood DC et al. Regional hemodynamic effects of dopamine in the sick preterm neonate. J Pediatr 1998; 133: 728–734. *Renal blood flow increased while mesenteric and cerebral blood flow remained unchanged during dopamine treatment. See also pp. 719-724.*

Shulman RJ, Schanler RJ, Lau C et al. Early feeding, feeding tolerance, and lactase activity in preterm infants. J Pediatr 1998; 133: 645–649. *Early feeding increases intestinal lactase activity in preterm infants.*

Stiskal JA, Dunn MS, Shennan AT et al. α1-Proteinase inhibitor therapy for the prevention of chronic lung disease of prematurity: a randomized, controlled trial. Pediatrics 1998; 101: 89–94. *The incidence of pulmonary haemorrhage was lower in the treated group.*

Tan KL. Decreased response to phototherapy for neonatal jaundice in breast-fed infants. Arch Pediatr Adolesc Med 1998; 152: 1187–1190. *The addition of formula for breast fed infants would enhance the efficacy of phototherapy.*

Tarnow-Mordi WO. Room air or oxygen for asphyxiated babies? Lancet 1998; 352: 341–342. *Editorial review.*

Truog WE. Inhaled nitric oxide: a tenth anniversary observation. Pediatrics 1998; 101: 696–697. *Review.*

Wolke D. Psychological development of prematurely born children. Arch Dis Child 1998; 78: 567–570. *Review.*

Wood CM, Rushforth JA, Hartley R et al. Randomised double blind trial of morphine versus diamorphine for sedation of preterm neonates. Arch Dis

Child 1998; 79: F34–F39. *Diamorphine's more rapid onset of sedation and morphine's hypotensive tendency suggest that diamorphine is preferable.*

Yetman RJ, Parks DK, Huseby V et al. Rebound bilirubin levels in infants receiving phototherapy. J Pediatr 1998; 133: 705–707. *Infants completing phototherapy for hyperbilirubinemia who are otherwise healthy do not require follow-up solely to identify a rebound bilirubin level.*

NEPHROLOGY

Arant Jr BS. Screening for urinary abnormalities: worth doing and worth doing well. Lancet 1998; 351: 307–308. *Review.*

Postlethwaite RJ, Eminson DM, Reynolds JM et al. Growth in renal failure: a longitudinal study of emotional and behavioural changes during trials of growth hormone treatment. Arch Dis Child 1998; 78: 222–229. *Parents appreciate the efforts but children preferred results.*

Taylor CM, Mommens LAH. Advances in haemolytic uraemic syndrome. Arch Dis Child 1998; 78: 190–193. *Review.*

NEUROLOGY

Barlow CF, Priebe CJ, Mulliken JB et al. Spastic diplegia as a complication of interferon treatment of hemangiomas of infancy. J Pediatr 1998; 132: 527–530. *An alarming but unconfirmed complication.*

Cabana MD, Crawford TO, Winkelstein JA et al. Consequences of the delayed diagnosis of ataxia-telangiectasia. Pediatrics 1998; 102: 98–100. *Recommends the use of routine serum α-fetoprotein testing for all children with persistent ataxia.*

Freeman JM, Vining EPG, Pillas DJ et al. The efficacy of the ketogenic diet – 1998: a prospective evaluation of intervention in 150 children. Pediatrics 1998; 102: 1358–1359. *More effective than many of the new anticonvulsant medications and well tolerated by children and families.*

Garvey MA, Gaillard WD, Rusin JA et al. Emergency brain computed tomography in children with seizures: who is most likely to benefit? J Pediatr 1998; 133: 664–669. *A first seizure in the setting of a fever rarely indicates the presence of an unexpected CT scan lesion requiring intervention.*

Gemke RJBJ, Tasker RC. Clinical assessment of acute coma in children. Lancet 1998; 351: 926–928. *Review.*

Hoyte P. Awards for handicapped children. Arch Dis Child 1998; 79: 516–519. *Review.*

Jacobson RD. Approach to the child with weakness or clumsiness. Pediatr Clin North Am 1998; 45: 145–168. *Review.*

Panayiotopoulos CP. Significance of the EEG after the first afebrile seizure. Arch Dis Child 1998; 78: 575–577. *Review and commentary.*

Rosenow F, Wyllie E, Kotagal P et al. Staring spells in children: descriptive features distinguishing epileptic and nonepileptic events. J Pediatr 1998; 133: 660–663. *Preserved responsiveness to touch, lack of interruption of playing, and initial identification by a teacher or health professional were more frequent in nonepileptic staring than in absence seizures.*

Scott RC, Surtees RAH, Neville BGR. Status epilepticus: pathophysiology, epidemiology, and outcomes. Arch Dis Child 1998; 79: 73–77. *Review.*

Sillanpaa M, Jalava M, Kaleva O et al. Long-term prognosis of seizures with onset in childhood. N Engl J Med 1998; 338: 1715–1722. *Although the majority of patients with epilepsy in childhood are free of seizures by the time they become adults, they are at increased risk for social and educational problems.*

Smith PEM. The teenager with epilepsy. BMJ 1998; 317: 960–962. *Has special needs.*

Soler D, Cox T, Bullock P et al. Diagnosis and management of benign intracranial hypertension. Arch Dis Child 1998; 78: 89–94. *Review.*

Tasker RC. Emergency treatment of acute seizures and status epilepticus. Arch Dis Child 1998; 79: 78–83. *Review.*

Van Stuijvenberg M, Moll HA, Steyerberg EW et al. The duration of febrile seizures and peripheral leukocytosis. J Pediatr 1998; 133: 557–558. *No correlation.*

Verity CM, Greenwood R, Golding J. Long-term intellectual and behavioural outcomes of children with febrile convulsions. N Engl J Med 1998; 338: 1723–1728. *Children who had febrile convulsions performed as well as other children in terms of their academic progress, intellect, and behaviour at 10 years of age.*

Verity CM. Do seizures damage the brain? The epidemiological evidence. Arch Dis Child 1998; 78: 78–84. *Review.*

Viswanathan V, Bridges SJ, Whitehouse W et al. Childhood headaches: discrete entities or continuum? Dev Med Child Neurol 1998; 40: 544–550. *Tension and migraine type headaches are at extreme ends of a symptom spectrum.*

Wood NW. Diagnosing Friedreich's ataxia. Arch Dis Child 1998; 78: 204–207. *Review.*

OPHTHALMOLOGY

Abramson DH, Frank CM, Susman M et al. Presenting signs of retinoblastoma. J Pediatr 1998; 132: 505–508. *The most common were leukocoria, strabismus, poor vision and family history.*

Rahi JS, Dezateux C. Epidemiology of visual impairment in Britain. Arch Dis Child 1998; 78: 381–386. *Review.*

Russell-Eggitt I, Harris CM, Kriss A. Delayed visual maturation: an update. Dev Med Child Neurol 1998; 40: 130–136. *Review.*

Glorieux FH, Bishop NJ, Plotkin H et al. Cyclic administration of pamidronate in children with severe osteogenesis imperfecta. N Engl J Med 1998; 339: 947–952. *Results in increased bone density. See also pp. 986-987 and Acta Paediatr 1998; 87: 64–68.*

Godward S, Dezateux C. Surgery for congenital dislocation of the hip in the UK as a measure of outcome of screening. Lancet 1998; 351: 1149–1152. *The incidence of a first operative procedure for congenital dislocation of the hip in the UK was similar to that reported before screening was introduced.*

Saito N, Ebara S, Ohotsuka K et al. Natural history of scoliosis in spastic cerebral palsy. Lancet 1998; 351: 1687–1692. *The risk factors for progression of scoliosis in spastic cerebral palsy are: having a spinal curve of 40 degrees before age 15 years; having total body involvement; being bedridden; and having a thoracolumbar curve.*

PSYCHIATRY

Black D. The dying child. BMJ 1998; 316: 1376–1378. *Children with life threatening illness often know that they are dying but seldom have the opportunity to talk about it.*

Black D. Bereavement in childhood. BMJ 1998; 316: 931–933. *Review.*

Block SL. Attention-deficit disorder. Pediatr Clin North Am 1998; 45: 1053–1082. *Review.*

Cannon M, Murray RM. Neonatal origins of schizophrenia. Arch Dis Child 1998; 78: 1–3. *Review.*

DeLong GR, Teague LA, Kamran MM. Effects of fluoxetine treatment in young children with idiopathic autism. Dev Med Child Neurol 1998; 40: 551–562. *Worthy of further study – may help some cases.*

Harrington R, Whittaker J, Shoebridge P et al. Systematic review of efficacy of cognitive behaviour therapies in childhood and adolescent depressive disorder. BMJ 1998; 316: 1559–1563. *Cognitive behaviour therapy may be of benefit for depressive disorder of moderate severity but cannot be recommended for severe depression.*

Hill P. Attention deficit hyperactivity disorder. Arch Dis Child 1998; 79: 381–385. *Review. See also Lancet 1998; 351: 429–433.*

Kewley GD. Attention deficit hyperactivity disorder is underdiagnosed and undertreated in Britain. BMJ 1998; 316: 1594–1595. *Review.*

Krilov LR, Fisher M, Friedman SB et al. Course and outcome of chronic fatigue in children and adolescents. Pediatrics 1998; 102: 360–366. *Children and adolescents with chronic fatigue have a syndrome that is similar to that described in adults.*

Mars AE, Mauk JE, Dowrick PW. Symptoms of pervasive developmental disorders as observed in prediagnostic home videos of infants and toddlers. J Pediatr 1998; 132: 500–504. *A decreased frequency of looks at faces, points with gaze at another, shows objects, and alternating gaze was associated with a later diagnosis of PDD.*

Pearce JB, Thompson AE. Practical approaches to reduce the impact of bullying. Arch Dis Child 1998; 79: 528–531. *Review. See also BMJ 1998; 317: 924–925.*

Scott S. Aggressive behaviour in childhood. BMJ 1998; 316: 202–206. *Review.*

RESPIRATORY

Carey JA, Hamilton JRL, Spencer DA et al. Empyema thoracis: a role for open thoractomy and decortication. Arch Dis Child 1998; 79: 510–513. *Treatment must be tailored to the disease stage.*

Cochran D. Diagnosing and treating chesty infants. BMJ 1998; 316: 1546–1548. *A short trial of inhaled corticosteroid is probably the best approach.*

Fahey T, Stocks N, Thomas T. Systematic review of the treatment of upper respiratory tract infection. Arch Dis Child 1998; 79: 225–230. *Antibiotic treatment of URTI is not supported by evidence from randomised trials.*

Jardine E, Wallis C. Core guidelines for the discharge home of the child on long term assisted ventilation in the United Kingdom. Thorax 1998; 53: 762–767. *Detailed presentation of guidelines.*

Johnson DW, Jacobson S, Edney PC et al. A comparison of nebulized budesonide, intramuscular dexamethasone, and placebo for moderately severe croup. N Engl J Med 1998; 339: 498–503. *Dexamethasone offered the greatest improvement. See also pp. 553-555.*

Johnston IDA, Strachan DP, Anderson HR. Effect of pneumonia and whooping cough in childhood on adult lung function. N Engl J Med 1998; 338: 581–587. *Childhood pneumonia is associated with reduced ventilatory function in adults.*

Kadatis AG, Wald ER. Viral croup: current diagnosis and treatment. Pediatr Infect Dis J 1998; 17: 827–834. *Review.*

Milner AD. Effects of 15% oxygen on breathing patterns and oxygenation in infants. BMJ 1998; 316: 873–874. *Infants are probably safe in aircraft. See also pp. 887-894.*

Richter H, Seddon P. Early nebulised budesonide in the treatment of bronchiolitis and the prevention of postbronchiolitic wheezing. J Pediatr 1998; 132: 849–853. *Did not reduce the symptoms of acute bronchiolitis or prevent postbronchiolitic wheezing.*

The IMpact-RSV Study Group. Palivizumab, a humanized respiratory syncytial virus monoclonal antibody, reduces hospitalization from respiratory syncytial virus infection in high-risk infants. Pediatrics 1998; 102: 531–537.

Monthly intramuscular administration of palivizumab is safe and effective for prevention of serious RSV illness in premature children and those with BPD. See also pp. 1211-1215 and J Pediatr 1998; 133: 492–499.

Asthma

Banner AS. Non-steroidal anti-inflammatory therapy for bronchial asthma. Lancet 1998; 351: 5–7. *Review of methotrexate, cyclosporin, gold, immunoglobulin and others.*

Ducharme FM, Davis M. Randomized controlled trial of ipratropium bromide and frequent low doses of salbutamol in the management of mild and moderate acute pediatric asthma. J Pediatr 1998; 133: 479–485. *Hourly salbutamol 0.15 mg/kg worked as well.*

Everard ML. Asthma in the emergency department. J Pediatr 1998; 133: 469–470. *Review. For preventable admission see Arch Dis Child 1998; 78: 143–147.*

Faniran AO, Peat JK, Woolcock AJ. Persistent cough: is it asthma? Arch Dis Child 1998; 79: 411–414. *Cough variant asthma is probably a misnomer for most children in the community who have persistent cough.*

Garrett J, Williams S, Wong C et al. Treatment of acute asthmatic exacerbations with an increased dose of inhaled steroid. Arch Dis Child 1998; 79: 12–17. *Increasing the dose of inhaled steroids at the onset of an exacerbation is ineffective.*

Peat JK. Can asthma be prevented? Evidence from epidemiological studies of children in Australia and New Zealand in the last decade. Clin Exp Allergy 1998; 28: 261–265. *Review.*

Plotnick LH, Ducharme FM. Should inhaled anticholinergics be added to β2 agonists for treating acute childhood and adolescent asthma? A systematic review. BMJ 1998; 317: 971–977. *Adding multiple doses of anticholinergics to β2 agonists seems safe, improves lung function, and may avoid hospital admission in 1 of 11 such treated patients. See also N Engl J Med 1998; 339: 1030–1035.*

Yung M, South M. Randomised controlled trial of aminophyline for severe acute asthma. Arch Dis Child 1998; 79: 405–410. *Aminophylline continues to have a place in severe acute asthma.*

Cystic fibrosis

Aris RM, Renner JB, Winders AD et al. Increased rate of fractures and severe kyphosis: sequalae of living into adulthood with cystic fibrosis. Ann Intern Med 1998; 128: 186–193. *Osteoporosis is universal in adults with late-stage cystic fibrosis, and its complications include increased fracture rates and severe kyphosis. See also J Pediatr 1998; 133: 18–27.*

Conway SP, Stableforth DE, Webb AK. The failing health care system for adult patients with cystic fibrosis. Thorax 1998; 53: 3–4. *The few adult centres cannot cope. More are needed.*

Dodge JA. Gene therapy for cystic fibrosis: what message for the recipient? Thorax 1998; 53: 157–158. *Gene therapy has been oversold.*

Heine RG, Button BM, Olinsky A et al. Gastro-oesophageal reflux in infants under 6 months with cystic fibrosis. Arch Dis Child 1998; 78: 44–48. *About one in five newly diagnosed infants had reflux.*

Jaffe A, Francis J, Rosenthal M et al. Long-term azithromycin may improve lung function in children with cystic fibrosis. Lancet 1998; 351: 420–421. *Uncontrolled data.*

Jelalian E, Stark LJ, Reynolds L et al. Nutrition intervention for weight gain in cystic fibrosis: a meta analysis. J Pediatr 1998; 132: 486–492. *Behavioural intervention was as effective as more invasive procedures. See also pp. 265–269.*

Krebs NF, Sontag M, Accurso FJ et al. Low plasma zinc concentrations in young infants with cystic fibrosis. J Pediatr 1998; 133: 761–764. *Data suggest that many of the infants were zinc deficient at the time of diagnosis.*

Lai HC, Kosorok MR, Sondel SA et al. Growth status in children with cystic fibrosis based on the national cystic fibrosis patient registry data: evaluation of various criteria used to identify malnutrition. J Pediatr 1998; 132: 478–485. *20% of all patients were less than 5th centile for height or weight.*

Mahadeva R, Webb K, Westerbeck RC et al. Clinical outcome in relation to care in centres specialising in cystic fibrosis: cross sectional study. BMJ 1998; 316: 1771–1775. *Claims benefit of CF centres but conclusion undermined by selection bias.*

Moran A, Doherty L, Wang X et al. Abnormal glucose metabolism in cystic fibrosis. J Pediatr 1998; 133: 10–17. *Review.*

Ring E, Eber E, Erwa W et al. Urinary N-acetyl-β-D-glucosaminidase activity in patients with cystic fibrosis on long term gentamicin inhalation. Arch Dis Child 1998; 78: 540–543. *Long term gentamicin inhalation risks renal toxicity.*

Rivlin J, Lerner A, Augarten A et al. Severe Clostridium difficile-associated colitis in young patients with cystic fibrosis. J Pediatr 1998; 132: 177–179. *Report of 4 cases.*

Rosenstein BJ, Cutting GR. The diagnosis of cystic fibrosis: a consensus statement. J Pediatr 1998; 132: 589–595. *Review. See also pp. 563-564 and 596–599.*

Rosenstein BJ, Zeitlin PL. Cystic fibrosis. Lancet 1998; 351: 277–282. *Review.*

Santamaria F, Grillo G, Guido G et al. Cystic fibrosis: when should high-resolution computed tomography of the chest be obtained? Pediatrics 1998; 101: 908–913. *The role of CT is unclear.*

Schechter MS, Margolis PA. Relationship between socioeconomic status and disease severity in cystic fibrosis. J Pediatr 1998; 132: 260–264. *Disadvantaged children do less well.*

Sidhu H, Hoppe B, Hesse A et al. Absence of Oxalobacter formigenes in cystic fibrosis patients: a risk factor for hyperoxaluria. Lancet 1998; 352: 1026–1029. *Helps to explain risk of urolithiasis.*

Stallings VA, Fung EB, Hofley PM et al. Acute pulmonary exacerbation is not associated with increased energy expenditure in children with cystic fibrosis. J Pediatr 1998; 132: 493–499. *No increase above baseline resting energy expenditure.*

Vic P, Ategbo S, Turck D et al. Efficacy, tolerance, and pharmacokinetics of one daily tobramycin for pseudomonas exacerbations in cystic fibrosis. Arch Dis Child 1998; 78: 536–539. *One or three times daily tobramycin were equally effective (or equally useless).*

SURGERY

Baker A, Dhawan A, Heaton N. Who needs a liver transplant? (new disease specific indications). Arch Dis Child 1998; 79: 460–464. *Review.*

Borkowski S. Pediatric stomas, tubes, and appliances. Pediatr Clin North Am 1998; 45: 1419–1435. *Review.*

Bruns TB, Robinson BS, Smith RJ et al. A new tissue adhesive for laceration repair in children. J Pediatr 1998; 132: 1067–1070. *Octylcyanoacrylate is an acceptable method of wound repair.*

Davis CF, Sabharwal AJ. Management of congenital diaphragmatic hernia. Arch Dis Child 1998; 79: F1–F3. *Review. See also Pediatrics 1998; 101: 289–295.*

Ghosh A, Griffiths DM. Rectal biopsy in the investigation of constipation. Arch Dis Child 1998; 79: 266–268. *If the age at onset of constipation is after the neonatal period, a rectal biopsy is unnecessary.*

Harrington L, Connolly B, Hu X et al. Ultrasonographic and clinical predictors of intussusception. J Pediatr 1998; 132: 836–839. *Supports the use of ultrasound screening for the child with nonclassic predictors of intussusception.*

Hendren WH. Pediatric rectal and perineal problems. Pediatr Clin North Am 1998; 45: 1353–1372. *Review.*

Rao PM, Rhea JT, Novelline RA et al. Effect of computed tomography of the appendix on treatment of patients and use of hospital resources. N Engl J Med 1998; 338: 141–146. *Routine appendiceal CT in patients with suspected appendicitis improves patient care and reduces the use of hospital resources. See also pp. 190-191.*

To T, Agha M, Dick PT et al. Cohort study on circumcision of newborn boys and subsequent risk of urinary-tract infection. Lancet 1998; 352: 1813–1816. *Circumcision may protect, but less than previously estimated.*

THERAPEUTICS

Hill SL, Evangelista JK, Pizzi AM et al. Proarrhythmia associated with cisapride in children. Pediatrics 1998; 101: 1053–1056. *Cisapride may cause prolongation of ventricular repolarization in children. See also Arch Dis Child 1998; 79: 469–471.*

Rowe C, Koren T, Koren G. Errors by paediatric residents in calculating drug doses. Arch Dis Child 1998; 79: 56–58. *Errors are common.*

Tang SF, Sherwood MC, Miller OI. Randomised trial of three doses of inhaled nitric oxide in acute respiratory distress syndrome. Arch Dis Child 1998; 79: 415–418. *A low concentration is as effective as higher concentrations.*

Turner S, Longworth A, Nunn AJ et al. Unlicensed and off label drug use in paediatric wards: prospective study. BMJ 1998; 316: 343–345. *Unlicensed and off label use is widespread.*

Watts D. Pain relief in children. BMJ 1998; 316: 1552. *Doing simple things better will enhance efficacy.*

Zempsky WT, Anand KJS, Sullivan KM, et al. Lidocaine iontophoresis for topical anesthesia before intravenous line placement in children. J Pediatr 1998; 132: 1061–1063. *Lidocaine iontophoresis provides rapid and effective topical anaesthesia for intravenous access in children.*

TROPICAL MEDICINE

Bhatnagar S, Singh KD, Sazawal S et al. Efficacy of milk versus yogurt offered as part of a mixed diet in acute noncholera diarrhea among malnourished children. J Pediatr 1998; 132: 999–1003. *No benefit.*

Duke T. Fluid management of bacterial meningitis in developing countries. Arch Dis Child 1998; 79: 181–185. *Review.*

Glezen WP. Editorial: prevention of neonatal tetanus. Am J Public Health 1998; 88: 871–872. *Review.*

Graham SM, Daley HM, Banerjee A et al. Ethambutol in tuberculosis: time to reconsider? Arch Dis Child 1998; 79: 274–278. *Review.*

Hossain S, Biswas R, Kabir I et al. Single dose vitamin A treatment in acute shigellosis in Bangldeshi children: randomised double blind controlled trial. BMJ 1998; 316: 422–426. *Vitamin A reduces the severity of acute shigellosis in children living in areas where vitamin A deficiency is a major public health problem.*

Jha TK, Olliaro P, Thakur CPN et al. Randomised controlled trial of aminosidine (paromomycin) v sodium stibogluconate for treating visceral leishmaniasis in North Bihar, India. BMJ 1998; 316: 1200–1205. *Aminosidine 16 or 20 mg/kg/day first line treatment.*

Kurtzhals JAL, Adabayeri V, Goka BQ et al. Low plasma concentrations of interleukin 10 in severe malarial anaemia compared with cerebral and uncomplicated malaria. Lancet 1998; 351: 1768–1772. *Insufficient IL-10 response to high TNF concentrations may have a central role.*

Lell B, Luckner D, Ndjave M et al. Randomised placebo-controlled study of atovaquone plus proguanil for malaria prophylaxis in children. Lancet 1998; 351: 709–713. *Could replace current regimens.*

Sazawal S, Black RE, Jalla S et al. Zinc supplementation reduces the incidence of acute lower respiratory infections in infants and preschool children: a double-blind, controlled trial. Pediatrics 1998; 102: 1–5. *Interventions to improve zinc intake will improve the health and survival of children in developing countries.*

Stanley SL. Malaria vaccines: are seven antigens better than one? Lancet 1998; 352: 1163–1164. *Review.*

Straus WL, Qazi SA, Kundi Z et al. Antimicrobial resistance and clinical effectiveness of co-trimoxazole versus amoxycillin for pneumonia among children in Pakistan: randomised controlled trial. Lancet 1998; 352: 270–274. *For non-severe cases co-trimoxazole is effective. For life threatening infection amoxycillin is more likely to be effective.*

Usen S, Adegbola R, Mulholland K et al. Epidemiology of invasive pneumococcal disease in the Western Region, The Gambia. Pediatr Infect Dis J 1998; 17: 23–28. *A proposed 9-valent vaccine would cover 74% of cases in the Gambia. For pneumococcal vaccination see Lancet 1998; 351: 1600–1601.*

WHO/CHD Immunisation-Linked Vitamin A Supplementation Study Group. Randomised trial to assess benefits and safety of vitamin A supplementation linked to immunisation in early infancy. Lancet 1998; 352: 1257–1263. *No sustained benefits in terms of vitamin A status beyond age 6 months or infant morbidity.*

Winstanley P. Albendazole for mass treatment of asymptomatic trichuris infections. Lancet 1998; 352: 1080–1082. *Review. See also pp. 1103-1108.*

Index